Intelligent Polymers for Nanomedicine and Biotechnologies

First Edition

Intelligent Polymers for Nanomedicine and Biotechnologies

First Edition

Edited by
Magdalena Aflori

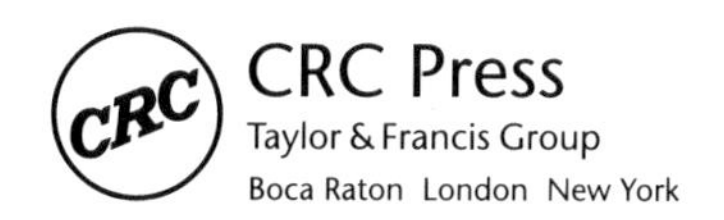

CRC Press is an imprint of the
Taylor & Francis Group, an **informa** business

CRC Press
Taylor & Francis Group
6000 Broken Sound Parkway NW, Suite 300
Boca Raton, FL 33487-2742

Printed on acid-free paper

International Standard Book Number-13: 978-1-1387-4645-9 (Paperback)
International Standard Book Number-13: 978-1-138-03522-5 (Hardback)

Library of Congress Cataloging-in-Publication Data

Names: Aflori, Magdalena, editor.
Title: Intelligent polymers for nanomedicine and biotechnologies / [edited by] Magdalena Aflori.
Description: Boca Raton : Taylor & Francis, 2018. | Includes bibliographical references.
Identifiers: LCCN 2017026587 | ISBN 9781138035225 (hardback : alk. paper) | ISBN 9781138746459 (pbk. : alk. paper) | ISBN 9781315268903 (ebook)
Subjects: | MESH: Polymers--chemistry | Surface Properties | Biocompatible Materials | Nanostructures | Theranostic Nanomedicine
Classification: LCC R857.P6 | NLM QT 37.5.P7 | DDC 610.28/4--dc23
LC record available at https://lccn.loc.gov/2017026587

Visit the Taylor & Francis Web site at
http://www.taylorandfrancis.com

and the CRC Press Web site at
http://www.crcpress.com

Contents

Preface

Nowadays, the study of intelligent polymers has become reference work in the fields of biotechnologies and nanomedicine, due to the ability of these materials to "adapt" their structure to the biological environment in which they are inserted. These polymers can undergo fast and reversible physical or chemical modifications in response to external stimuli action or change in environmental conditions: temperature, pH, redox potential, magnetic or electric field, ionic strength, light, enzyme, etc. Multistimuli responsive polymeric materials, which are sensitive to a combination of two or more external stimuli, attract much interest in designing biomaterials with tunable response in physiological conditions. Many efforts were made to ensure specificity, biocompatibility, biodegradability, and high efficacy in order to improve their life quality. In this context, the book attempts to cover a wide range of polymers that respond intelligently to physical, chemical, or biological stimuli, adopting a multidisciplinary approach to bridge chemistry, materials science, physics, pharmacology, engineering sciences, biology, and other related sciences. This work offers a convincing and understandable approach to such interesting and versatile materials in different forms—in solution, on surfaces, or as solids—reflecting the maturation of the field and the demand for the development of new, smart polymer systems. This book provides a comprehensive study of the designing and analysis of smart polymers, from nanocomposites to polymers with different functionalities for target applications like artificial implants, orthopedics, ocular devices, dental implants, drug delivery systems, and burns and wounds.

Chapter 1 focuses on the structure–property relationship, basic remarks on synthesis and applications on modern research fields of noble metal bionanoconjugates, with respect to the great numbers of scientific papers, books, and journal contributions on nanoscience and nanotechnology. For a fundamental understanding of the nanoparticles' effects on the cells, tissues, and organs, it is necessary to highlight their physicochemical properties, as each metal nanoparticle behaves differently and has specific properties depending on its size, shape, and composition. Chapter 2 is devoted to the study of designing and analysis of polymer nanofibers containing metal oxide nanoparticles, a new class of materials combining the advantages of both components and having special properties through reinforcing or modifying each other. The incorporation of undoped/doped metal oxide nanoparticles in a polymer matrix is obtained by using electrospinning for producing fibers with diameters in the range from a few microns to nanometers. Chapter 3 is focused on the preparation and properties of different polyurethane–ZnO nanomaterials, highlighting the mechanism of nanoparticles action as bactericidal and antifungal agents and their potential applications. Chapter 4 makes a brief rundown of the interest for synthesis and characterization of novel phosphorus-based materials and gold nanoparticles incorporated into electrospun polymeric matrices. The compounds containing phosphorus or nitrogen functionalities in the main and/or side chain are recommended for applications in top fields of biomedicine (biosensors, drug controlled release, tissue engineering). Chapter 5 deals with the synthesis, characterization, and biomedical applications of micro- and nanoparticles based on polysaccharides as an important kind of smart materials: drug delivery systems. These particulate systems can transport a drug to the desired place and maintain its concentration in the required therapeutic domain, the release rate being controlled by varying the surface/size/weight ratio. The flexibility of the route of administration is another major advantage; these particles can be administered by any route of access in an organism: oral inhalation, topical, intra-arterial, and intravenous. In addition, the use of bioadhesive properties of microparticulate systems gives them the possibility of other routes of administration: ocular, nasal, anal, vaginal, etc. In addition, Chapter 6 continues with an overview of the composites based on biopolymers and synthetic apatites used in the orthopedic and dental fields. These materials, shaped in various forms such as injectable hydrogel, pastes, or scaffolds, should be well integrated at the fracture site and must possess specific properties such as bioactivity, osteoconductivity, and osteoinductivity. These composites can also be used as drug delivery systems able to treat bone infections or to slow down bone resorption in some pathologies. The composites can be made by controlling not only the size and morphology of the components but also their physicochemical properties, ultimately being able to incorporate specific elements such as bioactive principles, bone cells, or growth factors to guide bone repair. Chapter 7 presents the most recent and relevant investigations on natural and synthetic intelligent polymer systems that respond to different stimuli, mainly temperature and pH conditions. Also, multiple stimuli-responsive polymeric materials are reviewed and discussed. Chapter 8 attempts to touch on some deep insights into the considerable potential of polymeric materials based on amidic and imidic building blocks in several biomedical areas by reviewing some of the new concepts of molecular design, physical and chemical features of interest for the envisaged area, functionalization potential, processing opportunities, and some clinical trials. Chapter 9 illustrates the contribution of natural materials and natural materials–based protein delivery systems to regenerative medicine research and their application for cell growth and growth factor delivery in skin regeneration research. In Chapter 10, topics like passive transport, active transport, endocytic processes, pore transport, persorption, and mass transfer models are discussed as they bring huge benefits to the investigation, prevention, treatment, and even optimization and design of implants, artificial organs, and testing and investigation instruments.

With contributions from leading researchers as well as extensive end-of-chapter references, this book offers a comprehensive overview of the current state of the art in the field and the potential for future developments. The topics presented in this book are addressed to those working as researchers, PhD students in doctoral or postdoctoral schools, and engineers, and they can be considered as a source of information on all mentioned aspects.

The editor and the authors acknowledge the financial support for this research through the European Regional Development Fund, Project POINGBIO, ID P_40_443, Contract no. 86/8.09.2016.

Editor

Magdalena Aflori is a scientific researcher in the Department of Polymer Materials Physics at Petru Poni Institute of Macromolecular Chemistry, Iasi, Romania. She received her PhD in physics in 2005 at the Alexandru Ioan Cuza University Faculty of Physics. She has made remarkable scientific contributions in polymer chemistry, plasma physics, surface science, x-ray diffraction, and small-angle x-ray scattering. Her interdisciplinary research is published in more than 70 papers in peer-reviewed journals, eight books or book chapters, and one patent. She is coordinator or member of many research projects with national and international funding and referee for a number of international journals with high impact factors.

Contributors

Magdalena Aflori
Laboratory of Polymer Physical Chemistry
Petru Poni Institute of Macromolecular Chemistry
Iasi, Romania

Anton Airinei
Laboratory of Polymeric Materials Physics
Petru Poni Institute of Macromolecular Chemistry
Iasi, Romania

Maria Bercea
Laboratory of Electroactive Polymers and Plasmochemistry
Petru Poni Institute of Macromolecular Chemistry
Iasi, Romania

Maria Butnaru
Department of Biomedical Sciences
Gr. T. Popa University of Medicine and Pharmacy
Iasi, Romania

Constantin Ciobanu
Laboratory of Polyaddition and Photochemistry
Petru Poni Institute of Macromolecular Chemistry
Iasi, Romania

Catalin Paul Constantin
Laboratory of Polycondensation and Thermostable Polymers
Petru Poni Institute of Macromolecular Chemistry
Iasi, Romania

Marieta Constantin
Laboratory of Natural Polymers, Bioactive and Biocompatible Material
Petru Poni Institute of Macromolecular Chemistry
Iasi, Romania

Mariana Dana Damaceanu
Laboratory of Polycondensation and Thermostable Polymers
Petru Poni Institute of Macromolecular Chemistry
Iasi, Romania

Petronela Dorneanu
Laboratory of Polymeric Materials Physics
Petru Poni Institute of Macromolecular Chemistry
Iasi, Romania

Mioara Drobota
Laboratory of Polymeric Materials Physics
Petru Poni Institute of Macromolecular Chemistry
Iasi, Romania

Gheorghe Fundueanu
Laboratory of Natural Polymers, Bioactive and Biocompatible Material
Petru Poni Institute of Macromolecular Chemistry
Iasi, Romania

Luiza M. Gradinaru
Laboratory of Polyaddition and Photochemistry
Petru Poni Institute of Macromolecular Chemistry
Iasi, Romania

Robert V. Gradinaru
Department of Chemistry
Al. I. Cuza University
Iasi, Romania

Mihaela Mandru
Laboratory of Polyaddition and Photochemistry
Petru Poni Institute of Macromolecular Chemistry
Iasi, Romania

Simona Morariu
Laboratory of Electroactive Polymers and Plasmochemistry
Petru Poni Institute of Macromolecular Chemistry
Iasi, Romania

Nicolae Olaru
Laboratory of Natural Polymers, Bioactive and Biocompatible Material
Petru Poni Institute of Macromolecular Chemistry
Iasi, Romania

Irina M. Pelin
Laboratory of Natural Polymers, Bioactive and Biocompatible Material
Petru Poni Institute of Macromolecular Chemistry
Iasi, Romania

Radu Dan Rusu
Laboratory of Polycondensation and Thermostable Polymers
Petru Poni Institute of Macromolecular Chemistry
Iasi, Romania

Diana Serbezeanu
Laboratory of Polycondensation and Thermostable Polymers
Petru Poni Institute of Macromolecular Chemistry
Iasi, Romania

Maria Spiridon
Laboratory of Polymeric Materials Physics
Petru Poni Institute of Macromolecular Chemistry
Iasi, Romania

Dana M. Suflet
Laboratory of Natural Polymers, Bioactive and Biocompatible Material
Petru Poni Institute of Macromolecular Chemistry
Iasi, Romania

Mirela Teodorescu
Laboratory of Electroactive Polymers and Plasmochemistry
Petru Poni Institute of Macromolecular Chemistry
Iasi, Romania

Stelian Vlad
Laboratory of Polyaddition and Photochemistry
Petru Poni Institute of Macromolecular Chemistry
Iasi, Romania

Tachita Vlad-Bubulac
Laboratory of Polycondensation and Thermostable Polymers
Petru Poni Institute of Macromolecular Chemistry
Iasi, Romania

1

Opportunities and Challenges in Polymer–Noble Metal Nanocomposites

Luiza M. Gradinaru, Mihaela Mandru, Constantin Ciobanu, and Magdalena Aflori

CONTENTS

1.1 Introduction

Nanotechnology, especially used in biomedical applications, is a new field that has been developing exponentially in the last decade, which may have a positive impact on the population health care system. The most important biomedical applications of nanotechnology that may have potential clinical applications include targeted drug delivery, detection, diagnosis, imaging, and treatment.

Noble metal nanoparticles (NMNPs) have attracted growing interest in recent years because of their unique chemical and physical properties, which can be exploited in a wide range of biomedical applications, including antibacterial applications (Hajipour et al. 2012), cancer therapy (Minelli et al. 2010, Bhattacharyya et al. 2011, Conde et al. 2012, Jeyaraj et al. 2013, Mollick et al. 2015), bioimaging (Thurn et al. 2007), biosensing (Saha et al. 2012), wound dressing management (Parani et al. 2016), etc. Research in this field has demonstrated that the optical, electrical, magnetic, and catalytic properties of NMNPs are influenced by shape, size, and size distribution, which in turn are strongly influenced by the synthesis methods (Kuppusamy et al. 2016), reducing agents (Castro et al. 2013), and stabilizers used.

NMNPs such as silver, gold, and platinum are particularly interesting due to their ease of synthesis, characterization, and surface functionalization (Abou El-Nour et al. 2010, Dhand et al. 2015); their size- and shape-dependent properties (Pal et al. 2007, Badwaik et al. 2012); and ease of drugs loaded by using methods, such as encapsulation, surface attachment, or entrapment (Duncan et al. 2010). Thereby, the research in this field of nanomaterials, including NPs, will continue to grow in the next years.

A rapidly growing application is the use of the NPs as antibacterial agents because of the increase in the resistance of bactericides and antibiotics due to the development of resistant strains. For example, AgNPs, owing to their broad-spectrum antimicrobial action against bacteria, viruses, and other eukaryotic microorganisms, are widely used in antiseptics, wound dressings, food containers, detergents, cosmetics, and many other products (Rai et al. 2009, Haider and Kang 2015).

Since biological processes occur at the nanometer scale and inside the cells, nanotechnology offers tools that may be able to detect various diseases in a very small volume of cells or tissue. Thus, the optical properties of NMNPs are a promising approach in the development of new bioimaging and biosensing strategies (Thurn et al. 2007). Due to the fact that the absorption, scattering, and fluorescence of NMNPs are orders of magnitude stronger than that of organic dyes, they can act as excellent sensors and contrast agents for optical detection. In this regard, AuNPs and PtNPs can be explored in nanomedicine as nanoplatforms and biomarkers for diagnosis and treatment of different types of cancers (Uehara and Nagaoka 2010, Tanaka et al. 2011).

A wide range of NMNP materials could be used as therapeutic delivery agents to accelerate the regeneration of acute or chronic wounds or to control their infection (Parani et al. 2016). Both natural and synthetic polymers embedded with different NMNPs could be utilized to prepare such systems (Garcia-Orue et al. 2016).

This chapter is focused on structure–property relationships, basic remarks on the synthesis and applications in modern research fields of noble metal bionanoconjugates with respect to the great numbers of scientific papers, books, and journal contributions on nanoscience and nanotechnology. For a fundamental understanding of the effects of nanoparticles (NPs) on the cells, tissues, and organs, it is necessary to highlight their physicochemical properties, with each metal nanoparticle behaving differently and having specific properties depending on its size, shape, and the dose and composition of the reducing compound.

Thus, this chapter is intended to provide a valuable background for researchers in nanobiotechnology, chemistry, biology, and biomedical engineering, especially those with an interest in the manipulation of polymer–noble metal nanocomposites. Their biomedical applications as antimicrobial agents in cancer therapy, biosensors, bioimaging, and wound dressings are discussed highlighting current opportunities, limitations, and challenges with respect to the structure–property relationship.

1.2 Biomedical Applications of NMNP Nanocomposites

Due to the unique physicochemical properties of the NPs, such as small size, large surface area to volume ratio, high surface reactivity, biocompatibility, and ease of surface functionalization, they are widely used in biomedical applications. A variety of NPs with the possibility of being diversely modified with biomolecules have been investigated over the years. The combination of various polymeric materials with noble metals has led to the fabrication of different metal nanocomposites with unique physicochemical properties. To date, several reviews, book chapters, and books have been dedicated to the application of NP nanocomposites.

1.2.1 Antibacterial Applications

Over the years, resistance of bactericides and antibiotics has increased due to the development of resistant strains. Significant effort has been dedicated by researchers during the past years in order to obtain new antibacterial materials. The most promising strategy for overcoming microbial resistance is the use of NPs, due to their unique properties arising from the small volume to big surface area ratio.

1.2.1.1 AgNPs

AgNPs show an enhanced broad-range activity against bacteria, representing a promising potential for pharmaceutical and biomedical industries (Prabhu and Poulose 2012). Therefore, AgNPs have been used extensively as antibacterial agents in a wide range of applications such as disinfecting medical devices, wound dressings, water and air treatment, textile coatings, food storage, paints and pigments, etc. (Franci et al. 2015). Although the antibacterial action of AgNPs is still not completely understood, AgNPs remain the subject of various bionanomaterials that are widely used especially in medicine. Thereby, a compressed overview of the antibacterial mechanism of AgNPs is rendered in the following text.

1.2.1.1.1 Antibacterial Mechanism of AgNPs

It is well known that Gram-positive and Gram-negative bacteria have differences in their membrane structure, the most distinctive being the thickness of the peptidoglycan layer (Hajipour et al. 2012, Eckhardt et al. 2013). The antimicrobial mechanism of AgNPs is still not completely understood but the studies have revealed several theories. First, AgNPs adhere to the surface of the bacteria due to the electrostatic interactions between the positively charged particles and the negatively charged cell membrane (Morones et al. 2005, Kim et al. 2007, Mahmoudi et al. 2014). This can cause membrane damage to the contacting domains leading to the formation of pits and gaps on the cell wall surface of the bacteria (Sondi and Salopek-Sondi 2004). Thus, the membrane morphology changes, exhibiting a significant increase in permeability, which affects the proper transport through the cell wall (Morones et al. 2005, Li et al. 2010). Other reports suggest that silver forms some complexes with electron donors, such as nitrogen, oxygen, and especially sulfur atoms from membrane wall proteins, resulting in protein denaturation and, thus, inactivation of bacteria (Sondi and Salopek-Sondi 2004, Morones et al. 2005, Dallas et al. 2011, Paul et al. 2013). Then, AgNPs are able to penetrate the inside of the bacteria and to interact with phosphorus-containing compounds in its interior like DNA, enzymes, etc. (Morones et al. 2005). Thus, AgNPs interact and bind with double-stranded DNA molecules and influence their ability for replication and transcription. This affects the respiratory chain and cell division, and as a consequence, the metabolic pathways are interrupted, resulting finally in the death of the cell (Kurek et al. 2011, Durán et al. 2016). Some studies have reported that the toxicity effects of AgNPs could be ascribed to the silver ions that can be released from NPs. This induces the formation of some reactive oxygen species (ROS) via the Fenton-type reaction, leading to oxidative stress (Magdolenova et al. 2014). ROS (singlet oxygen, hydrogen peroxide, and hydroxyl radicals) are produced as a by-product during the metabolism of cell growth under aerobic conditions from molecular oxygen. These species react mainly with lipids, proteins, and DNA and determine serious consequences (Kim et al. 2007, Eckhardt et al. 2013, Rizzello and Pompa 2014, Wei et al. 2015).

The antibacterial activity of AgNPs was also associated with the size and shape of NPs (Rai et al. 2009). Thus, very small AgNPs (<10 nm) penetrate the cells more easily and exert more pronounced toxicity because of their higher surface area (Liu et al. 2010, Rizzello and Pompa 2014). Another factor is the shape of NPs and it was reported that AgNPs with different shapes have different effects on bacterial cells (Morones et al. 2005, Pal et al. 2007, Zhang et al. 2016).

In conclusion, numerous studies have shown that the antibacterial mechanism of AgNPs is very complex and silver acts in a multidirectional fashion.

The synthesis (Behra et al. 2013, Zhang et al. 2014), properties, and antibacterial applications (Salem et al. 2015) of AgNPs are extensively described in the literature. For instance, Sheikh et al. (2009) reported a simple method to synthesize the AgNPs in/on polyurethane (PU) nanofibers. They exploited the reduction ability of *N*,*N*-dimethylformamide (DMF) to decompose silver nitrate to silver NPs. The orientation of PU nanofibers and the dispersion of AgNPs were confirmed using SEM. The diameter of AgNPs was in the range of 5–20 nm. The crystallinity of the AgNPs in the electrospun PU nanofiber mats was determined by XRD measurements. The antimicrobial activities against two Gram-negative test microorganisms have been evaluated, and the results indicate that the prepared AgNP–PU matrix can be used as an antimicrobial wound dressing material. A similar study using the ability of DMF to reduce the silver nitrate was also reported by Lakshman et al. (2010), but they also prepared AgNPs via an aqueous route. They found that the AgNP–PU nanofibers constructed via the aqueous route were cytocompatible, while those synthesized via the organic route were cytotoxic. The antibacterial activity of the nanofibers was proved using the Kirby disc diffusion method performed on *Klebsiella* bacteria.

Silver-containing thermoplastic hydrogel nanofibrous webs based on PU have been developed by Wu et al. (2009). They synthesized the polyurethane hydrogel using poly(ethylene glycol) (PEG), polyhedral oligosilsesquioxane, and lysine methyl ester diisocyanate and electrospun into nanofibrous webs with a diameter of ~150 nm, with or without $AgNO_3$. They focused their study on the ability of the electrospun hydrogel webs to inhibit biofilm formation in a sustained manner over time.

Qu et al. (2014) presented a dry spinning process to prepare PU/nanosilver fibers. They focused their study on the influence of the AgNPs on the structure and mechanical properties of PU fibers, and the antibacterial activities were assessed against both *S. aureus* and *E. coli*. Their research showed that the introduction of AgNPs improves the thermogravimetric and mechanical properties of PU and also inhibits the growth of bacteria even at low concentrations (0.030% Ag) of AgNPs embedded in the PU fibers.

Recently, Wang et al. (2015) have developed an eco-friendly, direct, one-step, dual-spinneret, electrospinning fabrication method to obtain nanofibers from waterborne polyurethane, poly(vinyl alcohol) (PVA), and AgNPs with ultrasmall sizes (~5 nm). In this study, the high number of hydroxyl groups of

PVA plays the two roles of a reducing agent and an efficient stabilizing agent for the fabrication of PVA/AgNP composite nanofibers. Wang et al. obtained a uniform distribution of hybrid nanofibers by optimization of electrospinning parameters, such as applied voltage, tip–collector distance, and viscosity of the solution and feed mass ratio. The thermal stability and biocidal activity of the hybrid nanofibers were enhanced by the addition of waterborne polyurethane and incorporation of AgNPs without increase of cytotoxicity.

Nanocomposites based on waterborne polyurethane with various small amounts of AgNPs were studied by Hsu et al. (2010). The chemical structure of PU was modified by the presence of AgNPs, which influenced the chemical, thermal, and biological stabilities. They found that the PU with a concentration of 30 ppm of AgNPs showed superior physicochemical properties, cellular response (of fibroblasts, endothelial cells, platelets, monocytes), and bacteriostatic effect.

Chen et al. (2014) synthesized a series of antibacterial coatings through redox reactions between Ag (I) and catechol functional groups of polyurethane containing tannin. The authors used the catechol groups to induce the reduction of Ag (I) to Ag (0) as well as induce antibacterial properties into polyurethane. They synthesized PUs via a two-step method using PEG of different molecular weights, isophorone diisocyanate, and tannin (M_n = 1700). The AgNP–polyurethane composite coatings showed several times increased ability to inhibit both Gram-positive (*S. aureus*) and Gram-negative (*E. coli*) bacteria.

Cellulose-based semi-interpenetrating polymer network hydrogels loaded with AgNPs have been designed as a new antimicrobial biomaterial by Babu et al. (2013). They used the free radical polymerization technique to obtain sodium carboxymethyl cellulose/poly(acrylamide-*co*-2-acrylam-ido-2-methylpropane sulfonic acid) hydrogels by varying the doses of the polymer, comonomer, and crosslinking agent. AgNPs were formed by reduction of silver nitrate in semi-IPN hydrogels with sodium borohydrate at room temperature, and different techniques were used to characterize the formation of AgNPs in hydrogels. The size of AgNPs was in the range of 10–20 nm as was evidenced by SEM and TEM microscopy results. The developed AgNP–semi-IPN hydrogels confirmed that the small size of AgNPs determine the antibacterial activity against *Bacillus subtilis*.

In another recent study (Hussain et al. 2015), hydroxypropylcellulose was used as a template nanoreactor, stabilizer, and capping agent to obtain stable AgNPs (25–55 nm) with significant antimicrobial activity against different bacterial and fungal strains.

1.2.1.2 AuNPs

Even if the AuNP-containing materials are not used on a large scale as those containing AgNPs, the antimicrobial activity of AuNPs has been recently demonstrated (Cui et al. 2012). As for AgNPs, their antimicrobial activity strongly depends on the size, shape, concentration, and surface modifications of AuNPs (Badwaik et al. 2012, Zhou et al. 2012).

For example, a recent study of Regiel-Futyra et al. (2015) reported the synthesis, antibacterial activity, and cytotoxicity of an innovative chitosan–gold nanocomposite. They used chitosan as both a reducing and a stabilizing agent and prepared AuNPs in situ (10–20 nm) by direct reduction of tetrachloroauric acid in chitosan solutions. The chitosan–Au nanocomposites demonstrated total bactericidal effect against two antibiotic-resistant strains *S. aureus* and *P. aeruginosa* and also no cytotoxic effect on human cells.

1.2.1.3 PtNPs

Platinum-based compounds have been widely used in the treatment of cancer, and various studies are available for their anticancer activity. To this date, very few reports are available about the antibacterial activity of PtNPs. Recently, Ahmed et al. (2016) reported the synthesis of PtNPs (2–5 nm) using pectin and sodium borohydride as capping and reducing agents, respectively. They demonstrated an *in vivo* antibacterial activity of the synthesized PtNPs using an adult zebrafish that was infected with different bacteria as an animal model. Their results suggested that the PtNPs could control the bacterial proliferation and enhanced survival of infected zebrafish. Moreover, they demonstrated the mechanism of antibacterial activity and found that PtNPs decreased the bacterial cell viability through the mechanism of ROS generation and loss of membrane integrity.

1.2.2 Cancer Therapy

Because cancer is believed to be one of the most challenging diseases, scientists are trying to find different ways to improve its diagnosis and treatment. Cancer nanotechnology will lead to the discovery of useful research tools, advanced drug delivery systems, and new ways to diagnose and treat cancer disease or repair damaged tissues and cells. To reduce or eliminate many of the side effects of the standard methods used for cancer treatment (surgical removal of malignant tumors, chemotherapy, and radiotherapy), it is necessary to develop efficient and targeted cancer treatments. Thereby, nanotechnology is considered a promising tool for the construction of such molecular agents that could help in the detection and localization of many cancers. In the last decade, various studies were conducted using this approach (Praetorius and Mandal 2007, Cherukuri et al. 2010, Minelli et al. 2010, Akhter et al. 2011).

The properties of noble metal NPs, such as high surface-to-volume ratio, broad optical properties, ease of synthesis, and facile surface functionalization chemistry, make them extensively used in cancer therapeutics (Conde et al. 2012). The exact mechanism of MNPs interaction with cancer cells is not yet fully known, but studies have reported their interaction with cells and intracellular macromolecules such as DNA and proteins. The cellular uptake of MNPs leads to the generation of ROS that provoke oxidative stress (Manke et al. 2013, Miethling-Graff et al. 2014). In cancer medicine, NPs are used for the development of various bionanoconjugates in diagnosis, sustained and targeted drug delivery systems, imaging, etc. (Díaz and Vivas-Mejia 2013).

1.2.2.1 AgNPs

The synthesis of AgNPs with controlled size and shape using biological entities like plant extracts (Shah et al. 2015), bacteria (Han et al. 2014), fungi (Ballottin et al. 2016), or algae (Xie et al. 2007) has offered an alternative to chemical or physical methods. The use of the green pathway for the synthesis of different NPs is desired because it is simple, safe, cost-effective, and eco-friendly. Research in this field has confirmed that the different polyphenols, glucosides, alkaloids, aminoacids, or vitamins of the respective plant extracts are responsible for biosynthesis and they are mainly used as reducing or stabilizing agents (El-Deeb et al. 2015). Various plant extracts have been used in anticancer studies due to their high efficacy and limited side effects (Jeyaraj et al. 2013). The studies on different cancer cell lines have shown that AgNPs induce cellular damage in terms of loss of cell membrane integrity, oxidative stress, and apoptosis.

For example, Kumar et al. (2016) reported the biosynthesis of AgNPs using the Andean Mora (*Rubus glaucus* Benth.) leaf (ML), a blackberry leaf with astringent, antidiarrheal, hypoglycemic, and anti-inflammatory activities due to the higher amount of flavonoids, tannins, and ellagic acid. This extract may act as both a reducing and a capping agent and provides growth conditions for the synthesis of NPs. The size range of the synthesized ML-AgNPs was between 12 and 50 nm, and they have a quasi-spherical shape as was revealed by TEM, DLS, and XRD measurements. The prepared NPs showed no cytotoxicity at the concentration between 0.01 and 1.0 μM on the hepatic cancer (Hep-G2) cell line. Many other papers and reviews regarding the biogenic synthesis of AgNPs and the potential anticancer activity are available (Shawkey et al. 2013, Rao et al. 2016).

1.2.2.2 AuNPs

Over the past decade, AuNPs have been extensively studied for potential applications in different cancer therapies (Akhter et al. 2011, Jain et al. 2012, Muddineti et al. 2015). Like AgNPs, AuNPs can be also synthesized via a biogenic pathway from various plant extracts: guava leaf and clove bud (Raghunandan et al. 2011), *Acalypha indica* Linn. leaves (Krishnaraj et al. 2014), *Eucalyptus macrocarpa* leaves (Shah et al. 2015), and many others (Ahmed and Ikram 2015, Ramaswamy et al. 2015). These studies demonstrated the anticancer effect of these functionalized AuNPs using a variety of human cancer cell lines (Muthukumar et al. 2016, Rao et al. 2016).

To date, various papers and reviews have been focused on the preparation and targeted delivery of different anticancer drugs (Duncan et al. 2010, Rana et al. 2012). For example, the study of Paciotti et al. (2004) described the formulation of AuNPs for the targeted delivery of the potent yet highly toxic anticancer protein, tumor necrosis factor (TNF), to a solid tumor. The vector included molecules of thiol-derivatized polyethylene glycol (PEG-THIOL) that were bound with molecules of TNF on a gold NP surface. The systemic administration of this vector potentiated the immunotherapeutic effects of TNF by sensitizing immune cells to recognize and destroy cancer cells.

The optical properties of AuNPs could be used in the biosensor development for the diagnosis and investigation of cancer cells. Thus, El-Sayed et al. (2005) evaluated the optical properties of colloidal AuNPs and conjugated AuNPs with monoclonal anti–epidermal growth factor receptor antibodies incubated in single living cancerous and noncancerous cells using surface plasmon resonance (SPR) scattering images and SPR absorption spectra. They observed that conjugated AuNPs have a greater affinity (600%) for binding to the surface of cancerous cells than noncancerous cells. Therefore, future investigations will focus on developing antibody-coated gold NPs for targeted delivery.

Another study was focused on the synthesis and utilization of Au nanocages (hollow and porous Au nanostructures with edge lengths <100 nm) for cancer detection and treatment (Skrabalak et al. 2007).

Other studies have described the use of AuNP enhancer solutions coupled with a noninvasive radiofrequency machine to thermally ablate tissue and cancer cells in both in vitro and in vivo systems (Cardinal et al. 2008). They demonstrated that AuNPs are not directly cytotoxic but can, upon exposure to the radiowave field, become heated to a degree that results in cell death.

The versatility of AuNPs leads to the production of a large family of drug delivery compounds with enhanced properties and offers a different approach to cancer therapy. Combination chemotherapy has been demonstrated to be better than single agents for many solid tumors. Thus, AuNPs were used to reduce the side effects of other anticancer drugs such as platinum-based drugs. In this context, Brown et al. (2010) reported in their study the synthesis of platinum-tethered AuNPs for improved anticancer drug delivery. They showed that these NPs had better cytotoxicity than oxaliplatin (a platinum-based drug) alone in all of the cell lines and also the ability to penetrate the nucleus in lung cancer cells.

1.2.2.3 PtNPs

Platinum-based anticancer drugs have been widely used in cancer chemotherapy for the management of different types of tumors in cancers of the lung, head, neck, esophagus, bladder, etc. (Oberoi et al. 2013) It was also accepted as an alternative option in therapies of other solid tumors, including liver, gastric, and brain tumors, melanoma, and soft-tissue sarcomas. The most commonly used platinum-based anticancer drugs are cisplatin and its analogs carboplatin and oxaliplatin that act by binding to DNA, thereby preventing its transcription and replication and then inducing cellular apoptosis. However, they have several limitations, such as dose-limiting toxicities, partial antitumor response, drug resistance, tumor relapse, etc. These limitations have motivated the researchers to develop new strategies for improving platinum chemotherapy. Nowadays, various formulations based on the delivery of platinum compounds like polymer–platinum bionanoconjugates (liposomes, nanocapsules, dendrimers, nanotubes, micelles, etc.) have been studied (Oberoi et al. 2013). These new carrier-based deliveries were chosen to improve the drug efficacy, reduce the side effects, and prevent cellular accumulation.

The studies performed on a DNA model system, a system used by researchers in biological conditions, have shown that the combination of fast ion radiation (hadron therapy) with PtNPs should strongly improve the cancer therapy protocols. Thus, Porcel et al. (2010) observed that PtNPs (~3 nm) enhance lethal damage in the DNA system when they are used in combination with irradiation by fast ions. They used this type of radiation (fast ion irradiation) because it is more efficient and less traumatic than the conventional types of radiations. Their study has shown that the DNA damage is due to the autoamplification of electronic cascades generated inside NPs together with charge transfer processes.

The use of NPs to improve detection of cancer will undoubtedly continue to expand.

The development of NP formulations used in diagnosis, drug delivery systems, and imaging has greatly improved the stability and therapeutic effectiveness of several anticancer agents.

1.2.3 Bioimaging and Biosensing

Noble metal NPs such as gold and silver have strong, size- and shape-dependent optical properties with an absorbance of SPR. This property makes the NPs highly photo-stable with a narrow emission spectra and possibility for high-resolution imaging of samples. Due to this unique property, it can be exploited for use in a variety of different applications including medical imaging (Thurn et al. 2007) and biosensing (Doria et al. 2012). Over time, many studies have highlighted several strategies and techniques for improvements in the fabrication and characterization of NP arrays (Willets et al. 2007, Zhang et al. 2012).

1.2.3.1 AgNPs

The plasmonic properties of AgNPs also enable them to be employed as an *in vivo* therapeutic tool when they are conjugated to biological targets. To be used for bioimaging, AgNPs could be incubated with cells or the surfaces could be functionalized with some biomolecules that bind to the sites on the cell membranes (Sotiriou and Pratsinis 2011). SPR depends on the size and shape of AgNPs and the dielectric environment that surrounds them. For example, triangular AgNPs were deposited on substrates using nanosphere lithography to monitor the interactions between two biomolecules, amyloid β-derived diffusible ligands (ADDLs) and the anti-ADDL antibody, molecules possibly involved in the development of Alzheimer's disease (Haes et al. 2004).

Controlling the particle size and structure is a powerful strategy to modulate electronic structures and optical properties of metal NPs. Thus, Zheng et al. (2008) reported the observation that polycrystalline AgNPs with grain sizes down to the electron Fermi wavelength exhibit both bright luminescence and a large enhancement effect of the Raman scattering signals. They synthesized luminescent and Raman active AgNPs (2–30 nm) by thermal reduction of silver ions in a glycine matrix. An interesting remark is that these glycine-AgNPs remained stable in aqueous solution for more than 2 years under ambient conditions.

1.2.3.2 AuNPs

Even though silver has a higher plasmonic performance than gold, gold is typically used for biosensing because silver oxidizes and easily forms plasmonically unattractive compounds like halides in biological solutions (Sotiriou and Pratsinis 2011). AuNPs possess alternative properties that enhance their imaging capabilities in cells that are fixed or live and can also be used as multifunctional analysis systems of single samples using different forms of detection.

The ability to modify the surface chemistry and to conjugate with various biological molecules allows them to be used successfully in different bionanoconjugate systems.

Tang et al. (2007) demonstrated the ability of 60 nm AuNPs to provide high spatial resolution data within individual fixed or live cancer cells using near-infrared surface-enhanced Raman scattering (SERS). The AuNPs were present inside of the living cell, in the cytoplasm, and also in the nucleus, allowing a detailed SERS characterization of cellular components throughout. In the same direction, Wilson and Willets (2013) reviewed the fundamental principles of SER spectroscopy imaging regarding the careful selection of NP substrates because the NPs were required to produce the necessary signal enhancements.

Their distinct physical and optical properties make AuNPs excellent scaffolds for the fabrication of a variety of biosensors for *in vitro* diagnosis. Many studies based on different AuNP-bionanomaterials used to create high-sensitivity systems for *in vitro* diagnosis biomarkers have been reported in the review of Zhou et al. (2015). In this review, they restrict their discussions to the detection strategies including localized surface plasmon resonance (LSPR), fluorescence, electronic, and SER spectroscopy, and their integration with point-of-care systems, rather than synthesis and surface modification.

The review of Saha et al. (2012) had focused on the application of AuNPs in the fabrication of chemical and biological sensors mainly used in biomedical, environmental, and legal sciences. Thus, they highlighted a variety of synthesis routes and properties of AuNPs that make them excellent probes for different sensing strategies. These sensors have a very widespread applicability, providing a broad spectrum of innovative approaches for the detection of various metal ions, cancer cells, proteins, small molecules, microorganisms, biomarkers, etc., in a rapid and efficient manner. They can be used as both molecular receptors and signal transducers in a single sensing element leading to the miniaturization of the sensor.

1.2.3.3 PtNPs

Like other NPs, PtNPs show optical properties and can be successfully used in preparation of fluorescent markers. Thereby, Tanaka et al. (2011) reported the synthesis of water-soluble, blue-emitting, atomically monodispersed Pt_5 nanoclusters that could act as fluorescent probes for bioimaging and subcellular targeting. In order to retain the nanometer-scale size of PtNPs, they used as the template a fourth-generation polyamidoamine dendrimer with a uniform structure comprising an internal core containing tertiary amines that can form coordination bonds with the Pt ions and an external shell. Another example in this direction is the work of Yao et al. (2008) who focused their study on the fabrication of biosensors based on dendrimer-encapsulated PtNPs and glucose oxidase, for direct glucose concentration analysis.

The catalytic activity of PtNPs can be used in combination with a volumetric bar-chart chip (V-Chip) to specifically detect cancer biomarkers both in the serum and on the cell surface. Song et al. (2014) reported the integration of PtNPs into a V-Chip using the microfluidics technology to measure the production of oxygen gas volumetrically. They demonstrated that the PtNPs (~30 nm) had catalytic stability at high H_2O_2 concentrations over long reaction periods, and this activity was maintained in a broad temperature range in the presence of catalase inhibitors.

1.2.4 Wound (Dressing) Management

A wound dressing should have some properties, such as ability for wound exudate absorption, ability for releasing antimicrobial and tissue regeneration agents, high gas permeability, etc., to protect the wound from infection. Many natural and synthetic polymers, with or without NPs have been used over the year to prepare wound dressings and various publications are available (Parani et al. 2016). Nowadays, various types of dressings are available on the biomedical market. Nanofiber dressings are the most significant because of their large surface-to-volume ratios, high porosity, and softness and have led to the use of a wide variety of natural and synthetic polymers. The natural polymers that have been used to obtain electrospun nanofiber mats for wound care can include collagen, gelatin, silk, hyaluronic acid, cellulose, and chitin. The advantage of using them in the fabrication of nanofiber dressings is that they are highly biocompatible, but they also have some drawbacks such as low stiffness and mechanical strength (Zhong et al. 2010). From the class of synthetic polymers used for the development of electrospun dressing, the following can be listed: poly(vinyl alcohol), poly(caprolactone), poly(lactide), polyurethanes, poly(ethylene oxide), and different copolymers. In addition, the dressings used to treat wounds could be in the form of gels, sponges, films, etc.

1.2.4.1 AgNPs

Although silver has been recognized for centuries to inhibit infection (Klasen 2000), its use in wound care, particularly in burns, is relatively recent. There are a growing number of silver dressings in the form of creams, foams, hydrogels, meshes, and polymeric films that are already available on the market (Leaper 2006). Most of the studies performed to obtain different dressing materials were based on the determination of their antibacterial activity and have been described earlier.

In addition to its recognized antibacterial properties, which have been discussed previously, some studies have reported the healing properties of silver (Marcato et al. 2015). Thus, these results suggested that the nanosilver might play a significant role in decreasing the inflammatory response in wounds and facilitating the early phase of wound healing (Atiyeh et al. 2007).

For example, in our study, we demonstrated that the polyurethane gels enriched with AgNPs in a concentration of 10 ppm has led to the treatment of a dermatosis of unknown etiology after 78 days (Ciobanu et al. 2009). AgNPs were synthesized *in situ*, in a poly(hydroxy urethane-acrylate) matrix (Ciobanu et al. 1987), and were added to RGD (Arg-Gly-Asp) sequences. First, the antibacterial activity of the samples was tested and it was found that different amounts of AgNPs (10.907, 15.96, 31.92, 39.5, 56.88 ppm) were able to suppress the bacterial colonization rate with a good efficiency against *E. coli*, *S. aureus*, or *Candida albicans*, which were destroyed after 24 or 48 h. Then, we examined the healing behavior of skin dermatosis before (Figure 1.1a) and after treatment (Figure 1.1b) with poly(hydroxy urethane-acrylate) gel. We found the complete disappearance of the hyperkeratosis between the 8th and the 19th days and a decrease of the hyperpigmented zone with a gradual regeneration of the skin between the 24th and the 65th days. A visible regeneration of the skin without scars was also observed, especially of the hair follicle between the 57th and the 78th days, Figure 1.1b. Nanometric silver and RGD sequences contributed substantially to the healing of the dermatosis and led to the suggestion that

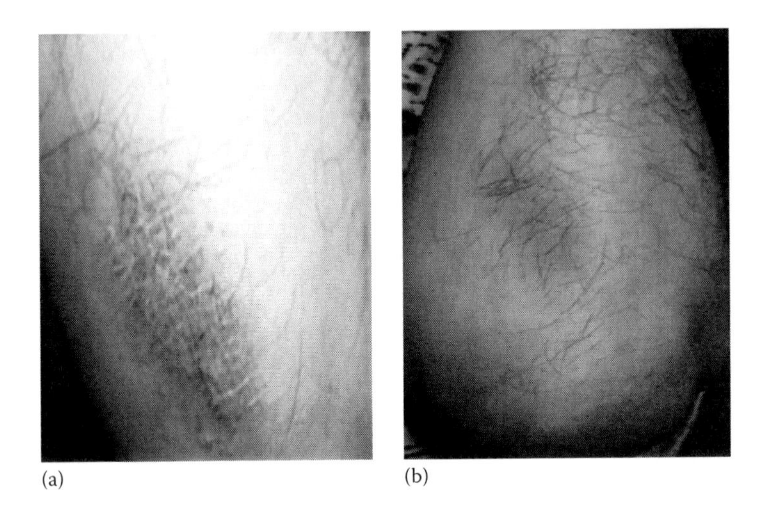

FIGURE 1.1
The patient skin (a) before treatment and (b) after 78 days of treatment with AgNPs polyurethane gel. (Courtesy of C. Ciobanu.)

a stimulation of the stem cells took place and the derma cells could appear from mesenchymal stem cells or from fibroblasts (Morasso and Tomic-Canic 2005, Bellis 2011).

Other *in vivo* studies reported that AgNPs could promote wound healing and reduce the appearance of the scar depending on the dose used (Tian et al. 2007). The decrease of inflammatory response was due to the ability of silver to modulate the cytokines involved in wound healing.

1.2.4.2 AuNPs

The unique properties of AuNPs, such as antimicrobial properties, and easy incorporation of peptides, antibody, and growth factors at the surface, make them suitable for the preparation of various wound dressings in the form of gels, sponges, films, etc.

Leu et al. (2012) showed that the AuNPs mixed with two antioxidants accelerated wound healing in mice by a mechanism that may involve anti-inflammatory and antioxidation actions in the cutaneous wound and, moreover, led to the proliferation and migration of Hs68 and HaCaT cells. The toxicity of spherical AuNPs (25–50 nm) on cell viability and on biomarkers involved in wound healing was tested by Pivodová et al. (2015). The resulting data revealed that AuNPs were not toxic to fibroblasts and keratinocytes and also decreased the production of pro-inflammatory cytokines and proteins involved in angiogenesis.

Recently, Akturk et al. (2016) evaluated the role of AuNPs (13–55 nm) embedded in collagen sponges on wound healing. First, they evaluated the properties of these cross-linked nanocomposites and the data showed that the AuNP–collagen scaffolds have higher resistance against hydrolytic and enzymatic degradation and higher tensile strength. *In vivo* studies showed that the AuNP–collagen nanocomposite sponge had a higher wound closure percentage, reduced inflammatory response, and increased tensile strength, elastic modulus, neovascularization, and granulation tissue formation, than untreated control group.

1.2.4.3 PtNPs

The catalytic activity of platinum (Pt) and palladium (Pd) NPs highlights their possibility for being used as antioxidants and promising compounds in materials science and engineering.

But, the number of the studies in this field is very small compared to those carried out for AgNPs. Thus, the antioxidant properties were evaluated in several research studies (Kim et al. 2008, Shiny et al. 2014, Yusof and Ismail 2015). For example, the work of Shibuya et al. (2014) revealed that a mixture of Pt and Pd NPs could have protective effects against aging-related skin pathologies in mice. To highlight the mechanisms of the *in vivo* effects of this mixture, they analyzed the expression profiles of skin-related genes, including those involved in matrix biosynthesis, inflammation, and aging, and they found that this treatment had few adverse effects on the skin morphology.

1.3 Conclusions and Future Directions

Due to the unique characteristics and properties, metal NPs, especially NMNPs, have allowed the development of a broad range of applications in the medical, electronic, and industrial fields. Nanotechnology represents a modern and innovative approach to develop and test new formulations based on NMNPs used in biomedical applications. Thus, nanotechnology is a promising tool to obtain more cost-effective therapies to improve, in the end, the patient's quality of life.

The physicochemical properties of MNPs depend on their size, shape, surface properties, and also the mode of synthesis. Any change in them, even very small, leads to an exponential change in the properties and biological activity of NPs. The decrease in the particle size to the nanometer length scale increases the surface-to-volume ratio and makes them very good candidates for obtaining different antibacterial materials. The optical properties of NMNPs are a promising approach in the development of new bioimaging and biosensing strategies, especially in cancer therapy. A wide range of NMNP materials could be used as delivery agents to accelerate the regeneration of various wounds or to control their infection.

Therefore, a clear understanding of the polymer–noble metal nanocomposites structures, synthesis, and interaction with the biological environment, including toxicological considerations, is very important.

This chapter has attempted to summarize the fundamental understanding of the effect of NMNPs on the cells by highlighting their physicochemical properties in their current and potential applications such as antimicrobials, cancer detection, diagnosis and treatment, bioimaging and biosensing, and wound healing management. This subject needs extensive collaboration between researchers with expertise in chemistry, biology, medicine, nanoscience, and nanotechnology to provide new fundamental insights into a deep understanding of the interaction of NMNPs with the biological environment. A major challenge for the researchers consists in achieving the large-scale preparation of these types of biomaterials, because most of them are mainly for laboratory use on a research level. In conclusion, a wide variety of structures, properties, and applications are available for the preparation of polymer–noble metal nanocomposites that could be successfully used in nanotechnology.

Acknowledgments

The authors acknowledge the financial support of this research through the European Regional Development Fund, Project POINGBIO, ID P_40_443, Contract no. 86/8.09.2016.

References

Abou El-Nour, K. M. M., Eftaiha, A., Al-Warthan, A., and Ammar, R. A. A. 2010. Synthesis and applications of silver nanoparticles. *Arab J Chem* 3:135–140.

Ahmed, K. B. A., Raman, T., and Anbazhagan, V. 2016. Platinum nanoparticles inhibits bacteria proliferation and rescue zebrafish from bacterial infection. *RSC Adv* 6:44415–44424.

Ahmed, S. and Ikram, S. 2015. Synthesis of gold nanoparticles using plant extract: An overview. *Nano Res Appl* 1:1–6.

Akhter, S., Ahmad, M. Z., Singh, A. et al. 2011. Cancer targeted metallic nanoparticle: Targeting overview, recent advancement and toxicity concern. *Curr Pharm Des* 17(18):1834–1850.

Akturk, O., Kismet, K., Yasti, A. C. et al. 2016. Collagen/gold nanoparticle nanocomposites: A potential skin wound healing biomaterial. *J Biomater Appl* 31(2):283–301.

Atiyeh, B. S., Costagliola, M., Hayek, S. N., and Dibo, S. A. 2007. Effect of silver on burn wound infection control and healing: Review of the literature. *Burns* 33:139–148.

Babu, A. C., Prabhakar, M. N., Babu, A. S. et al. 2013. Development and characterization of semi-IPN silver nanocomposite hydrogels for antibacterial applications. *Int J Carbohydr Chem* 2013:8. ID 243695. doi:http://dx.doi.org/10.1155/2013/243695.

Badwaik, V. D., Vangala, L. M., Pender, D. S. et al. 2012. Size-dependent antimicrobial properties of sugar-encapsulated gold nanoparticles synthesized by a green method. *Nanoscale Res Lett* 7:623–634.

Ballottin, D., Fulaz, S., Souza, M. L. et al. 2016. Elucidating protein involvement in the stabilization of the biogenic silver nanoparticles. *Nanoscale Res Lett* 11:313–322.

Behra, R., Sigg, L., Clift, M. J. D. et al. 2013. Bioavailability of silver nanoparticles and ions: From a chemical and biochemical perspective. *J R Soc Interface* 10(87):20130396. doi:10.1098/rsif.2013.0396.

Bellis, S. L. 2011. Advantages of RGD peptides for directing cell association with biomaterials. *Biomaterials* 32(18):4205–4210.

Bhattacharyya, S., Kudgus, R. A., Bhattacharya, R., and Mukherjee, P. 2011. Inorganic nanoparticles in cancer therapy. *Pharm Res* 28(2):237–259.

Brown, S. D., Nativo, P., Smith, J.-A. et al. 2010. Gold nanoparticles for the improved anticancer drug delivery of the active component of oxaliplatin. *J Am Chem Soc* 132:4678–4684.

Cardinal, J., Klune, J. R., Chory, E. et al. 2008. Noninvasive radiofrequency ablation of cancer targeted by gold nanoparticles. *Surgery* 144:125–132.

Castro, L., Blázquez, M. L., González, F., Muñoz, J. A., and Ballester, A. 2013. Gold, silver and platinum nanoparticles biosynthesized using orange peel extract. *Adv Mater Res* 825:556–559.

Chen, J., Peng, Y., Zheng, Z., Sun, P., and Wang, X. 2014. Silver-releasing and antibacterial activities of polyphenol-based polyurethanes. *J Appl Polym Sci* 131:41349–41358.

Cherukuri, P., Glazer, E. S., and Curley, S. A. 2010. Targeted hyperthermia using metal nanoparticles. *Adv Drug Deliv Rev* 62:339–345.

Ciobanu, C., Farcas, A., Badea, N. et al. 1987. Process for preparing some poly(hidroxyurethan-acrylates). RO 93572/1987.

Ciobanu, C., Gavriliu, S., Lungu, M., Gavriliu, L., and Ciobanu, L. C. 2009. Polyurethane gel with silver nanoparticles for the treatment of skin diseases. *Open Chem Biomed Methods J* 2:86–90.

Conde, J., Doria, G., and Baptista, P. 2012. Noble metal nanoparticles applications in cancer. *J Drug Deliv* 2012:751075. doi:10.1155/2012/751075.

Cui, Y., Zhao, Y., Tian, Y. et al. 2012. The molecular mechanism of action of bactericidal gold nanoparticles on *Escherichia coli*. *Biomaterials* 33:2327–2333.

Dallas, P., Sharma, V. K., and Zboril, R. 2011. Silver polymeric nanocomposites as advanced antimicrobial agents: Classification, synthetic paths, applications, and perspectives. *Adv Colloid Interface Sci* 166:119–135.

Dhand, C., Dwivedi, N., Loh, X. J. et al. 2015. Methods and strategies for the synthesis of diverse nanoparticles and their applications: A comprehensive overview. *RSC Adv* 5:105003–105037.

Díaz, M. R. and Vivas-Mejia, P. E. 2013. Nanoparticles as drug delivery systems in cancer medicine: Emphasis on RNAi-containing nanoliposomes. *Pharmaceuticals* 6:1361–1380.

Doria, G., Conde, J., Veigas, B. et al. 2012. Noble metal nanoparticles for biosensing applications. *Sensors* 12:1657–1687.

Duncan, B., Kim, C., and Rotello, V. M. 2010. Gold nanoparticle platforms as drug and biomacromolecule delivery systems. *J Control Release* 148:122–127.

Durán, N., Durán, M., Bispo de Jesus, M. et al. 2016. Silver nanoparticles: A new view on mechanistic aspects on antimicrobial activity. *Nanomedicine: NBM* 12:789–799.

Eckhardt, S., Brunetto, P. S., Gagnon, J. et al. 2013. Nanobio silver: Its interactions with peptides and bacteria, and its uses in medicine. *Chem Rev* 113:4708–4754.

El-Deeb, N. M., El-Sherbiny, I. M., El-Aassara, M. R., and Hafez, E. E. 2015. Novel trend in colon cancer therapy using silver nanoparticles synthesized by honey bee. *J Nanomed Nanotechnol* 6:265. doi:10.4172/2157-7439.1000265.

El-Sayed, I. H., Huang, X., and El-Sayed, M. A. 2005. Surface plasmon resonance scattering and absorption of anti-EGFR antibody conjugated gold nanoparticles in cancer diagnostics: Applications in oral cancer. *Nano Lett* 5(5):829–834.

Franci, G., Falanga, A., Galdiero, S. et al. 2015. Silver nanoparticles as potential antibacterial agents. *Molecules* 20:8856–8874.

Garcia-Orue, I., Gainza, G., Villullas, S. et al. 2016. Nanotechnology approaches for skin wound regeneration using drug-delivery systems. In *Nanobiomaterials in Soft Tissue Engineering: Applications of Nanobiomaterials*, A. Grumezescu (Ed.), pp. 31–55. Oxford, U.K.: Elsevier Inc.

Haes, A. J., Hall, W. P., Chang, L., Klein, W. L., and Van Duyne, R. P. 2004. A localized surface plasmon resonance biosensor: First steps toward an assay for Alzheimer's disease. *Nano Lett* 4(6):1029–1034.

Haider, A. and Kang, I.-K. 2015. Preparation of silver nanoparticles and their industrial and biomedical applications: A comprehensive review. *Adv Mater Sci Eng* 2015:16. ID 165257. doi:http://dx.doi.org/10.1155/2015/165257.

Hajipour, M. J., Fromm, K. M., Ashkarran, A. A. et al. 2012. Antibacterial properties of nanoparticles. *Trends Biotechnol* 30:499–511.

Han, J. W., Gurunathan, S., Jeong, J.-K. et al. 2014. Oxidative stress mediated cytotoxicity of biologically synthesized silver nanoparticles in human lung epithelial adenocarcinoma cell line. *Nanoscale Res Lett* 9:459–473.

Hsu, S.-H., Tseng, H.-J., and Lin, Y.-C. 2010. The biocompatibility and antibacterial properties of waterborne polyurethane-silver nanocomposites. *Biomaterials* 31:6796–6808.

Hussain, M. A., Shah, A., Jantan, I. et al. 2015. Hydroxypropylcellulose as a novel green reservoir for the synthesis, stabilization, and storage of silver nanoparticles. *Int J Nanomedicine* 10:2079–2088.

Jain, S., Hirst, D. G., and O'Sullivan, J. M. 2012. Gold nanoparticles as novel agents for cancer therapy. *Br J Radiol* 85:101–113.

Jeyaraj, M., Sathishkumar, G., Sivanandhan, G. et al. 2013. Biogenic silver nanoparticles for cancer treatment: An experimental report. *Colloids Surf B Biointerfaces* 106:86–92.

Kim, J., Takahashi, M., Shimizu, T. et al. 2008. Effects of a potent antioxidant, platinum nanoparticle, on the lifespan of *Caenorhabditis elegans*. *Mech Ageing Dev* 129:322–331.

Kim, J. S., Kuk, E., Yu, K. N. et al. 2007. Antimicrobial effects of silver nanoparticles. *Nanomedicine: NBM* 3:95–101.

Klasen, H. J. 2000. Historical review of the use of silver in the treatment of burns. I. Early uses. *Burns* 26:117–130.

Krishnaraj, C., Muthukumaran, P., Ramachandran, R., Balakumaran, M. D., and Kalaichelvan, P. T. 2014. *Acalypha indica* Linn.: Biogenic synthesis of silver and gold nanoparticles and their cytotoxic effects against MDA-MB-231, human breast cancer cells. *Biotechnol Rep* 4:42–49.

Kumar, B., Smita, K., Seqqat, R. et al. 2016. In vitro evaluation of silver nanoparticles cytotoxicity on Hepatic cancer (Hep-G2) cell line and their antioxidant activity: Green approach for fabrication and application. *J Photochem Photobiol B: Biol* 159:8–13.

Kuppusamy, P., Yusoff, M. M., Maniam, G. P., and Govindan, N. 2016. Biosynthesis of metallic nanoparticles using plant derivatives and their new avenues in pharmacological applications—An updated report. *Saudi Pharm J* 24(4):473–484.

Kurek, A., Grudniak, A. M., Kraczkiewicz-Dowjat, A., and Wolska, K. I. 2011. New antibacterial therapeutics and strategies. *Pol J Microbiol* 60(1):3–12.

Lakshman, L. R., Shalumon, K. T., Nair, S. V., Jayakumar, R., and Nair, S. V. 2010. Preparation of silver nanoparticles incorporated electrospun polyurethane nanofibrous mat for wound dressing. *J Macromol Sci: Pure Appl Chem* 47:1012–1018.

Leaper, D. J. 2006. Silver dressings: Their role in wound management. *Int Wound J* 3(4):282–294.

Leu, J.-G., Chen, S.-A., Chen, H.-M. et al. 2012. The effects of gold nanoparticles in wound healing with antioxidant epigallocatechin gallate and α-lipoic acid. *Nanomedicine: NBM* 8:767–775.

Li, W.-R., Xie, X.-B., Shi, Q.-S. et al. 2010. Antibacterial activity and mechanism of silver nanoparticles on *Escherichia coli*. *Appl Microbiol Biotechnol* 85:1115–1122.

Liu, H.-L., Dai, S. A., Fu, K.-Y., and Hsu, S.-H. 2010. Antibacterial properties of silver nanoparticles in three different sizes and their nanocomposites with a new waterborne polyurethane. *Int J Nanomedicine* 5:1017–1028.

Magdolenova, Z., Collins, A. R., Kumar, A. et al. 2014. Mechanisms of genotoxicity: Review of recent in vitro and in vivo studies with engineered nanoparticles. *Nanotoxicology* 8(3):233–278.

Mahmoudi, M., Meng, J., Xue, X. et al. 2014. Interaction of stable colloidal nanoparticles with cellular membranes. *Biotechnol Adv* 32:679–692.

Manke, A., Wang, L., and Rojanasakul, Y. 2013. Mechanisms of nanoparticle-induced oxidative stress and toxicity. *Biomed Res Int* 2013:15. ID 942916. doi:http://dx.doi.org/10.1155/2013/942916.

Marcato, P. D., De Paula, L. B., Melo, P. S. et al. 2015. In vivo evaluation of complex biogenic silver nanoparticle and enoxaparin in wound healing. *J Nanomater* 2015:10. ID 439820. doi:http://dx.doi.org/10.1155/2015/439820.

Miethling-Graff, R., Rumpker, R., Richter, M. et al. 2014. Exposure to silver nanoparticles induces size- and dose-dependent oxidative stress and cytotoxicity in human colon carcinoma cells. *Toxicol In Vitro* 28:1280–1289.

Minelli, C., Lowe, S. B., and Stevens, M. M. 2010. Engineering nanocomposite materials for cancer therapy. *Small* 6:2336–2357.

Mollick, M. M. R., Rana, D., Dash, S. K. et al. 2015. Studies on green synthesized silver nanoparticles using *Abelmoschus esculentus* (L.) pulp extract having anticancer (in vitro) and antimicrobial applications. *Arab J Chem*. doi:http://dx.doi.org/10.1016/j.arabjc.2015.04.033.

Morasso, M. I. and Tomic-Canic, M. 2005. Epidermal stem cells: The cradle of epidermal determination, differentiation and wound healing. *Biol Cell* 97(3):173–183.

Morones, J. R., Elechiguerra, J. L., Camacho, A. et al. 2005. The bactericidal effect of silver nanoparticles. *Nanotechnology* 16:2346–2353.

Muddineti, O. S., Ghosh, B., and Biswas, S. 2015. Current trends in using polymer coated gold nanoparticles for cancer therapy. *Int J Pharm* 484:252–267.

Muthukumar, T., Sudhakumari, B., Sambandam, B. et al. 2016. Green synthesis of gold nanoparticles and their enhanced synergistic antitumor activity using HepG2 and MCF7 cells and its antibacterial effects. *Process Biochem* 51:384–391.

Oberoi, H. S., Nukolova, N. V., Kabanov, A. V., and Bronich, T. K. 2013. Nanocarriers for delivery of platinum anticancer drugs. *Adv Drug Deliv Rev* 65:1667–1685.

Paciotti, G. F., Myer, L., Weinreich, D. et al. 2004. Colloidal gold: A novel nanoparticle vector for tumor directed drug delivery. *Drug Deliv* 11:169–183.

Pal, S., Tak, Y. K., and Song, J. M. 2007. Does the antibacterial activity of silver nanoparticles depend on the shape of the nanoparticle? A study of the Gram-negative bacterium *Escherichia coli*. *Appl Environ Microbiol* 73(6):1712–1720.

Parani, M., Lokhande, G., Singh, A., and Gaharwar, A. K. 2016. Engineered nanomaterials for infection control and healing acute and chronic wounds. *ACS Appl Mater Interfaces* 8(16):10049–10069.

Paul, D., Paul, S., Roohpour, N., Wilks, M., and Vadgama, P. 2013. Antimicrobial, mechanical and thermal studies of silver particle-loaded polyurethane. *J Funct Biomater* 4:358–375.

Pivodová, V., Franková, J., Galandáková, A., and Ulrichová, J. 2015. In vitro AuNPs' cytotoxicity and their effect on wound healing. *Nanobiomedicine* 2:7, doi:10.5772/61132.

Porcel, E., Liehn, S., Remita, H. et al. 2010. Platinum nanoparticles: A promising material for future cancer therapy? *Nanotechnology* 21:085103.

Prabhu, S. and Poulose, E. K. 2012. Silver nanoparticles: Mechanism of antimicrobial action, synthesis, medical applications, and toxicity effects. *Int Nano Lett* 2:32–42.

Praetorius, N. P. and Mandal, T. K. 2007. Engineered nanoparticles in cancer therapy. *Recent Pat Drug Deliv Formul* 1:37–51.

Qu, R., Gao, J., Tang, B. et al. 2014. Preparation and property of polyurethane/nanosilver complex fibers. *Appl Surf Sci* 294:81–88.

Raghunandan, D., Ravishankar, B., Sharanbasava, G. et al. 2011. Anti-cancer studies of noble metal nanoparticles synthesized using different plant extracts. *Cancer Nanotechnol* 2:57–65.

Rai, M., Yadav, A., and Gade, A. 2009. Silver nanoparticles as a new generation of antimicrobials. *Biotechnol Adv* 27:76–83.

Ramaswamy, S. V. P., Sivaraj, R., Suji, M., and Vanathi, P. 2015. Role of biogenic synthesis of biocompatible nano gold particles and their potential applications—A review. *J Pharm Chem Biol Sci* 3(1):104–113.

Rana, S., Bajaj, A., Mout, R., and Rotello, V. M. 2012. Monolayer coated gold nanoparticles for delivery applications. *Adv Drug Deliv Rev* 64:200–216.

Rao, P. V., Nallappan, D., Madhavi, K. et al. 2016. Phytochemicals and biogenic metallic nanoparticles as anticancer agents. *Oxid Med Cell Longev* 2016:15. ID 3685671. doi:10.1155/2016/3685671.

Regiel-Futyra, A., Kus-Liśkiewicz, M., Sebastian, V. et al. 2015. Development of noncytotoxic chitosan–gold nanocomposites as efficient antibacterial materials. *ACS Appl Mater Interfaces* 7:1087–1099.

Rizzello, L. and Pompa, P. P. 2014. Nanosilver-based antibacterial drugs and devices: Mechanisms, methodological drawbacks, and guidelines. *Chem Soc Rev* 43:1501–1518.

Saha, K., Agasti, S. S., Kim, C., Li, X., and Rotello, V. M. 2012. Gold nanoparticles in chemical and biological sensing. *Chem Rev* 112(5):2739–2779.

Salem, W., Leitner, D. R., Zingl, F. G. et al. 2015. Antibacterial activity of silver and zinc nanoparticles against *Vibrio cholerae* and enterotoxic *Escherichia coli*. *Int J Med Microbiol* 305:85–95.

Shah, M., Poinern, G. E. J., Sharma, S. B., and Fawcett, D. 2015. Biogenic synthesis of gold and silver nanoparticles using the leaf extract from *Eucalyptus macrocarpa*. *Int J Sci* 4:27–33.

Shawkey, A. M., Rabeh, M. A., Abdulall, A. K., and Abdellatif, A. O. 2013. Green nanotechnology: Anticancer activity of silver nanoparticles using *Citrullus colocynthis* aqueous extracts. *Adv Life Sci Technol* 13:60–70.

Sheikh, F. A., Barakat, N. A. M., Kanjwal, M. A. et al. 2009. Electrospun antimicrobial polyurethane nanofibers containing silver nanoparticles for biotechnological applications. *Macromol Res* 17(9):688–696.

Shibuya, S., Ozawa, Y., Watanabe, K. et al. 2014. Palladium and platinum nanoparticles attenuate aging-like skin atrophy via antioxidant activity in mice. *PLoS One* 9(10):e109288. doi:10.1371/journal.pone.0109288.

Shiny, P. J., Mukherjee, A., and Chandrasekaran, N. 2014. Haemocompatibility assessment of synthesised platinum nanoparticles and its implication in biology. *Bioprocess Biosyst Eng* 37:991–997.

Skrabalak, S. E., Au, L., Lu, X., Li, X., and Xia, Y. 2007. Gold nanocages for cancer detection and treatment. *Nanomedicine* 2(5):657–668.

Sondi, I. and Salopek-Sondi, B. 2004. Silver nanoparticles as antimicrobial agent: A case study on *E. coli* as a model for Gram-negative bacteria. *J Colloid Interface Sci* 275:177–182.

Song, Y., Xia, X., Wu, X., Wang, P., and Qin, L. 2014. Integration of platinum nanoparticles with a volumetric bar-chart chip for biomarker assays. *Angew Chem Int Ed* 53:12451–12455.

Sotiriou, G. A. and Pratsinis, S. E. 2011. Engineering nanosilver as an antibacterial, biosensor and bioimaging material. *Curr Opin Chem Eng* 1(1):3–10.

Tanaka, S.-I., Miyazaki, J., Tiwari, D. K., Jin, T., and Inouye, Y. 2011. Fluorescent platinum nanoclusters: Synthesis, purification, characterization, and application to bioimaging. *Angew Chem Int Ed* 50:431–435.

Tang, H.-W., Yang, X. B., Kirkham, J., and Smith, D. A. 2007. Probing intrinsic and extrinsic components in single osteosarcoma cells by near-infrared surface-enhanced Raman scattering. *Anal Chem* 79:3646–3653.

Thurn, K. T., Brown, E. M. B., Wu, A. et al. 2007. Nanoparticles for applications in cellular imaging. *Nanoscale Res Lett* 2:430–441.

Tian, J., Wong, K. K. Y., Ho, C.-M. et al. 2007. Topical delivery of silver nanoparticles promotes wound healing. *Chem Med Chem* 2:129–136.

Uehara, N. and Nagaoka, T. 2010. Gold–polymer nanocomposites for bioimaging and biosensing. In *Nanomaterials for the Life Sciences*, C. S. S. R. Kumar (Ed.), pp. 199–240. Weinheim, Germany: Wiley-VCH Verlag GmbH & Co.

Wang, R., Wang, Z., Lin, S. et al. 2015. Green fabrication of antibacterial polymer/silver nanoparticle nanohybrids by dual-spinneret electrospinning. *RSC Adv* 5:40141–40147.

Wei, L., Lu, J., Xu, H. et al. 2015. Silver nanoparticles: Synthesis, properties, and therapeutic applications. *Drug Discov Today* 20(5):595–601.

Willets, K. A., Hall, W. P., Sherry, L. J. et al. 2007. Nanoscale localized surface plasmon resonance biosensors. In *Nanobiotechnology*, C. A. Mirkin and C. M. Niemeyer (Eds.), pp. 159–173. Weinheim, Germany: Wiley-VCH Verlag GmbH & Co.

Wilson, A. J. and Willets, K. A. 2013. Surface-enhanced Raman scattering imaging using noble metal nanoparticles. *Nanomed Nanobiotechnol* 5:180–189. doi:10.1002/wnan.1208.

Wu, J., Hou, S., Ren, D., and Mather, P. T. 2009. Antimicrobial properties of nanostructured hydrogel webs containing silver. *Biomacromolecules* 10:2686–2693.

Xie, J., Lee, J. Y., Wang, D. I. C., and Ting, Y. P. 2007. Silver nanoplates: From biological to biomimetic synthesis. *ACS Nano* 1(5):429–439.

Yao, K., Zhu, Y., Yang, X., and Li, C. 2008. ENFET glucose biosensor produced with dendrimer encapsulated Pt nanoparticles. *Mater Sci Eng C* 28:1236–1241.

Yusof, F. and Ismail, N. A. S. 2015. Antioxidants effects of platinum nanoparticles: A potential alternative treatment to lung diseases. *J Appl Pharm Sci* 5(7):140–145.

Zhang, T., Song, Y.-J., Zhang, X.-Y., and Wu, J.-Y. 2014. Synthesis of silver nanostructures by multistep methods. *Sensors* 14:5860–5889.

Zhang, X.-F., Liu, Z.-G., Shen, W., and Gurunathan, S. 2016. Silver nanoparticles: Synthesis, characterization, properties, applications, and therapeutic approaches. *Int J Mol Sci* 17:1534–1568.

Zhang, Y. J., Huang, R., Zhu, X. F., Wang, L. Z., and Wu, C. X. 2012. Synthesis, properties, and optical applications of noble metal nanoparticle-biomolecule conjugates. *Chin Sci Bull* 57:238–246.

Zheng, J., Ding, Y., Tian, B., Wang, Z. L., and Zhuang, X. 2008. Luminescent and Raman active silver nanoparticles with polycrystalline structure. *J Am Chem Soc* 130:10472–10473.

Zhong, W., Xing, M. M. Q., and Maibach, H. I. 2010. Nanofibrous materials for wound care. *Cutan Ocul Toxicol* 29(3):143–152.

Zhou, W., Gao, X., Liu, D., and Chen, X. 2015. Gold nanoparticles for in vitro diagnostics. *Chem Rev* 115(19):10575–10636.

Zhou, Y., Kong, Y., Kundu, S., Cirillo, J. D., and Liang, H. 2012. Antibacterial activities of gold and silver nanoparticles against *Escherichia coli* and bacillus Calmette-Guérin. *J Nanobiotechnol* 10:19–28.

2

Advances in Polymer Nanofibers Containing Metal Oxide Nanoparticles

Petronela Dorneanu, Anton Airinei, and Nicolae Olaru

CONTENTS

2.1 Introduction

In recent years, polymer–inorganic nanoparticle composites have gained great importance because of their unique properties, such as high mechanical strength and excellent electrical, magnetic, and optical properties, which are essentially different from those of the components taken separately or the physically combined properties of each component. These nanocomposites have attracted wide interest in both academic and industrial fields for their diverse potential applications in energy storage devices (Kim et al. 2009), electronics (Vacca et al. 2009), microwave absorbers (Guo et al. 2009), and sensors (Shimada et al. 2007). Generally, nanocomposites containing organic–inorganic components can be obtained by adding nanoparticles into polymer matrices or by the polymerization of monomers in the presence of metal nanoparticles. It is known that polymers are considered to be good host materials for metal (nonmagnetic/ferromagnetic) (Chen et al. 2011; Pascariu-Dorneanu et al. 2015) and semiconductor (Kim et al. 2010; Qin et al. 2013) nanoparticles, which exhibit exceptional optical and electrical properties. Also, because of their large surface-to-volume ratio, which results from their small sizes compared to the high surface-to-bulk ratio, nanoparticles significantly influence the matrix leading to some new properties that are not present in either of the pure materials. Therefore, the investigation of the influence of nanoparticles on the properties of a polymer matrix is necessary in order to be able to better predict the final properties of the composite.

Metal oxide nanoparticles have attracted much attention because they show a variety of properties (especially electrical and optical) from wide bandgap insulators and lasers to metallic, superconducting, and field emitting materials. These metal oxide nanoparticles can be obtained from different materials, such as zinc oxide (ZnO), tin oxide (SnO_2), nickel oxide (NiO), titanium dioxide (TiO_2), copper oxide (CuO), aluminum oxide (Al_2O_3), iron oxide (Fe_3O_4), magnesium oxide (MgO), etc. (Park et al. 2005; Zhao et al. 2007; Outokesh et al. 2011; Camtakan et al. 2012; Srivastava et al. 2013; Danial et al. 2015; Wu et al. 2015; Pascariu-Dorneanu et al. 2016). The properties of metal oxide nanoparticles depend on their preparation mode, dimensions, and good dispersion. The coupling of semiconductor metal oxides with matched bandgap configurations enhances the electrical, optical, and catalytic properties, and it has been extensively investigated for various potential applications, such as gas and humidity sensors (Li et al. 2014), solar cells (Wang et al. 2012), lithium batteries (Li and Li 2010), catalysis (Jamnongkan et al. 2014), and transparent conductive electrodes (Kim et al. 2010). Many different preparation methods have been applied to obtain nanofibers containing metal oxides. These methods include the coprecipitation procedure followed by the calcination (Outokesh et al. 2011), hydrothermal, or solvothermal route (Park et al. 2005), and the sol–gel process (Wu et al. 2015) combined with electrospinning techniques

(Camtakan et al. 2012). The electrospinning technique has the advantage of synthesizing nanostructures with larger surface-to-volume ratios, higher crystalline phase purities, and tunable morphologies like nanofibers, nanowires, nanoflowers, and nanorods.

2.2 Fundamental Considerations on Organic–Inorganic Nanofibers

Polymer nanofibers prepared by the electrospinning method are of industrial and scientific interest due to their long lengths, small diameters and pores, and high surface area per unit volume, which enable them to be used in several applications, such as tissue scaffolds, protective clothing, filters, sensors, etc. Also, metal oxide nanoparticles reinforced in polymer matrices produce nanocomposites known to improve mechanical strength, good conductivity, thermal stability, etc. Moreover, these nanostructures (organic/inorganic nanocomposites) represent an alternative way to obtain new materials with enhanced properties, which allow these nanocomposites to be used in various applications such as electronic, optical, and mechanical devices, magnetic recording media, catalysis, superconductors, ferrofluids, and magnetic refrigeration systems.

The incorporation of semiconducting oxides (undoped/doped with metal nanoparticles) into a polymer matrix using the electrospinning method has been used to produce inorganic/organic nanocomposites. Li et al. presented the structural, morphological, and optical properties of electrospun VO_2/PVP composite fibers (Li et al. 2014). ZnO has attracted much attention due to its chemical stability and good antimicrobial activity (Li and Li 2010; Wang et al. 2012). ZnO, being essentially nontoxic to humans and environmentally friendly, is especially suitable for biomedical applications. Therefore, electrospun poly(vinyl alcohol) (PVA) containing ZnO nanoparticles will have antibacterial properties with possible biomedical applications in wound dressings. In this regard, Jamnongkan et al. reported the effect of ZnO nanoparticles on the electrospinning characteristics of some PVA/ZnO nanofibers (Jamnongkan et al. 2014). Another metal oxide semiconductor is TiO_2, which has attracted increasing interest due to its optical and electrical applications, such as photocatalysis, gas sensors, and dye-sensitized solar cells and batteries. Furthermore, the mechanical stability of an electrospun nanofibrous mat can be improved by introducing interfiber bonding using a controlled electrospinning process or an after-treatment. Kim et al. reported the enhancement of mechanical properties of TiO_2 nanofibers by reinforcement in polysulfone fibers (Kim et al. 2010).

The incorporation of the magnetic nanoparticles into a polymer matrix using the electrospinning method is still rarely reported. Chen et al.

have investigated the morphology and thermal stability of some electrospun magnetic fibrillar polystyrene (PS)/Ni nanocomposites (Chen et al. 2010a,b). Recently, Pascariu et al. reported the morphological, photophysical (emission spectra, fluorescence quantum yields, and time-resolved fluorescence), and surface characteristics of electrospun polysulfone/nickel nanofibers (Pascariu-Dorneanu et al. 2015). Zhu et al. reported data on the morphology, thermal stability, and magnetic properties of electrospun Fe–FeO/polyimide nanocomposite fibers (Zhu et al. 2010). However, until now only a few reports were found on the construction of metal oxide/polysulfone composite nanofibers by electrospinning (Kim et al. 2010). Organic–inorganic fibrous composites are of great interest because of their promising environmental capabilities as oil sorbents, such as in oil spill cleanup, oil/water separation, and environmental remediation. The incorporation of a magnetic component in sorbent materials can be useful in the recovery process from the water surface (Liu et al. 2015; Cojocaru et al. 2017).

Jiang et al. reported the fabrication of PS/polyvinylidene fluoride (PVDF) nanofibers incorporating (Fe_3O_4 nanoparticles for oil-in-water separation (Jiang et al. 2015). The incorporation of a magnetic component in sorbent materials can be useful in the recovery process from the water surface. Also, Chen and Pan (2013) prepared different oil sorbent–reinforced magnetic materials to achieve the idea of easy repick after the sorbents are saturated. In 2015, Liu et al. synthesized Fe_3O_4/polyacrylonitrile composite nanofibers (Liu et al. 2015). These composites possess good absorption capacities and can have promising potential in wastewater treatment for the removal of antibiotics.

2.3 Electrospinning Method to Obtaining Polymer Nanofibers Containing Metal Oxide Nanoparticles

Electrospinning has been recognized as one of the most efficient techniques for the fabrication of micro- or nanoscale polymer fibers. Generally, the electrospinning method uses an electrically charged jet of polymer solution to produce polymer fibers by applying a high voltage potential of 10–40 kV between a syringe tip and a ground collector. The surface tension on the fluid droplet at the syringe tip is overcome by the strength of the electric field and a charged jet of fluid stretches from the syringe tip and deposits onto the ground collector, forming a mat of fibers with diameters in the micrometer and nanometer scale. As shown in Figure 2.1, the electrospinning system is composed of three main components: a high-voltage source, a syringe pump containing polymer solution/melt attached to a needle of small diameter, and a rotary collector disk (Cojocaru et al. 2017).

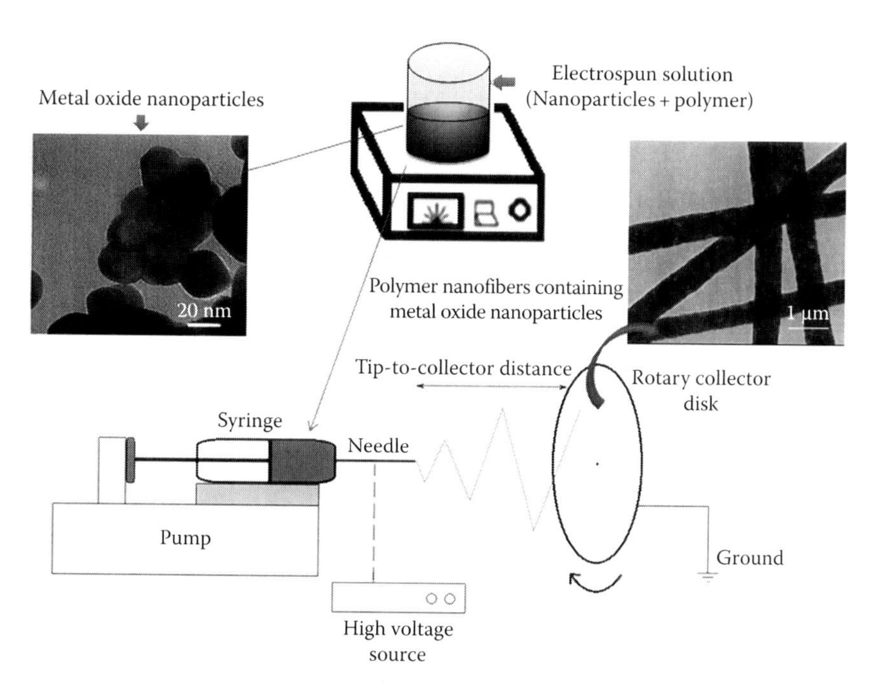

FIGURE 2.1
Schematic diagram of the electrospinning setup. (Adapted from Cojocaru, C. et al., *J. Taiwan Inst. Chem. Eng.*, 70, 267, 2017.)

The electrospinning process depends on the following parameters: (1) solution parameters (molecular weight of the polymer, viscosity, polymer concentration, conductivity, and surface tension); (2) working parameters (electric potential, flow rate, and distance between tip and collector), and (3) ambient parameters (temperature, humidity, and air velocity in the chamber).

2.3.1 Molecular Weight

Haghi et al. reported that the molecular weight of polymer has a significant effect on the rheological and electrical properties of the resulting nanofibers, such as viscosity, surface tension, conductivity, and dielectric strength (Haghi and Akbari 2007). It has been observed that too-low-molecular-weight solutions tend to form beads rather than fibers and high-molecular-weight nanofiber solutions form fibers with larger average diameters.

2.3.2 Polymer Solutions

Generally, the morphology of the nanofibers is directly influenced by viscosity and surface tension of the spinning solution. Razak et al. reported that for fiber formation to occur the viscosity of the solution must have values

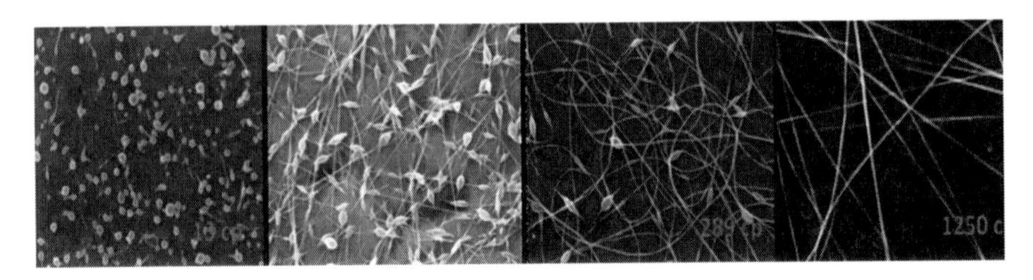

FIGURE 2.2
Evolution of the morphology of poly(ethyleneoxide) fibers upon increase of solution viscosity (viscosity values are given in gray). (Adapted from Fong, H. et al., *Polymer*, 40, 4585, 1999.)

between 1 and 20 poises and surface tension values of 35–55 dynes/cm^2 (Razak et al. 2015). If the viscosity of the solution is greater than 20 poises, the electrospinning process is hindered and the fibrous structure presents a nonuniform morphology with various sizes of fiber diameter. The fibers produced from the lower viscosity (below 1 poise) show a fibrous structure with more beads. Also, solvent volatility is a fundamental criterion in the electrospinning method. Bahrami et al. analyzed the effect of using solvents of different polarities, such as glacial acetic acid, dimethylformamide, glacial formic acid, and acetone, on the morphology of polymer nanofibers (Bahrami and Kanani 2011). Also, Fong et al. reported beaded fibers spun from poly(ethylene oxide) with the addition of NaCl in ethanol and water as solvents (Figure 2.2) (Fong et al. 1999). They found out that the viscosity plays an important role in nanofiber formation.

2.3.3 Feed Rate

Another important factor in the electrospinning process is the feed rate of the solution, which influences the diameter and morphology of fibers. The charge density decreases with the increase of the feed rate of the solution. Mitchell and Sanders (2006) and Son et al. (2004) showed that the high charge density might lead to the electrospinning jet undergoing secondary bending instabilities and cause the formation of small-diameter fibers. Fibers with larger diameters can be obtained if the feed rate of the solution increases. Fibers with high nonuniform diameters with the formation of bead defects in the fibers are formed when the feed rate of solution is too high due to there being not enough time for solvent evaporation (Zuo et al. 2005).

2.3.4 Applied Voltage

This parameter may affect the fiber diameter but sometimes varies with the other parameters (polymer solution concentration and distance between the tip and the collector) (Yordem et al. 2008). Generally, fiber formation occurs only when the applied voltage surpasses the threshold voltage (about ~1 kV/cm, dependent on the gel solution), and an increase in the applied voltage leads to reduction in the fiber diameter. Baumgarten demonstrated experimentally that the shape of the initiating drop changes with the applied voltage, resulting in a variation in the structure and morphology of the nanofibers (Baumgarten 1971).

2.4 Polymer Nanofibers Containing Metal Oxide Nanoparticles

2.4.1 Morphology

A favorable alternative for the development of new polymeric materials is to use inorganic nanoparticles reinforced in polymer matrices with enhanced physical properties that are not present in either of the pure materials. Chen et al. reported that the Ni nanoparticles were uniformly dispersed in the PS matrix, which was proven by SEM observations of the nanocomposite fibers (Chen et al. 2010). Figure 2.3 illustrates the SEM images of PS/Ni nanocomposite fibers with a Ni nanoparticle loading of 20 wt% observed under different accelerating voltages.

The effect of Ni nanoparticles (in 4%–8% amounts) added into the polysulfone matrix using the electrospinning procedure was discussed (Pascariu-Dorneanu et al. 2015). The authors show that Ni nanoparticles reinforced in polymer nanofibers have interesting optical properties due to their morphology and composition. SEM and TEM micrographs of electrospun polysulfone/Ni nanocomposite fibers with 8% Ni nanoparticles dispersed onto polymer fibers are shown in Figure 2.4.

Reitzenstein and coauthors produced electrospun polyvinylpyrrolidone or PS nanofibers by adding indium, iron, or titanium oxide nanoparticles (Von Reitzenstein et al. 2016). They showed that metal oxide nanoparticles

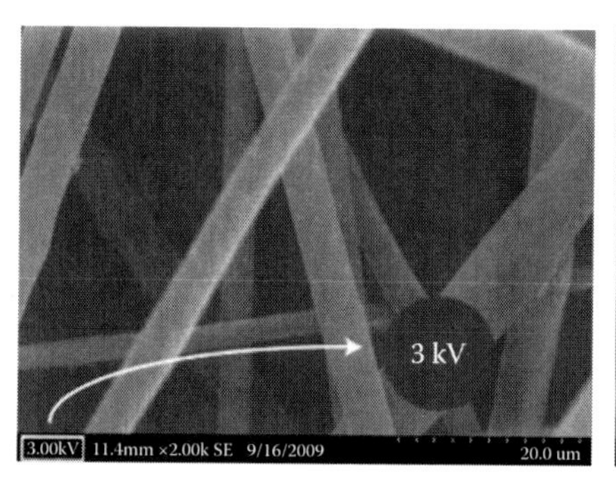

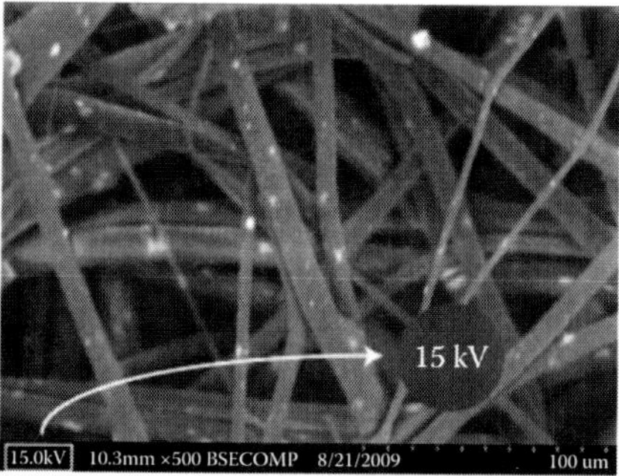

FIGURE 2.3
SEM microstructures of PS/Ni nanocomposite fibers. (Adapted from Chen, X. et al., *Macromol. Chem. Phys.*, 211, 1775, 2010b.)

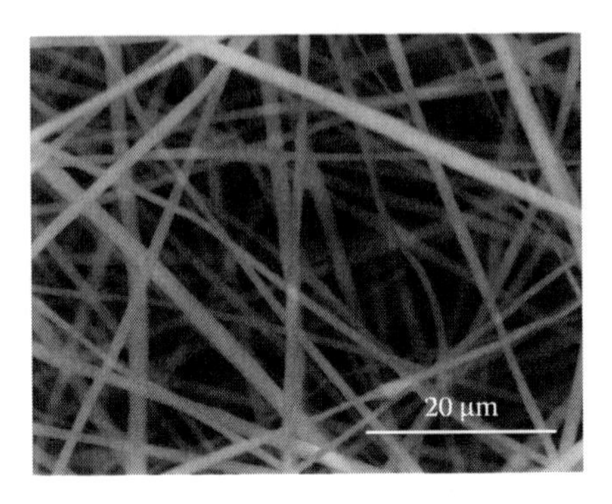

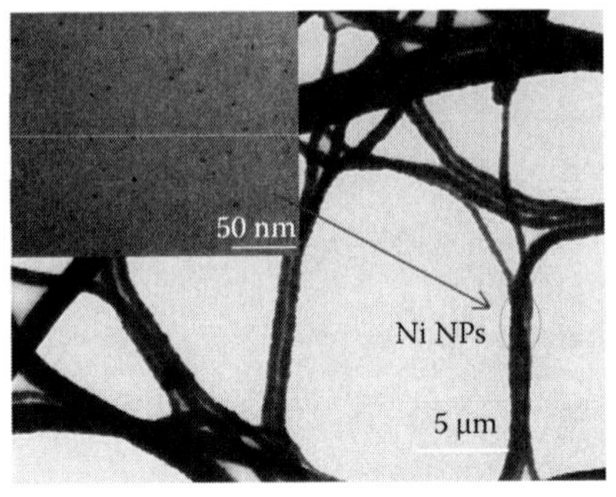

FIGURE 2.4
SEM and TEM images of the electrospun PSU/Ni composite fibers. (Adapted from Pascariu-Dorneanu, P. et al., *Mater. Res. Bull.*, 64, 306, 2015.)

do not affect the thickness and macroscopic morphology at less than 5 wt% because the critical voltage does not change; after this value the viscosity increased leading to the subsequent decrease of the fiber diameter (Figure 2.5).

Generally, there are three methods to disperse the inorganic nanoparticles into polymer matrices. The first method is the top-down process, which consists in the direct mixing of the inorganic nanoparticles into a polymer matrix in the melt or in solution. In the melt mixing, the agglomerated nanoparticles are broken down to the nanoscale by the shear stress induced in the polymer melt. The inorganic nanoparticles in the polymer melt are dispersed depending largely on the shear stresses induced in the polymer melt during mixing. Meanwhile, in the solution mixing, the nanoparticles are predispersed in a solution of polymer and solvent, followed by evaporation of the solvent from a solution of polymer and nanoparticles. The shear stress in a solution of polymer and nanoparticles during the solution mixing is much lower than that in a polymer melt during the melt mixing, and thus it is necessary for the nanoparticles to be predispersed in a solution of polymer and solvent using an external force such as ultrasonication.

Polymer composites comprising nanoparticles (including nanofibers where the fiber diameter is in the nano-dimensional range) are often investigated when the reinforcement of the polymer matrix is achieved. While the reinforcement aspects are a major part of the nanocomposite investigations reported in the literature, many other variants and property enhancements are under active study leading to different applications. The advantages of nanoscale particle incorporation can lead to a myriad of application possibilities where the analogous larger-scale particle incorporation would not yield the sufficient property profile for utilization. These areas include barrier properties, membrane separation, UV screens, flammability resistance, polymer blend compatibilization, electrical conductivity, impact modification, and biomedical applications.

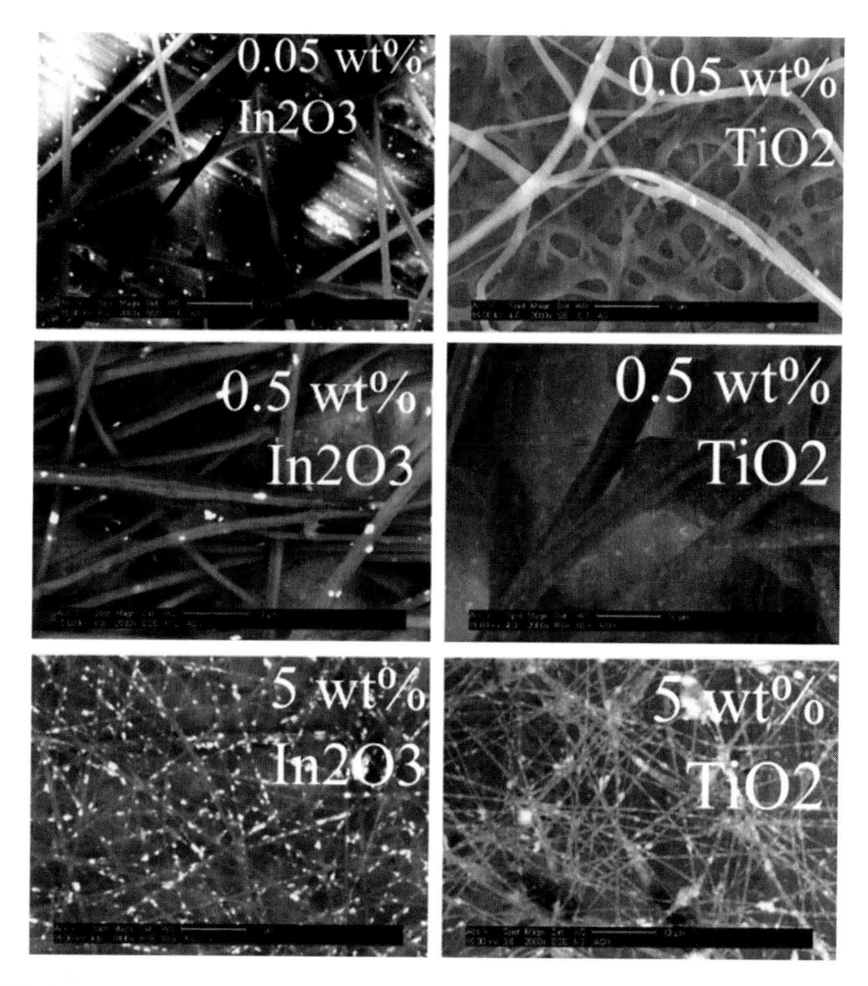

FIGURE 2.5
SEM images of polystyrene fibers with In_2O_3 and TiO_2. (Adapted from Von Reitzenstein, N.H. et al., *J. Appl. Polym. Sci.*, 43811, 1, 2016.)

2.4.2 Photocatalytic Activity

Since the discovery of the photocatalytic water splitting on TiO_2 electrodes by Fujishima and Honda (1972), semiconductor-based photocatalysts have attracted increasing interest due to their potential applications in obtaining photoelectrochemical hydrogen, sensitization dyes, solar energy conversion, reactor design, and process kinetics, and photochemical treatment of air and water. For the first time, the application of TiO_2 in the photocatalytic oxidation of CN^- and SO_3^{2-} in aqueous medium under sunlight was reported by Frank and Bard (1977). Moreover, Inoue et al. reported on the photocatalytic reduction of CO_2 in aqueous suspensions of titania (Inoue et al. 1979).

Several studies have focused on semiconducting metal oxides such as TiO_2, ZnO, Fe_2O_3, WO_3, Bi_2WO_6, and CuO, and these materials have been widely used as oxidative photocatalysts for the effective removal of industrial pollutants and wastewater treatment (Alves et al. 2009; Kumar et al. 2012; Lee et al. 2012; Sundaramurthy et al. 2012; Szilagyi et al. 2013). Chuangchote et al. synthesized TiO_2 nanofibers by electrospinning and they observed that one-dimensional electrospun nanofibers with highly aligned bundled nanofibrils are beneficial for the enhancement of crystallinity, large surface area, and high photocatalytic activity (Chuangchote et al. 2009). Li et al. synthesized anatase TiO_2 nanofibers by utilizing a simple electrospinning technique and then they followed the photocatalytic degradation of rhodamine B in water under visible light irradiation (Li et al. 2012). They observed that TiO_2 nanofibers obtained by calcination at 500°C for 3 h exhibited an excellent photocatalytic activity. Singh et al. were able to prepare highly mesoporous ZnO nanofibers with high crystallinity and large surface area by electrospinning (Singh et al. 2013). The fibers presented a better interaction with polycyclic aromatic hydrocarbons, such as naphthalene and anthracene, due to the higher surface-to-volume ratio of the nanofibers, and thereby higher rate constants for the UV light photodegradation of the aromatic compounds were obtained.

However, the utilization of metal oxides such as TiO_2, ZnO, SnO_2, and Fe_2O_3 for practical applications is still limited because of the fast electron–hole recombination and broad bandgaps that are sensitive to UV light. Therefore, it is essential to improve the visible light absorption and other shortcomings to ameliorate the photocatalytic activity by either combining them with other nanomaterials or just doping in order to tune their bandgap and shift their activity toward visible spectrum wavelengths. In recent years, the improvement in the efficiency of photocatalytic activity has been realized (Uddin et al. 2012; Zhu et al. 2013; Zheng and Wang 2014).

Zhang et al. reported TiO_2 nanofibers segregated by graphene oxide using the electrospinning technique, and they investigated the photocatalytic activity of methylene blue and 4-chlorophenol under visible light irradiation (Zhang et al. 2017). The photocatalytic activity was significantly improved after segregation with graphene oxide due to the enhanced separation efficiency of photogenerated electron–hole pairs.

Several studies have been performed on semiconductor metal oxides with matched bandgap configurations, which enhance the photocatalytic activity. The same results can be obtained by metallic nanoparticles combined with semiconducting metal oxides that possess synergetic properties and significantly improve the photocatalysis process (Madhavan et al. 2012; Alves et al. 2013; Song et al. 2013).

Semiconducting metal oxides have been used as photocatalysts upon irradiation with sunlight, creating electron–hole pairs, which in turn produce radicals in different pathways as shown in Figure 2.6. The photocatalytic mechanism is presented as follows: upon irradiation semiconductor metal

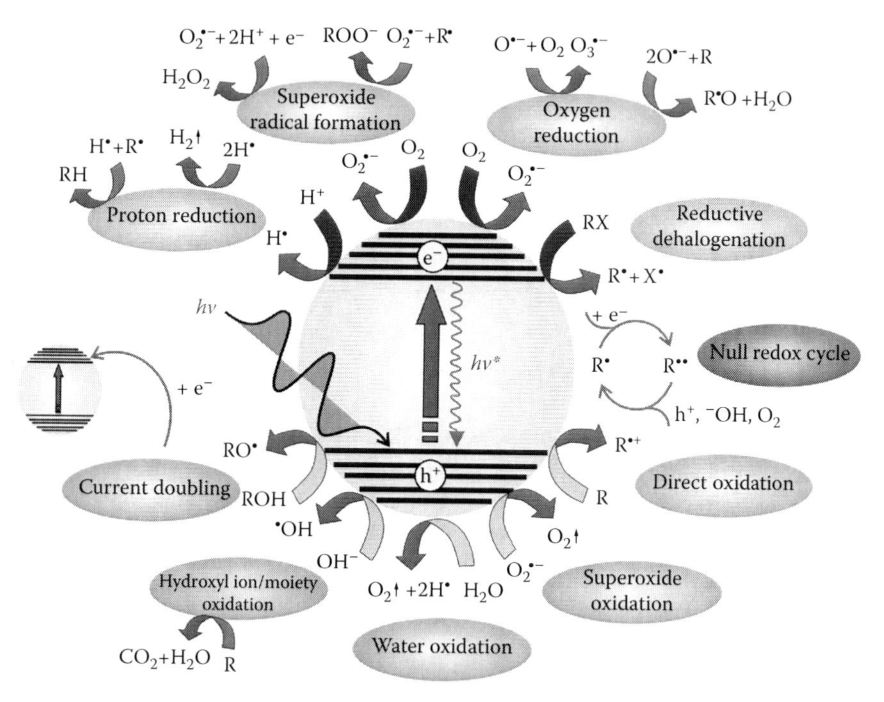

FIGURE 2.6
Photocatalytic mechanism of generating free radicals in the conduction band (CB) and valence band (VB) of semiconducting metal oxides. (Adapted from Teoh, W.Y. et al., *J. Phys. Chem. Lett.*, 3, 629, 2012.)

oxides eject an electron from the valence band to the conduction band, thereby leaving a hole in the valence band. The generated electrons and holes produce hydroxyl radicals to degrade the pollutants by reacting with chemisorbed oxygen on the catalyst surface and oxygen in the aqueous solution (Bhatkhande et al. 2002; Chong et al. 2010; Teoh et al. 2012).

In recent years, polymer nanofibers containing metal oxide nanoparticles have been developed as new materials, providing opportunities to create a new range of interests because they can combine the advantages of both components and lead to the improvement of many properties. Ryu et al. reported about the electrospun nylon 6,6 nanofiber composites in which Ag–TiO_2 was located either in the interior or on the surface of the nanofiber matrix, and the composites were tested for the degradation of methylene blue dye and antimicrobial activity (Ryu et al. 2015). The tests proved that these nanocomposites could be usefully applied as protective materials against various contaminants such as organic pollutants, harmful particles, bacteria, and viruses. Also, Panthi et al. synthesized polyacrylonitrile composites reinforced with Ag_2CO_3 nanoparticles, and they obtained enhanced antibacterial activity over *E. coli* and *S. aureus* under visible light due to photogenerated electron–hole pairs (Panthi et al. 2015).

2.5 Applications of Polymer Nanofibers Containing Metal Oxide Nanoparticles

2.5.1 Biomedical Applications

Many types of nanomaterials, such as nanowires, nanofibers, and nanoparticles, have been shown to present antimicrobial properties and some of them were embedded in polymer matrices using the electrospinning method. The most relevant studies have focused on silver, copper, zinc, and cobalt nanoparticles (Nguyen et al. 2011; Ahmad et al. 2012; Abdelgawad et al. 2014). In the case of these nanomaterials, the uniform dispersion of nanoparticles into polymer nanofibers influences their antibacterial efficiency and stability. Also, the fiber properties and processing parameters are strongly affected not only by the fiber structure, but also by the nanoparticle size and dispersion in a complex manner that is difficult to predict. Silver has been widely employed in various nanofibrous compositions. Several studies about the antifungal and antimicrobial activities of electrospun nanofiber composites have been reported in the last years. Rzayev et al. prepared and characterized nanofibrous films of poly(vinyl alcohol-*co*-vinyl acetate)/octadecyl amine-montmorillonite layered silicate nanocomposites with/without silver nanoparticles. They investigated antifungal and antimicrobial activities using *Candida* spp. fungals, Gram-positive and Gram-negative microorganisms and found that they strongly depended on chemical/physical structural factors, and loading of silver species (Rzayev et al. 2014). Song et al. reported data on PS nanofibers attached Ag nanoparticles on the fiber surface and tested antimicrobial activity for *Staphylococcus xylosus*. Electrospun polyacrylonitrile nanofibers externally loaded with silver nanoparticles presented excellent results for inhibiting the growth of bacteria and fungi (Song et al. 2012). Moreover, there are a variety of polymer materials obtained by the electrospinning method, such as natural polymers (silk, collagen, chitosan), synthetic polymers (PVA, polydioxanone), and nanocomposites (hydroxyapatite blends), which are utilized in tissue engineering. Kim et al. reported that the electrospun PVA/Hap nanocomposites can have a number of future applications related to hard tissue replacement and regeneration (bone and dentin), not limited to coating implants (Kim et al. 2008). Electrospun nanofiber composites composed from chitosan and thiolated chitosanin to which was added *Garcinia mangostana* (GM) extract were evaluated for the GM extract amount, mucoadhesion, in vitro release, antibacterial activity, and cytotoxicity. These nanocomposite materials have the potential to be in mucoadhesive dosage forms to maintain oral hygiene by reducing the bacterial growth that causes dental caries (Samprasit et al. 2015). Studies on the fabrication and characterization of poly(ε-caprolactone) can be beneficial for cartilage regeneration (Levorson et al. 2013; Samprasit et al. 2015; Thorvaldsson et al. 2008). Many materials have been used for dental implants, such as titanium and its alloys.

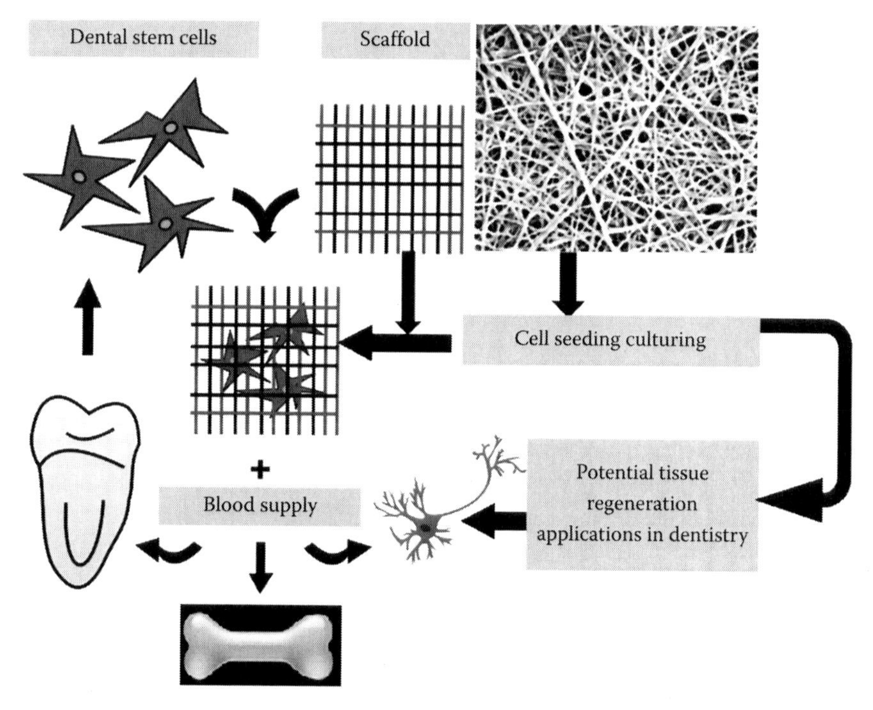

FIGURE 2.7
Schematic presentation of using electrospinning scaffolds for tissue engineering of various oral and dental tissues. (Adapted from Zafar, M. et al., *Materials*, 9, 73, 2016.)

Promising results were obtained for polymer nanocomposites, namely polyetheretherketone-reinforced zirconia (Najeeb et al. 2015). The dental tissue regeneration using electrospun materials is shown schematically in Figure 2.7.

Fibrous mats obtained by the electrospinning method have been extensively studied due to their antibacterial and regenerative properties that accelerate the healing process of wounds (Thakur et al. 2008; He et al. 2015). Also, wound dressings can be used as media to deliver analgesics and antibiotics such topical anesthesia, which can decrease the amount of systemic administration of these drugs needed. Electrospun mats can used to deliver topical anesthesia and antibiotics to surgical or traumatic wounds in dentistry. Noh et al. reported data on electrospun fiber mats that can be used as dressings for oral mucosal lesions, such as ulcers or surgical wounds, to relieve the patient's discomfort (Noh et al. 2006). In 2015, Tang et al. obtained silk fibroin using electrospinning techniques exhibiting potential to be used in human dermal matrices when tested against rat mucosal cells in vitro (Tang et al. 2015). Natural polymer nanofibers, such as collagen, chitosan, elastin, silk fibroin, chitin, and their combinations prepared by the electrospinning method can have numerous applications in vascular, cardiovascular, and tissue engineering (Matthews et al. 2002; Park et al. 2006; Chen et al. 2010).

Chen et al. reported that electrospun collagen–chitosan nanofibers can be a better candidate for vascular and nerve tissue engineering (Chen et al. 2010). Electrospun polyurethane nanofibers loaded with propolis could improve the hydrophilicity and the mechanical strength of the fibrous membrane. These composite nanofibers presented good antibacterial activity and potential for application in wound dressing and in skin tissue engineering (Kim et al. 2014). It is known that the most frequently used biodegradable polymers for the fabrication of novel materials for medical use and for tissue engineering applications are poly(a-hydroxy acids), especially lactic acids, glycolic acids, and their copolymers with 3-caprolactone. Recently, one of the most important topics of research has been devoted to hybrid nanofibers coming from the combinations of natural and synthetic polymers due to their potential applications in vascular (elastin–polylactic-*co*-glycolic acid), cardiovascular (elastin–gelatin–polycaprolactone), skin (collagen–polycaprolactone), and nerve (chitosan–polycaprolactone) regeneration (Zhang et al. 2005; Stitzela et al. 2006; Schnell et al. 2007; Bhattarai et al. 2009).

2.5.2 Supercapacitors

In recent years, energy crisis has been one of the vital problems in the society due to the excessive use of fossil-fuel resources and environmental pollution. Therefore, the development of very lightweight and environment-friendly proficient energy storage devices has become the priority of researchers and scientists for satisfying the demand for the modern consumer's hybrid electric and portable electronic devices. However, it is crucial to find ways to store energy in order to sustain a sufficient supply and to secure energy distribution. For this reason, supercapacitors have attracted considerable interest because of their high capacity, low internal resistance, fast charge and discharge, high power density, high energy density, and long life cycle, compared to conventional capacitors and batteries (Tang et al. 2012; Singh and Mandal 2015). A study of electrospun polyaniline nanofibers demonstrated that these materials are very stable and presented a superior performance with a specific capacitance of 267 F g^{-1} in 1 M H_2SO_4 at a current density of 0.35 A g^{-1} (Chaudhari et al. 2013). Also, Simotwo and coworkers published the data on electrospun nanofibers of pure polyaniline and poly(ethylene oxide) reinforced carbon nanotubes (Simotwo et al. 2016). They obtained good values for specific capacitance between 308 and 385 F g^{-1}, respectively, at a current density of 0.5 A g^{-1}.

2.5.3 Application of Nanofibers Containing Metal Oxide Nanoparticles in Oil-Related Pollution

Organic–inorganic fibrous composites play an important role in many fields, such as oil spill cleanup, oil/water separation, and environmental remediation. In recent years, there have been many studies on oil sorption capacities of different polymer and polymer composite nanofibers, such as PS, polyurethane (Lin et al. 2013), polyvinyl chloride (Zhu et al. 2011), cellulose acetate (Shang et al. 2012), PS/PVDF nanofiber–added Fe_3O_4 nanoparticles (Chen et al. 2013), and Fe_3O_4/polyacrylonitrile composite nanofibers (Liu et al. 2015). The incorporation of a magnetic component (e.g., Fe_3O_4) in the polymer matrix can be useful in the recovery process from the water surface. Recently, polymer nanofiber–reinforced Fe_3O_4 nanoparticles for the cleanup of oil/organic solvent polluted water bodies or antibiotic removal were reported (Liu et al. 2015). Also, Jiang et al. studied the oil sorption capacity of PVDF and PVDF/Fe_3O_4@PS nanofiber composites and they obtained low values of sorption capacity for PVDF (i.e., from 11 to 14 g g^{-1}) depending on the oil type: sunflower oil, soybean oil, motor oil (5W–30), and diesel oil (5W–40) (Jiang et al. 2015).

2.5.4 Photocatalytic Applications

Next-generation wastewater treatment involves membranes that contain organic and inorganic parts, and photocatalysis can be applied. A photocatalytic process is based on the activation of the photocatalyst after the absorption of light of a specific wavelength, correlated with its bandgap; the energy gained is used to create electrons and holes, which, after migrating to the surface, can induce the decomposition of various species of contaminants. In such applications, it is preferred that TiO_2 and ZnO nanoparticles are added in the polymer matrix because they are difficult to agglomerate and they present an easy recovery afterward. Recently, electrospun polymer nanofiber solutions containing photocatalytic nanomaterials (nanoparticles, nanowires, nanorods, nanotubes, etc.) have been employed as an alternative approach to reinforce nanofiber structures with the goal to increase the surface area and improve photocatalytic activity (Yun et al. 2010; Deniz et al. 2011; Prahsarn et al. 2011; Olaru et al. 2014; Cossich et al. 2015). Prahsarn and coauthors reported the photocatalytic activity of electrospun polyacrylonitrile nanofibers containing TiO_2 nanoparticles (Prahsarn et al. 2011). For this system, they obtained good photocatalytic activity by degradation of methylene blue under UV irradiation. Recently, Yu et al. studied photocatalytic activities by degradation of acid red 18 and methylene blue under visible light irradiation using Ag–AgI–TiO_2 nanoparticles embedded onto carbon nanofiber composites (Yu et al. 2015). He et al. investigated the photocatalytic activity and stability through degradation of methylene blue under UV irradiation for the TiO_2–fluoropolymer fiber nanocomposites obtained by the electrospinning method (He et al. 2009). The results show that these nanomaterials have a good photocatalytic activity and stability. In recent years, some of the most important materials used in photocatalytic applications are metal oxide semiconductor nanomaterials obtained using the electrospinning technique combined with calcination at different temperatures. Song et al. reported the photocatalytic activity of TiO_2-based composite films by a porous conjugated polymer coating of nanoparticles for degradation of phenol solution under visible light irradiation. The authors obtained a high efficiency for this system, which was attractive for applications in water purification (Song et al. 2016). The electrospun poly (methyl methacrylate) nanocomposites reinforced with TiO_2 nanotubes were evaluated by photocatalytic activity in methylene blue dye; the antibacterial activity was tested by measuring the survival rate of *E. coli*, as a model organism, after exposure to UV light–activated samples. Therefore, these materials could be applied as valid tools for the removal of organic and bacterial contaminants from water (Cantarella et al. 2016). Antimicrobial membranes based on silver-doped nanofibrous polyacrylonitrile were also tested for the filtration of microorganisms and dust particles and they were found to efficiently remove microorganisms and dust from hospitals or other places prone to bacterial infections (Chaudhary et al. 2014). There are many studies on the preparation of nanofibrous mats with antimicrobial functionality using different polymer-reinforced inorganic nanoparticles (Ag, Cu, ZnO, etc.), such as polyacrylonitrile/Ag nanoparticles (Zhang et al. 2011), polyamide/Ag nanoparticles (Vrieze et al. 2012), polyacrylonitrile/ZnO, polyvinylpyrrolidone/TiO_2 added with Cu nanoparticles (Yousef et al. 2015), and so on.

Acknowledgments

The authors acknowledge the financial support of this research through the European Regional Development Fund, Project POINGBIO, ID P_40_443, Contract no. 86/8.09.2016.

References

Abdelgawad A.M., Hudson S.M., Rojas O.J. Antimicrobial wound dressing nanofiber mats from multicomponent (chitosan/silver-NPs/polyvinyl alcohol) systems. *Carbohydr. Polym.* 100 (2014): 166–178.

Ahmad Z., Vargas-Reus M.A., Bakhshi R., Ryan F., Ren G.G., Oktar F., Allaker R.P. Antimicrobial properties of electrically formed elastomeric polyurethane-copper oxide nanocomposites for medical and dental applications. *Methods Enzymol.* 509 (2012): 87–99.

Alves A.K., Berutti F.A., Bergmann C.P. Visible and UV photocatalytic characterization of Sn-TiO_2 electrospun fibers. *Catal. Today* 208 (2013): 7–10.

Alves A.K., Berutti F.A., Clemens F.J., Graule T., Bergmann C.P. Photocatalytic activity of titania fibers obtained by electrospinning. *Mater. Res. Bull.* 44 (2009): 312–317.

Bahrami S.H., Kanani A.G. Effect of changing solvents on poly(ε-Caprolactone) nanofibrous webs morphology. *J. Nanomater.* 2011 (2011): 1–10, Article ID 724153.

Baumgarten P.K. Electrostatic spinning of acrylic microfibers. *J. Colloid Interface Sci.* 36 (1971): 71–79.

Bhatkhande D.S., Pangarkar V.G., Beenackers A.A.C.M. Photocatalytic degradation for environmental applications—A review. *J. Chem. Technol. Biotechnol.* 77 (2002): 102–116.

Bhattarai N., Li Z., Gunn J., Leung M., Cooper A., Edmondson D., Veiseh O. et al. Natural-synthetic polyblend nanofibers for biomedical applications. *Adv. Mater.* 21 (2009): 2792–2797.

Camtakan Z., Erenturk S.A., Yusan S.D. Magnesium oxide nanoparticles: Preparation, characterization, and uranium sorption properties. *Environ. Prog. Sustain. Energy* 31 (2012): 536–543.

Cantarella M., Sanz R., Buccheri M.A., Romano L., Privitera V. PMMA/TiO_2 nanotubes composites for photocatalytic removal of organic compounds and bacteria from water. *Mater. Sci. Semicond. Process.* 42 (2016): 58–61.

Chaudhari S., Sharma Y., Archana P.S., Jose R., Ramakrishna S., Mhaisalkar S., Srinivasan M. Electrospun polyaniline nanofibers web electrodes for supercapacitors. *J. Appl. Polym. Sci.* 129 (2013): 1660–1668.

Chaudhary A., Gupta A., Mathur R.B., Dhakate S.R. Effective antimicrobial filter from electrospun polyacrylonitrile-silver composite nanofibers membrane for conductive environment. *Adv. Mater. Lett.* 5 (2014): 562–568.

Chen J., Yang P., Wang C., Zhan S., Zhang L., Huang Z., Li W., Wang C., Jiang Z., Shao C. Ag nanoparticles/PPV composite nanofibers with high and sensitive opto-electronic response. *Nanoscale Res. Lett.* 6(121) (2011): 1–5.

Chen N., Pan Q.M. Versatile fabrication of ultralight magnetic foams and application for oil-water separation. *ACS Nano* 7 (2013): 6875–6883.

Chen X., Wei S., Gunesoglu C., Zhu J., Southworth C.S., Sun L., Karki A.B., Young D.P., Guo Z. Electrospun magnetic fibrillar polystyrene nanocomposites reinforced with nickel nanoparticles. *Macromol. Chem. Phys.* 211 (2010a): 1775–1783.

Chen Z.G., Wang P.W., Wei B., Mo X.M., Cui F.Z. Electrospun collagen-chitosan nanofiber: A biomimetic extracellular matrix for endothelial cell and smooth muscle cell. *Acta Biomater.* 6 (2010b): 372–382.

Chong M.N., Jin B., Chow C.W.K., Saint C. Recent developments in photocatalytic water treatment technology: A review. *Water Res.* 44 (2010): 2997–3027.

Chuangchote S., Jitputti J., Sagawa T., Yoshikawa S. Photocatalytic activity for hydrogen evolution of electrospun TiO_2 nanofibers. *ACS Appl. Mater. Interfaces* 1 (2009): 1140–1143.

Cojocaru C., Dorneanu P.P., Airinei A., Olaru N., Samoila P., Rotaru A. Design and evaluation of electrospun polysulfone fibers and polysulfone/$NiFe_2O_4$ nanostructured composite as sorbents for oil spill cleanup. *J. Taiwan Inst. Chem. Eng.* 70 (2017): 267–281.

Cossich E., Bergamasco R., Pessoa de Amorim M.T., Martins P.M., Marques J., Tavares C.J., Lanceros-Mendez S., Sencadas V. Development of electrospun photocatalytic TiO_2-polyamide-12 nanocomposites. *Mater. Chem. Phys.* 164 (2015): 91–97.

Danial A.S., Saleh M.M., Salih S.A., Awad M.I. On the synthesis of nickel oxide nanoparticles by sol-gel technique and its electrocatalytic oxidation of glucose. *J. Power Sources* 293 (2015): 101–108.

Deniz A.E., Celebioglu A., Kayaci F., Uyar T. Electrospun polymeric nanofibrous composites containing TiO_2 short nanofibers. *Mater. Chem. Phys.* 129 (2011): 701–704.
Fong H., Chun I., Reneker D.H. Beaded nanofibers formed during electrospinning, *Polymer* 40 (1999): 4585–4592.
Frank S.N., Bard A.J. Heterogeneous photocatalytic oxidation of cyanide and sulfite in aqueous solutions at semiconductor powders. *J. Phys. Chem.* 81 (1977): 1484–1488.
Fujishima A., Honda K. Electrochemical photolysis of water at a semiconductor electrode. *Nature* 238 (1972): 37–38.
Guo Z., Lee S.E., Kim H., Park S., Hahn H.T., Karki A.B., Young D.P. Fabrication, characterization and microwave properties of polyurethane nanocomposites reinforced with iron oxide and barium titanate nanoparticles. *Acta Mater.* 57 (2009): 267–277.
Haghi A.K., Akbari M. Trends in electrospinning of natural nanofibers. *Phys. Status Solidi* 204 (2007): 1830–1834.
He T., Wang J., Huang P., Zeng B., Li H., Cao Q., Zhang S., Luo Z., Deng D.Y., Zhang H. Electrospinning polyvinylidene fluoride fibrous membranes containing antibacterial drugs used as wound dressing. *Colloids Surf. B Biointerfaces* 130 (2015): 278–286.
He T., Zhou Z., Xu W., Ren F., Ma H., Wang J. Preparation and photocatalysis of TiO_2–fluoropolymer electrospun fiber nanocomposites. *Polymer* 50 (2009): 3031–3036.
Inoue T., Fujishima A., Konishi S., Honda K. Photoelectrocatalytic reduction of carbon dioxide in aqueous suspensions of semiconductor powders. *Nature* 277 (1979): 637–638.
Jamnongkan T., Shirota R., Sukumaran S.K., Sugimoto M., Koyama K. Effect of ZnO nanoparticles on the electrospinning of poly(vinyl alcohol) from aqueous solution: Influence of particle size. *Polym. Eng. Sci.* 54 (2014): 1969–1975.
Jiang Z., Tijing L.D., Amarjargal A., Park C.H., An K.J., Shon H.K., Kim C.S. Removal of oil from water using magnetic bicomponent composite nanofibers fabricated by electrospinning. *Compos Part B* 77 (2015): 311–318.
Kim G.M., Asran A.S., Michler G.H., Simon P., Kim J.S. Electrospun PVA/HAp nanocomposite nanofibers: Biomimetics of mineralized hard tissues at a lower level of complexity. *Bioinspir. Biomim.* 3 (2008): 1–12.
Kim J.I., Pant H.R., Sim H.J., Lee K.M., Kim C.S. Electrospun propolis/polyurethane composite nanofibers for biomedical applications. *Mater. Sci. Eng. C* 44 (2014): 52–57.
Kim P., Doss N.M., Tillotson J.P., Hotchkiss P.J., Pan M.J., Marder S.R., Li J., Calame J.P., Perry J.W. High energy density nanocomposites based on surface-modified $BaTiO_3$ and a ferroelectric polymer. *ACS Nano* 3 (2009): 2581–2592.
Kim Y.B., Cho D., Park W.H. Enhancement of mechanical properties of TiO_2 nanofibers by reinforcement with polysulfone fibers. *Mater. Lett.* 64 (2010): 189–191.
Kumar P.S., Sahay R., Aravindan V., Sundaramurthy J., Chui L.W., Thavasi V., Mhaisalkar S.G., Madhavi S., Seeram R. Free-standing electrospun carbon nanofibres—A high performance anode material for lithium-ion batteries. *J. Phys. D: Appl. Phys.* 45 (2012): 265302.
Lee S.S., Bai H., Liu Z., Sun D.D. Electrospun TiO_2/SnO_2 nanofibers with innovative structure and chemical properties for highly efficient photocatalytic H_2 generation. *Int. J. Hydrogen Energy* 37 (2012): 10575–10584.

Levorson E.J., Sreerekha P.R., Chennazhi K.P., Kasper F.K., Nair S.V., Mikos A.G. Fabrication and characterization of multiscale electrospun scaffolds for cartilage regeneration. *Biomed. Mater.* 8 (2013): 014103.

Li J., Qiao H., Du Y., Chen C., Li X., Cui J., Kumar D., Wei Q. Electrospinning synthesis and photocatalytic activity of mesoporous TiO_2 nanofibers. *Sci. World J.* 2012 (2012): 1–7, Article ID 154939.

Li S., Li Y., Qian K., Ji S., Luo H., Gao Y., Jin P. Functional fiber mats with tunable diffuse reflectance composed of electrospun VO_2/PVP composite fibers. *ACS Appl. Mater. Interfaces* 6 (2014): 9–13.

Li S.C., Li Y.N. Mechanical and antibacterial properties of modified nano-ZnO/high-density polyethylene composite films with a low doped content of nano-ZnO. *J. Appl. Polym. Sci.* 116 (2010): 2965.

Lin J., Tian F., Shang Y., Wang F., Ding B., Yu J., Guo Z. Co-axial electrospun polystyrene/polyurethane fibres for oil collection from water surface. *Nanoscale* 5 (2013): 2745–2755.

Liu Q., Zhong L.B., Zhao Q.B., Frear C., Zheng Y.M. Synthesis of Fe_3O_4/polyacrylonitrile composite electrospun nanofiber mat for effective adsorption of tetracycline. *ACS Appl. Mater. Interfaces* 7 (2015): 14573–14583.

Madhavan A.A., Kumar G.G., Kalluri S., Joseph J., Nagarajan S., Nair S., Subramanian K.R.V., Balakrishnan A. Effect of embedded plasmonic Au nanoparticles on photocatalysis of electrospun TiO_2 nanofibers. *J. Nanosci. Nanotechnol.* 12 (2012): 7963–7967.

Matthews J.A., Wnek G.E., Simpson D.G., Bowlin G.L. Electrospinning of collagen nanofibers. *Biomacromolecules* 3 (2002): 232–238.

Mitchell S.B., Sanders J.E. A unique device for controlled electrospinning. *J. Biomed. Mater. Res. Part A* 78 (2006): 110–120.

Najeeb S., Khurshid Z., Matinlinna J.P., Siddiqui F., Nassani M.Z., Baroudi K. Nanomodified peek dental implants: Bioactive composites and surface modification—A review. *Int. J. Dent.* 2015 (2015): 381759.

Nguyen T.H., Kim Y.H., Song H.Y., Lee B.T. Nano Ag loaded PVA nano-fibrous mats for skin applications. *J. Biomed. Mater. Res. B: Appl. Biomater.* 96 (2011): 225–233.

Noh H.K., Lee S.W., Kim J., Oh J., Kim K., Chung C., Choi S., Park W.H., Min B. Electrospinning of chitin nanofibers: Degradation behavior and cellular response to normal human keratinocytes and fibroblasts. *Biomaterials* 27 (2006): 3934–3944.

Olaru N., Calin G., Olaru L. Zinc oxide nanocrystals grown on cellulose acetate butyrate nanofiber mats and their potential photocatalytic activity for dye degradation. *Ind. Eng. Chem. Res.* 53 (2014): 17968–17975.

Outokesh M., Hosseinpour M., Ahmadi S.J., Mousavand T., Sadjadi S., Soltanian W. Hydrothermal synthesis of CuO nanoparticles: Study on effects of operational conditions on yield, purity, and size of the nanoparticles. *Ind. Eng. Chem. Res.* 50 (2011): 3540–3554.

Panthi G., Park S.J., Kim T.W., Chung H.J., Hong S.T., Park M., Kim H.Y. Electrospun composite nanofibers of polyacrylonitrile and Ag_2CO_3 nanoparticles for visible light photocatalysis and antibacterial applications. *J. Mater. Sci.* 50 (2015): 4477–4485.

Park K.E., Jung S.Y., Lee S.J., Min B.M., Park W.H. Biomimetic nanofibrous scaffolds: Preparation and characterization of chitin/silk fibroin blend nanofibers. *Int. J. Biol. Macromol.* 38 (2006): 165–173.

Park Y.K., Tadd E.H., Zubris M., Tannenbaum R. Size-controlled synthesis of alumina nanoparticles from aluminum alkoxides. *Mater. Res. Bull.* 40 (2005): 1506–1512.

Pascariu-Dorneanu P., Airinei A., Grigoras M., Fifere N., Sacarescu L., Lupu N., Stoleriu L. Structural, optical and magnetic properties of Ni doped SnO_2 nanoparticles. *J. Alloys Compd.* 668 (2016): 65–72.

Pascariu-Dorneanu P., Airinei A., Homocianu M., Olaru N. Photophysical and surface characteristics of electrospun polysulfone/nickel fibers. *Mater. Res. Bull.* 64 (2015): 306–311.

Prahsarn C., Klinsukhon W., Roungpaisan N. Electrospinning of PAN/DMF/H_2O containing TiO_2 and photocatalytic activity of their webs. *Mater. Lett.* 65 (2011): 2498–2501.

Qin W., Xu L., Song J., Xing R., Song H. Highly enhanced gas sensing materials of porous SnO_2-CO_2 composite nanofibers prepared by electrospinning. *Sens. Actuators B: Chem.* 185 (2013): 231–237.

Razak S.I.A., Wahab I.F., Fadil F., Dahli F.N., Khudzari A.Z.M., Adeli H. A review of electrospun conductive polyaniline based nanofiber composites and blends: Processing features, applications, and future directions. *Adv. Mater. Sci. Eng.* 2015 (2015): 1–19, Article ID 356286.

Ryu S.Y., Chung J.W., Kwak S.Y. Dependence of photocatalytic and antimicrobial activity of electrospun polymeric nanofiber composites on the positioning of Ag–TiO_2 nanoparticles. *Compos. Sci. Technol.* 117 (2015): 9–17.

Rzayev Z.M.O., Erdonmez D., Erkan K., Simsek M., Bunyatova U. Functional copolymer/organo-MMT nanoarchitectures. XXII. Fabrication and characterization of antifungal and antibacterial poly(vinyl alcohol-*co*-vinyl acetate)/ODA-MMT/AgNPs nanofibers and nanocoatings by e-spinning and c-spinning methods. *Int. J. Polym. Mater. Polym. Biomater.* 64 (2014): 267–278.

Samprasit W., Kaomongkolgit R., Sukma M., Rojanarata T., Ngawhirunpat T., Opanasopit P. Mucoadhesive electrospun chitosan-based nanofibre mats for dental caries prevention. *Carbohydr. Polym.* 117 (2015): 933–940.

Schnell E., Klinkhammer K., Balzer S., Brook G., Klee D., Dalton P., Mey J. Guidance of glial cell migration and axonal growth on electrospun nanofibers of poly-epsilon-caprolactone and a collagen/poly-epsilon-caprolactone blend. *Biomaterials* 28 (2007): 3012–3025.

Shang Y., Si Y., Raza A., Yang L., Mao X., Ding B., Yu J. An in situ polymerization approach for the synthesis of superhydrophobic and superoleophilic nanofibrous membranes for oil–water separation. *Nanoscale* 4 (2012): 7847–7854.

Shimada T., Ookubo K., Komuro N., Shimizu T., Uehara N. Blue-to-red chromatic sensor composed of gold nanoparticles conjugated with thermoresponsive copolymer for thiol sensing. *Langmuir* 23 (2007): 11225–11232.

Simotwo S.K., DelRe C., Kalra V. Supercapacitor electrodes based on high-purity electrospun polyaniline and polyaniline–carbon nanotube nanofibers. *ACS Appl. Mater. Interfaces* 8 (2016): 21261–21269.

Singh A.K., Mandal K. Engineering of high performance supercapacitor electrode based on Fe-Ni/Fe_2O_3-NiO core/shell hybrid nanostructures. *J. Appl. Phys.* 117 (2015): 1–8.

Singh P., Mondal K., Sharma A. Reusable electrospun mesoporous ZnO nanofiber mats for photocatalytic degradation of polycyclic aromatic hydrocarbon dyes in wastewater. *J. Colloid Interface Sci.* 394 (2013): 208–215.

Son W.K., Youk J.H., Lee T.S., Park W.H. The effects of solution properties and polyelectrolyte on electrospinning of ultrafine poly(ethylene oxide) fibers. *Polymer* 45 (2004): 2959–2966.

Song J., Wang C., Chen M., Regina V.R., Wang C., Meyer R.L., Xie E., Dong M., Besenbacher F. Safe and effective Ag nanoparticles immobilized antimicrobial nano-nonwovens. *Adv. Eng. Mater.* 14 (2012): B240–B246.

Song L., Xiong J., Jiang Q., Du P., Cao H., Shao X. Synthesis and photocatalytic properties of Zn^{2+} doped anatase TiO_2 nanofibers. *Mater. Chem. Phys.* 142 (2013): 77–81.

Song Y., Zhang J., Yang L., Cao S., Yang H., Zhang J., Jiang L., Dan Y., Rendu P.L., Nguyen T.P. Photocatalytic activity of TiO_2 based composite films by porous conjugated polymer coating of nanoparticles. *Mater. Sci. Semicond. Process.* 42 (2016): 54–57.

Srivastava V., Gusain D., Sharma Y.C. Synthesis, characterization and application of zinc oxide nanoparticles (n-ZnO). *Ceram. Int.* 39 (2013): 9803–9808.

Stitzela J., Liu J., Lee S.J., Komura M., Berry J., Soker S., Lim G. et al. Controlled fabrication of a biological vascular substitute. *Biomaterials* 27 (2006): 1088–1094.

Sundaramurthy J., Kumar P.S., Kalaivani M., Thavasi V., Mhaisalkar S.G., Ramakrishna S. Superior photocatalytic behaviour of novel 1D nanobraid and nanoporous α-Fe_2O_3 structures. *RSC Adv.* 2 (2012): 8201–8208.

Szilagyi I.M., Santala E., Heikkila M., Pore V., Kemell M., Nikitin T., Teucher G. et al. Photocatalytic properties of WO_3/TiO_2 core/shell nanofibers prepared by electrospinning and atomic layer deposition. *Chem. Vap. Depos.* 19 (2013): 149–155.

Tang J., Han Y., Zhang F., Ge Z., Liu X., Lu Q. Buccal mucosa repair with electrospun silk fibroin matrix in a rat model. *Int. J. Artif. Organs* 38 (2015): 105–112.

Tang Z., Tang C.H., Gong H. A high energy density asymmetric supercapacitor from nano-architectured $Ni(OH)_2$/carbon nanotube electrodes. *Adv. Funct. Mater.* 22 (2012): 1272–1278.

Teoh W.Y., Scott J.A., Amal R. Progress in heterogeneous photocatalysis: From classical radical chemistry to engineering nanomaterials and solar reactors. *J. Phys. Chem. Lett.* 3 (2012): 629–639.

Thakur R., Florek C., Kohn J., Michniak B. Electrospun nanofibrous polymeric scaffold with targeted drug release profiles for potential application as wound dressing. *Int. J. Pharm.* 364 (2008): 87–93.

Thorvaldsson A., Stenhamre H., Gatenholm P., Walkenstrom P. Electrospinning of highly porous scaffolds for cartilage regeneration. *Biomacromolecules* 9 (2008): 1044–1049.

Uddin Md.T., Nicolas Y., Olivier C., Toupance T., Servant L., Muller M.M., Kleebe H.J., Ziegler J., Jaegermann W. Nanostructured SnO_2–ZnO heterojunction photocatalysts showing enhanced photocatalytic activity for the degradation of organic dyes. *Inorg. Chem.* 51 (2012): 7764–7773.

Vacca P., Nenna G., Miscioscia R., Palumbo D., Minarini C., Sala D.D. Patterned organic and inorganic composites for electronic applications. *J. Phys. Chem. C* 113 (2009): 5777–5783.

Von Reitzenstein N.H., Bi X., Yang Y., Hristovski K., Westerhoff P. Morphology, structure, and properties of metal oxide/polymer nanocomposite electrospun mats. *J. Appl. Polym. Sci.* 43811 (2016): 1–9.

Vrieze S.D., Daels N., Lambert K., Decostere B., Hens Z., Hulle S.V., De Clerck K., Filtration performance of electrospun polyamide nanofibers loaded with bactericides. *Text. Res. J.* 82 (2012): 37–44.

Wang C., Liu L.L., Zhang A.T., Xie P., Lu J.J., Zou X.T. Antibacterial effects of zinc oxide nanoparticles on *Escherichia coli* K88. *Afr. J. Biotechnol.* 11 (2012): 10248.

Wu W., Wu Z., Yu T., Jiang C., Kim W.S. Recent progress on magnetic iron oxide nanoparticles: Synthesis, surface functional strategies and biomedical applications. *Sci. Technol. Adv. Mater.* 16 (2015): 023501.

Yordem O.S., Papila M., Menceloglu Y.Z. Effects of electrospinning parameters on polyacrylonitrile nanofiber diameter: An investigation by response surface methodology. *Mater. Des.* 29 (2008): 34–44.

Yousef A., El-Halwany M.M., Barakat N.A.M., Al-Maghrabi M.N., Kim H.Y. CuO-doped TiO_2 nanofibers as potential photocatalyst and antimicrobial agent. *J. Ind. Eng. Chem.* 26 (2015): 251–258.

Yu D., Bai J., Liang H., Wang J., Li C. Fabrication of a novel visible-light-driven photocatalyst Ag-AgI-TiO_2 nanoparticles supported on carbon nanofibers. *Appl. Surf. Sci.* 349 (2015): 241–250.

Yun J., Jin D., Lee Y.S., Kim H.I. Photocatalytic treatment of acidic waste water by electrospun composite nanofibers of pH-sensitive hydrogel and TiO_2. *Mater. Lett.* 64 (2010): 2431–2434.

Zafar M., Najeeb S., Khurshid Z., Vazirzadeh M., Zohaib S., Najeeb B., Sefat F. Potential of electrospun nanofibers for biomedical and dental applications. *Materials* 9 (2016): 73.

Zhang L., Luo J., Menkhaus T.J., Varadaraju H., Sun Y., Fong H. Antimicrobial nanofibrous membranes developed from electrospun polyacrylonitrile nanofibers. *J. Membr. Sci.* 369 (2011): 499–505.

Zhang L., Zhang Q., Xie H., Guo J., Lyu H., Li Y., Sun Z., Wang H., Guo Z. Electrospun titania nanofibers segregated by graphene oxide for improved visible light photocatalysis. *Appl. Catal. B: Environ.* 201 (2017): 470–478.

Zhang Y., Ouyang H., Lim C.T., Ramakrishna S., Huang Z.M. Electrospinning of gelatin fibers and gelatin/PCL composite fibrous scaffolds. *J. Biomed. Mater. Res. Part B: Appl. Biomater.* 72 (2005): 156–165.

Zhao Y., Li C., Liu X., Gu F., Jiang H., Shao W., Zhang L., He Y. Synthesis and optical properties of TiO_2 nanoparticles. *Mater. Lett.* 61 (2007): 79–83.

Zheng Y., Wang W. Electrospunnanofibers of Er^{3+}-doped TiO_2 with photocatalytic activity beyond the absorption edge. *J. Solid State Chem.* 210 (2014): 206–212.

Zhu C., Li Y., Su Q., Lu B., Pan J., Zhang J., Xie E., Lan W. Electrospinning direct preparation of SnO_2/Fe_2O_3 heterojunction nanotubes as an efficient visible-light photocatalyst. *J. Alloys Compd.* 575 (2013): 333–338.

Zhu H., Qiu S., Jiang W., Wu D., Zhang C. Evaluation of electrospun polyvinyl chloride/polystyrene fibres as sorbent materials for oil spill cleanup. *Environ. Sci. Technol.* 45 (2011): 4527–4531.

Zhu J., Wei S., Chen X., Karki A.B., Rutman D., Young D.P., Guo Z. Electrospun polyimide nanocomposite fibers reinforced with core-shell Fe-FeO nanoparticles. *J. Phys. Chem. C* 114 (2010): 8844–8850.

Zuo W., Zhu M., Yang W., Yu H., Chen Y., Zhang Y. Experimental study on relationship between jet instability and formation of beaded fibers during electrospinning. *Polym. Eng. Sci.* 45 (2005): 704–709.

3

Recent Developments in ZnO–Polyurethane Nanomaterials

Stelian Vlad, Luiza M. Gradinaru, Robert V. Gradinaru, and Constantin Ciobanu

CONTENTS

3.1 Introduction

The use of nanoparticles has increased successfully in various fields, such as agriculture (Prasad et al., 2014; Parisi et al., 2015), textiles (Vigneshwaran et al., 2010; Patra and Gouda, 2013), food packaging (Espitia et al., 2012; Bumbudsanpharoke et al., 2015), optics (Iskandar, 2009; Zhang et al., 2012), cosmetics (Wiechers and Musee, 2010; Silpa et al., 2012), optoelectronic devices (Godlewski et al., 2009), semiconductor devices (Bangal et al., 2005), aerospace (Dinca et al., 2012), construction (van Broekhuizen et al., 2011), and catalysis (Gawande et al., 2016), and nanoparticles have become, in recent years, a source of hope in medicine (Salata, 2004; Zhang et al., 2008).

Advanced research in nanotechnology has opened up new paths for effective solutions regarding the new treatments of diseases, which were until recently incurable (Schroeder et al., 2012).

Nanoparticles are useful not only in medicine—where they speak more than nanomedicine—but also in other technical fields, such as more efficient capture of solar energy (Yan et al., 2016), miniaturization of photonics devices (Forcherio and Roper, 2013), computers (Qiu et al., 2000), energy (Raimondi et al., 2005), food safety (quick detection of dangerous substances existing in extremely low amounts, which the current methods of analysis cannot detect) (Das et al., 2011), etc.

By embedding nanoparticles into polymers, nanocomposites are obtained with inorganic nanoparticles and organic polymers forming a new class of materials with improved performance. The properties of a polymer matrix can be significantly affected by incorporating inorganic nanoparticles. Thus, some properties, such as thermal, mechanical, optical, rheological, electrical, etc., could be improved.

Therefore, it is expected that this will improve, especially, the field of biomedical applications.

The characteristics of new composites depend on the types of nanoparticles that are embedded, their size and shape, their concentration, and their interaction with the polymer matrix.

Many studies have reported the influence of metal nanoparticles on the physical and mechanical properties of new composite materials, being focused especially on the use of these composites in the biomedical area (Blanco-Andujar et al., 2010; Volodina et al., 2013; Chatterjee et al., 2014). A significant number of studies on composites containing nanoparticles of Au, Ag, Zn, etc., have been tested for their anticancer but also antibacterial and antifungal effects (Pal et al., 2007; Thanh and Green, 2010; Wu et al., 2015).

On the other hand, some recent studies have highlighted the great potential of gold nanoparticles in cancer cell treatment and have opened new, alternative ways other than radiation therapy as the mode of treatment (Cai et al., 2008; Jain et al., 2012). The team attached gold nanoparticles and injected pH low insertion peptide (pHLIP) compounds and thus obtained samples of tumor tissue.

The new technique involves the use of pHLIP compounds that are attracted to acidic environments (Weerakkody et al., 2013; Tapmeier et al., 2015). It has been found that the particles accumulate around the pHLIP tumor sites because cancer cells tend to be more acidic in terms of pH than healthy ones. They showed that the cancer cells have a survival rate of 24% less than those irradiated without injection and with 21% less injection of individual gold particles without pHLIPs (Antosh et al., 2015).

The scientists hope that this technology will be soon tested in animal models of cancer, and this will lead to clinical application in order to be used in human pathology of cancer.

There is potential for more precise targeting of tumors and a significant reduction in the radiation dose in patients where pHLIPs are carried by nanoparticles.

Progress in new medical technologies relies heavily upon benefits provided by nanotechnologies.

Nanodrugs have many advantages compared to classical formulations: a particular action in the tissue, increased bioavailability, intracellular penetration, better protection from a degradation-induced biological environment, etc. Therefore, it is anticipated that applying a more effective pharmaceutical nanotechnology would increase the specificity of active substances, tolerability, and the therapeutic index.

From ancient times (Eckhardt et al., 2013), silver has been known to exhibit a strong toxicity to a wide range of microorganisms, such as bacteria (Paul et al., 2013), fungi (Monje and Reséndiz, 2013), viruses (Mori et al., 2013), etc. Silver nanoparticles show efficient antimicrobial properties due to their extremely large surface area, which provides better contact with the microorganisms. For this reason, silver-based compounds have been used extensively in many bactericidal applications like textile coatings, disinfecting sprays, wound dressings, food containers, etc. (Rai et al., 2009).

In the international scientific community, the idea that nanotechnology is the key for the new millennium appears more strongly. It is particularly relevant to this century, because it can provide a high quality of life.

Nanotechnology is a technique that controls and manipulates matter at the nanometer size and allows new hybrid materials with improved properties, by incorporating them in the polymer matrix, a filler with at least one dimension on the order of nanometers (Mansoori and Soelaiman, 2005; Tarafdar et al., 2013). Therefore, a number of morphologies for specific applications have been developed, such as nanoparticles, nanomatrices, dendrimers, nanotubes, etc. (Neelgund and Oki, 2011; Athar and Das, 2014; Mody et al., 2014).

This chapter aims to describe a review of the important recent advances in the nanoparticle domain, from the basics to their application.

The combination of polymers and nanoparticles represents a large pathway for engineering flexible composites, which exhibit advantageous electrical, optical, mechanical, and biological properties (Balazs et al., 2006).

Bacterial contamination shortens the life of foods, posing serious risks to human health.

Nanotechnology provides an opportunity for the research and development of new antibacterial and antifungal agents.

Antimicrobial packaging materials inhibit the growth of microorganisms present on the surface of food. Nanoparticles of zinc oxide (ZnO) are attractive especially in the food packaging industry due to their strong and broad-spectrum antimicrobial properties (Li et al., 2009; Espitia et al., 2013b).

Nanometal oxides have shown important potential in reducing bacterial contamination of foods and in many other applications with particular success. When the particle size of the material decreases to the nanometer level, some properties, such as diffusion, mechanical strength, chemical reactivity, and biological properties, are improved. Recently, the antimicrobial activity of ZnO nanoparticles and the feasibility of their inclusion in active antimicrobial packaging materials have been investigated. Many studies have shown that ZnO nanoparticles have enhanced antibacterial activity. The exact mechanism of action of antimicrobial ZnO nanoparticles is not yet clear, but this action has been considered to contribute to the release of antimicrobial ions.

Some authors (Hong and Rhim, 2008) presented nanoclays modified with quaternary ammonium salts and metals or metal oxides having a nanosize, which showed a strong antimicrobial activity against various groups of Gram-negative and Gram-positive bacteria or against pathogenic fungi.

Other authors prepared antimicrobial packaging materials using different types of nanostructured particles (Llorens et al., 2012; Kanmani and Rhim, 2014).

Because of their large surface-to-volume ratio, ZnO nanoparticles modify some physical, mechanical, and electrical properties, increasing surface reactivity and thermal properties (Becheri et al., 2007).

Many polymer materials have been doped with ZnO nanoparticles in order to prepare antimicrobial nanocomposite packaging films (de Azeredo, 2009; Espitia et al., 2013a).

In general, the antimicrobial nanocomposites act on the packaged product to reduce the growth of microorganisms present on the surface of foodstuff, prolonging the shelf life (Espitia et al., 2013b).

ZnO nanoparticles are more used by many researchers because of their wide potential applications in diverse domains such as nanotechnology, the microelectronic industry, aerospace, the food industry, and not the least in molecular medicine (Kanmani and Rhim, 2014).

The lower cost of ZnO compared to silver nanoparticles is an important reason for using them high on the ladder.

These nanoparticles can be used in different composites for UV-blocking (Becheri et al., 2007) and as absorbers for infrared light and infrared electromagnetic waves (Vigneshwaran et al., 2006). In some polymeric nanocomposites, ZnO produces a reinforcing and enhancement wear-resistant phase and an antisliding phase in composites as a consequence of their high elastic modulus and strength (Dastjerdi and Montazer, 2010).

The biomedical field is of growing interest for nanocomposites with antimicrobial and antifungal activity due to their active surface area, chemical reactivity, and biological activity, which is often radically different from that of particles of greater size. The size and high surface-to-volume ratio of the metallic nanoparticles are accepted as an important mechanism for antimicrobial activity, which allow them to interact closely with microbial membranes favoring an intense ionic exchange (Morones et al., 2005).

Nanocomposites based on metallic and other nanoparticles have potential antimicrobial and antiadhesive applications within the oral cavity (Allaker and Memarzadeh, 2014; Allaker and Douglas, 2015).

Polyurethane (PU) composites based on nanometal oxides can be used in various fields due to acquiring of new or special properties (Mittal et al., 2011).

3.2 ZnO–Polyurethane Nanocomposites as Antibacterial and Antifungal Agents

The manufacture of a biomaterial scaffold is of great importance for successful tissue engineering. PU-based composites are widely used in coatings (Chattopadhyay and Raju, 2007), paints (Gurunathan et al., 2013), foams (Baltopoulos et al., 2013), elastomers (Mothé and de Araújo, 2000; Vlad and Oprea, 2007; Zhang et al., 2007), adhesives (Volkova et al., 2013), and medical devices (Zdrahala and Zdrahala, 1999; Rahimi and Mashak, 2013; Maitz, 2015; Teo et al., 2016). The applications of PUs have been the objects of several of our studies aimed to produce advanced materials with high performances (Vlad, 2005; Macocinschi et al., 2010; Vlad et al., 2010a,b,c). ZnO nanoparticles (nano-ZnO) are useful as antibacterial and antifungal agents when incorporated into materials, such as surface coatings, textiles, and plastics (Sun et al., 2008). The enhanced surface area of ZnO nanoparticles allows increased interaction with bacteria (Premanathan et al., 2011; Vlad et al., 2011; Sirelkhatim et al., 2015). This aspect permits the use of a smaller amount of ZnO for the same or improved biostatic behavior. Furthermore, nanoparticles have a large surface area-to-volume ratio that results in a significant increase of the effectiveness in blocking UV radiation when compared to bulk materials (Hossain and Rahman, 2015).

The polymer utilized in this study was synthesized from 1,6-hexamethylene diisocyanate (HDI), a mixture of polyesters consisting of poly(1,4-butylene adipate) diol end capped (PBA, M 2000), and polycaprolactone diol (PCL, M 2000), with dimethylolpropionic acid (DMPA) as anionic center and 1,4-butane diol (BD) as the chain extender. Different concentrations of nano-ZnO powder were incorporated into the PU matrix solution in dimethylformamide (DMF). The PU/nano-ZnO membranes were prepared by precipitation in warm water, washed with distilled water, and then dried at room temperature for several days. Their structure was evidenced by Fourier transform infrared spectroscopy. Different techniques were used to evaluate surface and wetting properties (contact angle, DVS), morphological properties (SEM), and mechanical properties (tensile test). The antibacterial evaluation was performed for *Escherichia coli*, a Gram-negative bacterium. The results suggest that the PU membranes modified by nano-ZnO have important antibacterial properties and can be used as biocidal materials (Vlad et al., 2011, 2012, 2015).

3.2.1 Synthesis of ZnO–Polyurethane Nanomaterials

During the last decades, several procedures have been reported for the synthesis of ZnO–PU nanomaterials. In our study (Vlad et al., 2011, 2012), we synthesized some ZnO-containing polyesterurethane via a two-step reaction in which HDI, DMPA, PBA (Mn 2000), and PCL (Mn 2000) were

$2\ OCN\text{-}(CH_2)_6\text{-}NCO + HOH_2C\text{-}C(CH_3)(COOH)\text{-}CH_2OH \rightarrow OCN\text{-}(CH_2)_6\text{-}NH\text{-}C(=O)\text{-}O\text{-}CH_2\text{-}C(CH_3)(COOH)\text{-}CH_2O\text{-}C(=O)\text{-}NH\text{-}(CH_2)_6\text{-}NCO$

1,6-Hexamethylene diisocyanate; Dimethylpropionic acid (DMPA); DMPA Urethane Prepolymer—solution in DMF

3:1 PBA/PCL ↓

$OCN\text{-}(CH_2)_6\text{-}NH\text{-}C(=O)\text{-}O\text{-}CH_2\text{-}C(CH_3)(COOH)\text{-}CH_2O\text{-}C(=O)\text{-}NH\text{-}(CH_2)_6\text{-}NH\text{-}OC\text{-}PBA/PCL\text{-}OC\text{-}HN\text{-}(CH_2)_6\text{-}NH\text{-}C(=O)\text{-}O\text{-}CH_2\text{-}C(CH_3)(COOH)\text{-}CH_2O\text{-}C(=O)\text{-}NH\text{-}(CH_2)_6\text{-}NCO$

1,4-BD ↓

PUDMPA —ZnONp→ PUDMPA/ZnONp

SCHEME 3.1
Synthetic pathway to obtain PU-DMPA/ZnONp.

first polymerized, and the polymer was then chain extended with BD. Then, different concentrations of nano-ZnO powder were incorporated into PU matrix solution in DMF. The membranes were prepared by precipitation in warm distilled water, washed, and then dried at room temperature (Scheme 3.1).

In order to improve the biocompatibility and biodegradability of the PU, we also prepared some polycarbonate urethane–hydroxypropyl cellulose (PCU-HPC) in three simple steps (Vlad et al., 2015). In the first step, a urethane prepolymer based on poly(hexamethylene carbonate) diol (Mn 2000) and HDI was synthesized. Then, in the second step, another urethane prepolymer was prepared based on DMPA and HDI. In the last stage, these two prepolymers were mixed together, and the chain extender (BD) was added. ZnO-PCU-HPC materials were obtained by incorporating different amounts of ZnO powder in the PU matrix, in DMF. The steps taken for obtaining PCU-HPC with ZnO nanoparticles are shown schematically (Scheme 3.2).

Finally, a PCU solution in DMF of 25% (w/w), with a hard-segment content (HDI and BD) of 19% (w/w), was obtained. A solution from 4 g HPC in 6 g DMF was added to PCU solution and sonicated for 10 min. This final solution of PCU-HPC was used for preparation of samples with different amounts of ZnONp.

Other authors (Guo et al., 2007) used the in situ suspension polymerization technique in order to prepare ZnO–PU composites. They prepared a prepolymer using polypropylene glycol (Mn 1000), different concentrations of ZnO powders, and tolylene diisocyanate. Afterward, according to the isocyanate group content of PU prepolymer determined by dibutylamine titration, the exact amount of melting methylene-bis-ortho-chloroaniline was added as a chain extender.

Some authors (Jena et al., 2012) proposed some composite materials with the potential to be used for high-performance coatings as antimicrobial materials. These coatings were prepared by mixing hyperbranched

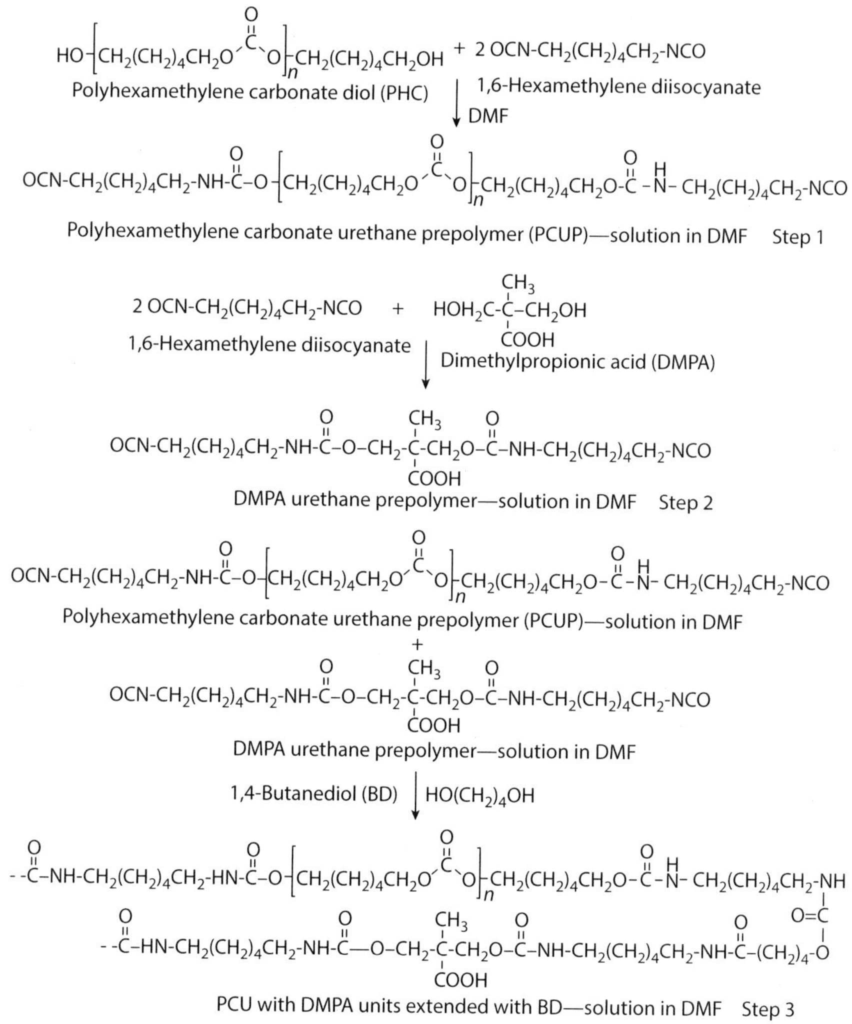

$$HO{-}[CH_2(CH_2)_4CH_2O{-}C(=O){-}O]_n{-}CH_2(CH_2)_4CH_2OH + 2\ OCN{-}CH_2(CH_2)_4CH_2{-}NCO$$

Polyhexamethylene carbonate diol (PHC) ↓ 1,6-Hexamethylene diisocyanate, DMF

$$OCN{-}CH_2(CH_2)_4CH_2{-}NH{-}C(=O){-}O{-}[CH_2(CH_2)_4CH_2O{-}C(=O){-}O]_n{-}CH_2(CH_2)_4CH_2O{-}C(=O){-}N(H){-}CH_2(CH_2)_4CH_2{-}NCO$$

Polyhexamethylene carbonate urethane prepolymer (PCUP)—solution in DMF Step 1

$$2\ OCN{-}CH_2(CH_2)_4CH_2{-}NCO + HOH_2C{-}C(CH_3)(COOH){-}CH_2OH$$

1,6-Hexamethylene diisocyanate ↓ Dimethylpropionic acid (DMPA)

$$OCN{-}CH_2(CH_2)_4CH_2{-}NH{-}C(=O){-}O{-}CH_2{-}C(CH_3)(COOH){-}CH_2O{-}C(=O){-}NH{-}CH_2(CH_2)_4CH_2{-}NCO$$

DMPA urethane prepolymer—solution in DMF Step 2

$$OCN{-}CH_2(CH_2)_4CH_2{-}NH{-}C(=O){-}O{-}[CH_2(CH_2)_4CH_2O{-}C(=O){-}O]_n{-}CH_2(CH_2)_4CH_2O{-}C(=O){-}N(H){-}CH_2(CH_2)_4CH_2{-}NCO$$

Polyhexamethylene carbonate urethane prepolymer (PCUP)—solution in DMF

\+

$$OCN{-}CH_2(CH_2)_4CH_2{-}NH{-}C(=O){-}O{-}CH_2{-}C(CH_3)(COOH){-}CH_2O{-}C(=O){-}NH{-}CH_2(CH_2)_4CH_2{-}NCO$$

DMPA urethane prepolymer—solution in DMF

1,4-Butanediol (BD) ↓ $HO(CH_2)_4OH$

$$--C(=O){-}NH{-}CH_2(CH_2)_4CH_2{-}HN{-}C(=O){-}O{-}[CH_2(CH_2)_4CH_2O{-}C(=O){-}O]_n{-}CH_2(CH_2)_4CH_2O{-}C(=O){-}N(H){-}CH_2(CH_2)_4CH_2{-}NH{-}C(=O){-}O{-}$$

$$--C(=O){-}HN{-}CH_2(CH_2)_4CH_2{-}NH{-}C(=O){-}O{-}CH_2{-}C(CH_3)(COOH){-}CH_2O{-}C(=O){-}NH{-}CH_2(CH_2)_4CH_2{-}NH{-}C(=O){-}(CH_2)_4{-}O$$

PCU with DMPA units extended with BD—solution in DMF Step 3

SCHEME 3.2
Synthesis of poly(hexamethylene carbonate) urethane.

polyurethane-urea (HBPUU) with ZnO nanoparticles. The HBPU used in this study was synthesized from glycerol-based, second-generation hyper-branched polyester and isophorone diisocyanate. DMF and methyl isobutyl ketone were chosen as solvents for the synthesis. HBPUU–ZnO nanocomposites were prepared by adding various amounts of ZnO nanoparticles into solutions of NCO-terminated HBPU.

Other researchers (Mishra et al., 2010) described the synthesis of aqueous ZnO–PU hybrid dispersions using DMPA as an ionic center. For this, NCO-terminated PU prepolymers with pendant acid groups were first prepared, and then different concentrations of ZnO nanopowder were incorporated into the PU matrix. The hybrid dispersions were prepared by adding the required amount of triethylamine, water, and chain extender.

3.2.2 Properties of ZnO–Polyurethane Nanomaterials

In this section, some of the properties of ZnO–PU nanomaterial will be briefly described.

3.2.2.1 Mechanical Properties

The incorporation of ZnO nanoparticles into PU composites is interesting because it has vast applications in various areas, such as optical, piezoelectric, magnetic, and gas sensing, and recently in the medical field. Besides these properties, the number of research topics on the mechanical properties of nanoparticles has increased in recent years as also the number of relevant publications. The mechanical properties of the PU samples obtained in our group (Vlad et al., 2011) were influenced by the proportion of the added ZnO nanoparticles.

The main characteristic values of the mechanical measurements of the polyesterurethane samples are shown in Figure 3.1. In general, the mechanical characteristics of the PU samples can be affected by factors such as the

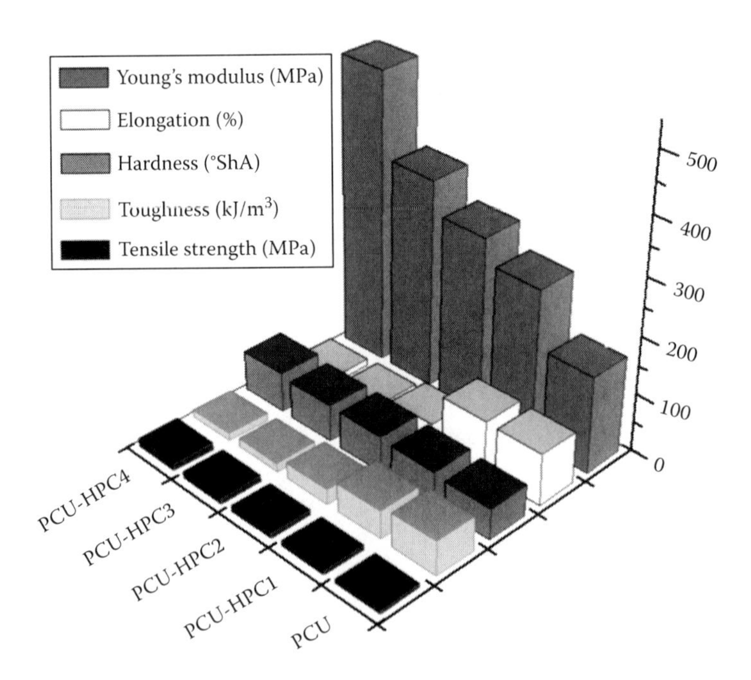

FIGURE 3.1
Main physico-mechanical characteristics of PCU-HPC with ZnONp.

content of soft and hard segments, their cohesion energy, packing degree of macromolecules, phase separation, cross-linking degree of PU samples, etc. (Vlad et al., 2010a,b,c). It was observed that the proportion of ZnO nanoparticles in the sample influenced the mechanical characteristics.

The Young's modulus and tensile strength of the materials are significantly improved by the addition of ZnONp, in detriment of elongation. In addition, hardness increases with the amount of ZnONp. The tensile toughness represents the quantity of energy per volume that can be absorbed by material before failure. It was estimated as the area under each stress–strain curve and can be indirectly correlated with the energy that could be released by an elastic material when the force that acted on it was removed, like in a harvesting energy system. PCU-HPC with lower amounts of ZnONp (PCU-HPC1 and PCU-HPC2) absorbs more energy per volume before failure as compared to samples comprising higher contents of ZnONp.

3.2.2.2 Wetting Properties

The physical properties of the nanomaterials, such as those related to the surface, depend strongly on the polymer chain mobility, conformation, and ordering. This influence further increases the interaction between the material surface and the biological environment. Therefore, any small change results in a dramatic change of the surface properties, leading to different biological responses. Thus, the knowledge of the wetting properties becomes an important factor for the characterization of biomaterials.

The easiest and most used method to describe the wettability of a surface is the determination of contact angles. The hydrophobic/hydrophilic character of the ZnO–PU nanomaterial films was evaluated by measuring the contact angle between the surface of the films and drops of the test liquid, using a KSV CAM 101 goniometer (Finland) and the sessile-drop technique. A contact angle less than 90° (low contact angle) usually indicates that wetting of the surface is very favorable and the surface is also known as hydrophilic. In contrast, a contact angle greater than 90° (high contact angle) indicates that wetting of the surface is unfavorable and the surface is known as hydrophobic. Our data showed that the ZnO–PU nanocomposite surfaces have a contact angle degree greater than 90°, and thereby the surfaces are hydrophobic. The variation of the contact angle with ZnONp concentration of our synthesized PUs is illustrated in Figure 3.2.

The amount of ZnONp had a significant influence on the surface wettability of the synthesized ZnO–PU films. Thus, for the samples with HPC in the structure an increase of the contact angle degree with the amount of ZnONp is observed, leading to an increase of the hydrophobic character of the films. This increase may be attributed to the lower amount of polar components in the structures due to the formation of more cross-linked structures in the PU matrix (Mishra et al., 2010) and also to the presence of an oxide layer on the solid surface (El-Sayed et al., 2016).

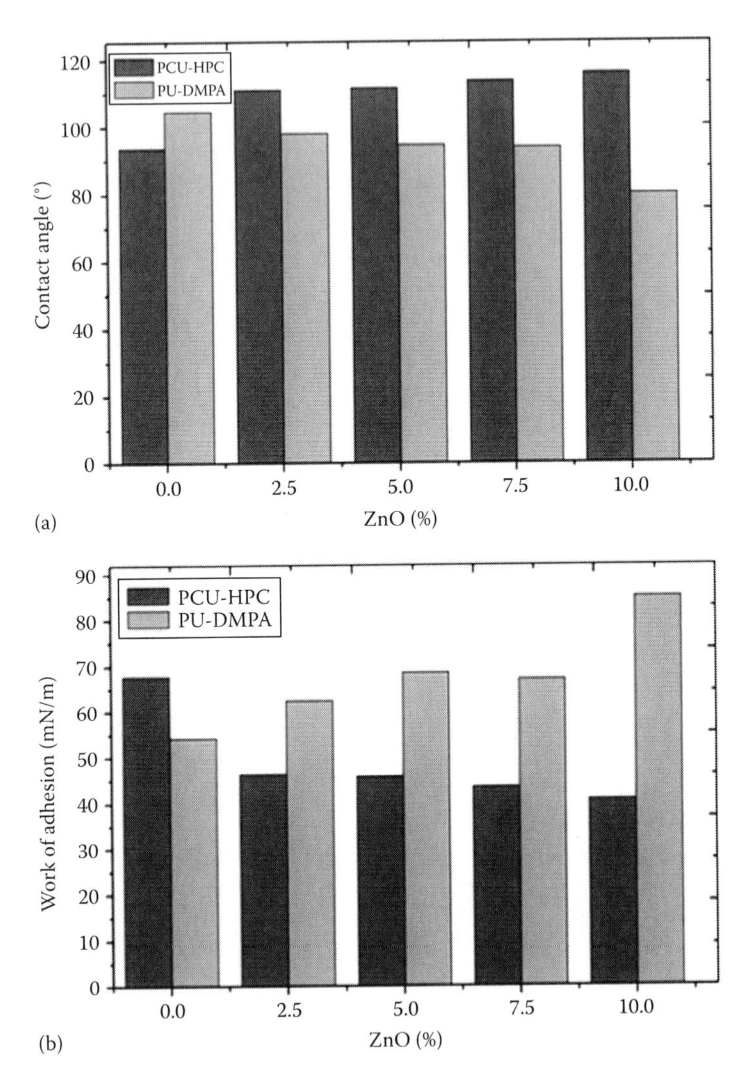

FIGURE 3.2
Influence of the ZnONp concentration on the (a) contact angle and (b) work of adhesion.

For the other samples, with DMPA in their structures, the values of the contact angles degree decrease with the increase of the amount of ZnONp. These surfaces therefore become hydrophilic.

Based on the measurements of the contact angle, some parameters such as work of adhesion, surface free energy, etc., could be also calculated using different mathematical equations (Erbil et al., 2002; Erbil, 2006; Mittal, 2006). For example, in Figure 3.2b is presented the dependence of the work of adhesion on the ZnONp concentration. The values of work of adhesion are decreased/increased, while the values of their contact angle increase/decrease for

PCU-HPC and PU-DMPA, respectively. The contact angles of the materials increase in the order PCU < PCU-HPC1 < PCU-HPC2 < PCU-HPC3 < PCU-HPC4, proving that the increase of the ZnONp amount increased the hydrophobicity, while for PUDMPA samples the effect is contrary.

In conclusion, the understanding of the interface between nanomaterials and biological systems is very important and should allow the researchers to control the preparation of such biomaterials with specific properties.

3.2.2.3 Water Absorption Capacity

Determination of the water vapor sorption capacity and physical stability of PU samples modified with nano-ZnO was done using the IGAsorp system. The interaction of materials with water vapor has attracted broad-spectrum research interest in science and industry. Almost all materials have some interaction with moisture that is present in their surroundings. The effects of water can be both harmful and beneficial depending on the material and how it is used. Isothermal studies can be performed as a function of humidity (0%–95%) in the temperature range 5°C–85°C, with an accuracy of ±1% for 0%–90% RH and ±2% for 90%–95% RH. The relative humidity (RH) is controlled by wet and dry nitrogen flow around the sample. The RH is held constant until equilibrium or until a given time is exceeded, before changing the RH to the next level. The water vapor sorption behavior of this sample was analyzed using moisture sorption isotherms. The role played by water molecules in the sample was interpreted on the basis of two models, Brunauer–Emmet–Teller (BET) (Brunauer et al., 1940) and Guggenheim–Anderson–de Boer (GAB) (Anderson, 1946; Guggenheim, 1966; De Boer, 1968), which allow a good fit of the water sorption data. The average pore size can be estimated based on desorption branch assuming a cylindrical pore geometry by using surface area calculated by BET or GAB equations. From the present study, it is evident that many parameters, such as the amount of ZnONp, the presence of the polar groups on the PU surface, pore size, and surface area, can influence in the complex mode the sorption capacity of the samples.

3.2.2.4 Antibacterial Behavior

Antibacterial activity was tested in Luria–Bertani broth, which was initially grown for 20 h at 28°C. The cell density was determined at 5 and 20 h by reading the absorbance (optical density [OD]) at 580 nm using a Libra UV/Vis spectrophotometer (Biochrom, UK). Analysis of the antimicrobial test was carried out by preparing samples from ZnONp-free PU membranes and ZnONp-containing ones in a solution of agar with *Escherichia coli* cells. Before using, the samples were sterilized by autoclaving at 120°C. The PU samples were screened for antibacterial activity using the turbidimetric method, and the turbidity produced was measured by comparing the

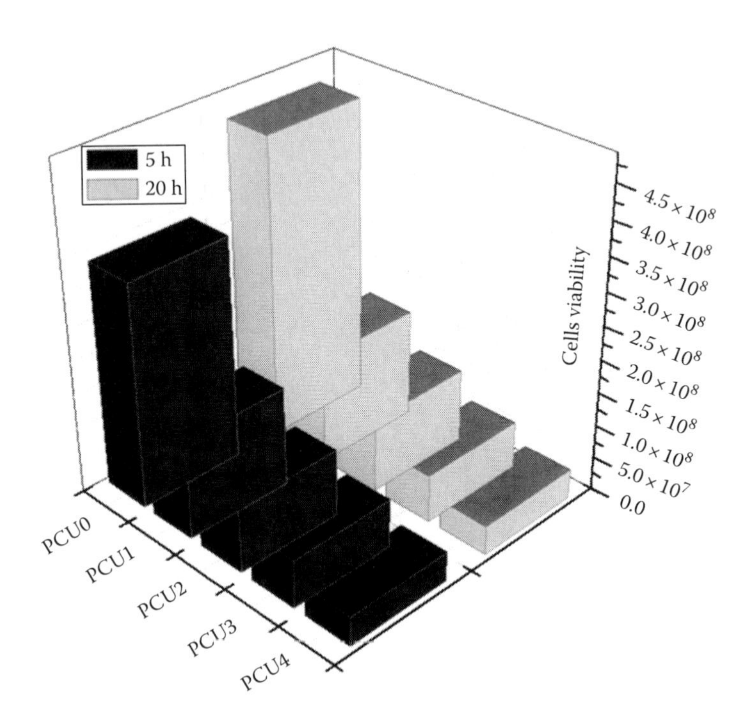

FIGURE 3.3
Cell viability of the studied materials after 5 and 20 h respectively.

absorbance with the turbidity produced by the standard probe. The antibacterial activity has been proven by the reduction in the OD of the cell culture test relative to controls.

In Figure 3.3 are presented the OD values and their correlation with the number of cells grown on PU membranes modified by ZnONp. The reduction in the OD of the cell culture test relative to controls proved to have a high antibacterial activity when the amount of ZnONp in the material was increased (Sawai et al., 1998).

3.2.2.5 ZnO–Polyurethane Nanocomposites as Antifungal Agents

In the same manner as in a previous paper (Vlad et al., 2012) , the sample was prepared for the antifungal tests. The PUDMPA samples, containing between 0 and 10 wt.% ZnO, were cut into small pieces of 10 × 15 mm and placed in the middle of sterile 9 cm plates containing Sabouraud agar medium. The medium was inoculated at four points with spores of *Aspergillus brasiliensis*. Other polymer samples having the same size were inoculated with fungal spores and placed in sterile Petri dishes without medium and used as the control.

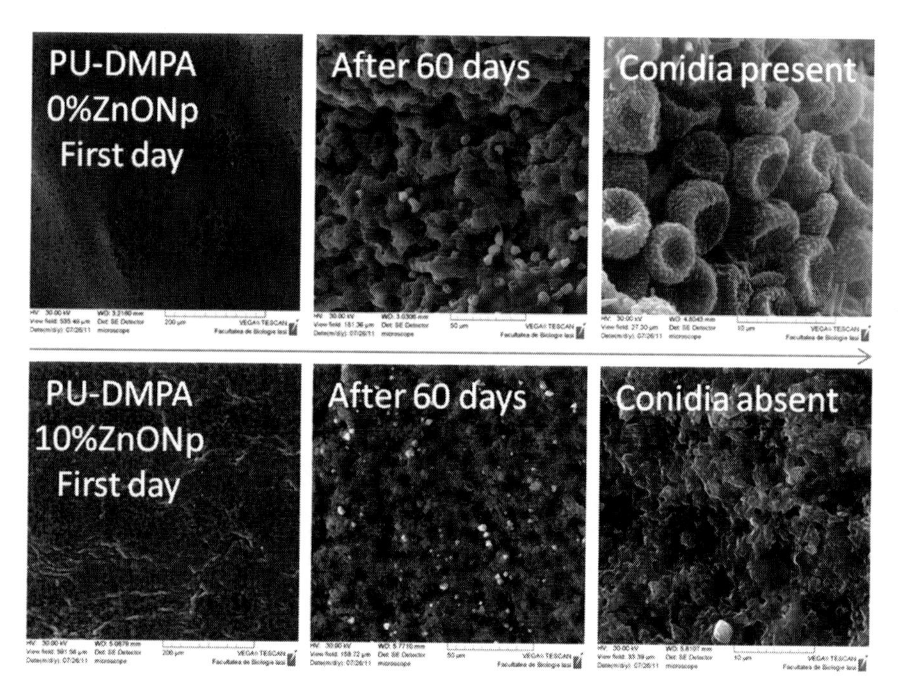

FIGURE 3.4
Fungal growing profiles of the samples.

All the samples were incubated at 23°C for 60 days in the dark. The dishes were visualized after 7, 14, 21, 28, and 60 days after inoculation. The surface morphology was performed studying the membrane samples using SEM.

The SEM observations were made starting from the overall analysis on a wide field (low resolution) to focus on a narrow field for observation details (high resolution). In the case of the sample without ZnONp, the adsorption of fungal conidia on the polymer surface was evidenced (Figure 3.4). These aspects are in agreement with the previous observations carried out by Sawai and Yoshikawa (2004).

3.3 Conclusions

Various metal nanoparticles embedded in polymer composites are of great interest to the scientific world because of new qualities acquired by these materials and the many perspectives of application in nanotechnology. The chapter briefly reviews the use of metal nanoparticles, highlighting new composite qualities in terms of antibacterial and antifungal activity compared to other research studies in the field. A few PU membranes, in whose matrix have been introduced different percentages of ZnO nanoparticles, were studied. The characteristics of these materials were influenced by the content of the metal nanoparticles used. Wetting characteristics are influenced by the ZnONp content of the material studied. The hydrophilicity of these PU membranes increased as a percentage increase of ZnONp in the sample. Based on the sorption/desorption isotherms registered by DSV, BET, and GAB, the surface area as well as average pore size were estimated, and these polymers, set by IUPAC, were placed between microporous and mesoporous materials. Humidity loss and drying speed of water from these PU samples depend on the amount of ZnONp. For some PU membranes with a progressive amount of ZnONp, the Young's modulus and tensile strength of the samples are improved significantly in detriment of elongation. In addition, the hardness too increases with the amount of ZnONp. Tensile toughness increased when a low amount of ZnONp was incorporated into the sample. Hydrophobicity of these membranes increased as the percentage of ZnONp increased. Antibacterial activity was evaluated by determining the degree of turbidity, measuring the OD of the analyzed solutions. The antibacterial activity of these membranes against *E. coli* increases as the ZnONp content increases. The antifungal behavior for a set of ZnO nanoparticles–based PUs was envisaged. For this study was used *Aspergillus brasiliensis*, a very widespread aggressive fungal species from the environment. The evaluation of biological activity of these membranes against the attack of these fungi has been done through inoculation onto Sabouraud agar nutrient medium. The fungal growth was monitored visually by zone diameter inhibition method and by SEM images. The presence of fungi conidia was observed for the sample without ZnO nanoparticles. It is notable that at relatively low concentrations of nano-ZnO, the polymers studied show antifungal behavior. In general, the results suggest that the PU membranes modified by nano-ZnO have important antibacterial properties, respectively, antifungal properties, and can be successfully used in biomedical applications.

Acknowledgments

The authors acknowledge the financial support of this research through the European Regional Development Fund, Project POINGBIO, ID P_40_443, Contract no. 86/8.09.2016.

References

Allaker, R.P. and Douglas, C.W. 2015. Non-conventional therapeutics for oral infections. *Virulence* 6(3):196–207.

Allaker, R.P. and Memarzadeh, K. 2014. Nanoparticles and the control of oral infections. *Int J Antimicrob Agents* 43(2):95–104.

Anderson, R.B. 1946. Modifications of the Brunauer, Emmett and Teller Equation. *J Am Chem Soc* 68:686–691.

Antosh, M.P., Wijesinghe, D.D., Shrestha, S. et al. 2015. Enhancement of radiation effect on cancer cells by gold-pHLIP. *Proc Natl Acad Sci USA* 112(17):5372–5376.

Athar, M. and Das, A.J. 2014. Therapeutic nanoparticles: State-of-the-art of nanomedicine. *Adv Mater Rev* 1(1):25–37.

Balazs, A.C., Emrick, T., and Russell, T.P. 2006. Nanoparticle polymer composites: Where two small worlds meet. *Science* 314(5802):1107–1110.

Baltopoulos, A., Athanasopoulos, N., Fotiou, I., Vavouliotis, A., and Kostopoulos, V. 2013. Sensing strain and damage in polyurethane-MWCNT nano-composite foams using electrical measurements. *Express Polym Lett* 7(1):40–54.

Bangal, M., Ashtaputre, S., Marathe, S. et al. 2005. Semiconductor nanoparticles. *Hyperfine Interact* 160:81–94.

Becheri, A., Durr, M., Nostro, P.L., and Baglioni, P. 2007. Synthesis and characterization of zinc oxide nanoparticles: Application to textiles as UV-absorbers. *J Nanopart Res* 10:679–689.

Blanco-Andujar, C., Tungc, L.D., and Thanh, N.T.K. 2010. Synthesis of nanoparticles for biomedical applications. *Annu Rep Prog Chem A* 106:553–568.

Brunauer, S., Deming, L.S., Deming, W.E., and Teller, E. 1940. On a theory of the van der Waals adsorption of gases. *J Am Chem Soc* 62(7):1723–1732.

Bumbudsanpharoke, N., Choi, J., and Ko, S. 2015. Applications of nanomaterials in food packaging. *J Nanosci Nanotechnol* 15(9):6357–6372.

Cai, W., Gao, T., Hong, H., and Sun, J. 2008. Applications of gold nanoparticles in cancer nanotechnology. *Nanotechnol Sci Appl* 1:17–32.

Chatterjee, K., Sarkar, S., Rao, K.J., and Paria, S. 2014. Core/shell nanoparticles in biomedical applications. *Adv Colloid Interface Sci* 209:8–39.

Chattopadhyay, D.K. and Raju, K.V.S.N. 2007. Structural engineering of polyurethane coatings for high performance applications. *Prog Polym Sci* 32(3):352–418.

Das, M., Ansari, K.M., Tripathi, A., and Dwivedi, P.D. 2011. Need for safety of nanoparticles used in food industry. *J Biomed Nanotechnol* 7(1):13–14.

Dastjerdi, R. and Montazer, M. 2010. A review on the application of inorganic nano-structured materials in the modification of textiles: Focus on anti-microbial properties. *Colloids Surf B Biointerfaces* 79:5–18.

De Azeredo, H.M.C. 2009. Nanocomposites for food packaging applications. *Food Res Int* 42:1240–1253.

De Boer, J.H. 1968. *The Dynamical Character of Adsorption*. Clarendon Press, Oxford, U.K., pp. 200–219.

Dinca, I., Ban, C., Stefan, A., and Pelin, G. 2012. Nanocomposites as advanced materials for aerospace industry. *INCAS Bull* 4(4):73–83.

Eckhardt, S., Brunetto, P.S., Gagnon, J. et al. 2013. Nanobio silver: Its interactions with peptides and bacteria, and its uses in medicine. *Chem Rev* 113:4708–4754.

El-Sayed, M.A., Hassanin, H., and Essa, K. 2016. Bifilm defects and porosity in Al cast alloys. *Int J Adv Manuf Technol* 86:1173–1179.

Erbil, H.Y. 2006. *Surface Chemistry of Solid and Liquid Interfaces*. Blackwell Publishing, Oxford, U.K.

Erbil, H.Y., McHale, G., and Newton, M.I. 2002. Drop evaporation on solid surfaces: Constant contact angle mode. *Langmuir* 18(7):2636–2641.

Espitia, P.J.P., Pacheco, J.J.R., de Melo, N.R., Soares, N.F.F., and Durango, A.M. 2013a. Packaging properties and control of *Listeria monocytogenes* in bologna by cellulosic films incorporated with pediocin. *Braz J Food Technol Campinas* 16(3):226–235.

Espitia, P.J.P., Soares, N.F.F., Coimbra, J.S.R. et al. 2012. Zinc oxide nanoparticles: Synthesis, antimicrobial activity and food packaging applications. *Food Bioprocess Technol* 5:1447–1464.

Espitia, P.J.P., Soares, N.F.F., Teófilo, R.F. et al. 2013b. Physical–mechanical and antimicrobial properties of nanocomposite films with pediocin and ZnO nanoparticles. *Carbohydr Polym* 94(1):199–208.

Forcherio, G.T. and Roper, D.K. 2013. Optical attenuation of plasmonic nanocomposites within photonic devices. *Appl Opt* 52(25):6417–6427.

Gawande, M.B., Goswami, A., Felpin, F.X. et al. 2016. Cu and Cu-based nanoparticles: Synthesis and applications in catalysis. *Chem Rev* 116(6):3722–3811.

Godlewski, M., Yatsunenko, S., Nadolska, A. et al. 2009. Nanoparticles doped with TM and RE ions for applications in optoelectronics. *Opt Mater* 31(3):490–495.

Guggenheim, E.A. 1966. *Application of Statistical Mechanics*. Clarendon Press, Oxford, U.K., pp. 186–206.

Guo, C., Zheng, Z., Zhu, Q., and Wang, X. 2007. Preparation and characterization of polyurethane/ZnO nanoparticle composites. *Polym Plast Technol Eng* 46(12):1161–1166.

Gurunathan, T., Rao, C.R.K., Narayan, R., and Raju, K.V.S.N. 2013. Polyurethane conductive blends and composites: Synthesis and applications perspective. *JMater Sci* 48:67–80.

Hong, S.I. and Rhim, J.W. 2008. Antimicrobial activity of organically modified nanoclays. *J Nanosci Nanotechnol* 8:5818–5824.

Hossain, M.A. and Rahman, M. 2015. A review of nano particle usage on textile material against ultra violet radiation. *J Text Sci Technol* 1(3):93–100.

Iskandar, F. 2009. Nanoparticle processing for optical applications—A review. *Adv Powder Technol* 20:283–292.

Jain, S., Hirst, D.G., and O'Sullivan, J.M. 2012. Gold nanoparticles as novel agents for cancer therapy. *Br J Radiol* 85(1010):101–113.

Jena, K.K., Rout, T.K., Narayan, R., and Raju, K.V.S.N. 2012. Novel organic–inorganic hybrid coatings prepared by the sol–gel process: Corrosion and mechanical properties. *Polym Int* 61(7):1101–1107.

Kanmani, P. and Rhim, J.W. 2014. Properties and characterization of bionanocomposite films prepared with various biopolymers and ZnO nanoparticles. *Carbohydr Polym* 106:190–199.

Li, X., Xing, Y., Jiang, Y., Ding, Y., and Li, W. 2009. Antimicrobial activities of ZnO powder-coated PVC film to inactivate food pathogens. *Int J Food Sci Technol* 44:2161–2168.

Llorens, A., Lloret, E., Picouet, P.A., Trbojevich, R., and Fernandez, A. 2012. Metallic-based micro and nanocomposites in food contact materials and active food packaging. *Trends Food Sci Technol* 24:19–29.

Macocinschi, D., Filip, D., and Vlad, S. 2010. Surface and mechanical properties of some new biopolyurethane composites. *Polym Compos* 31(11):1956–1964.

Maitz, M.F. 2015. Applications of synthetic polymers in clinical medicine. *Biosurface Biotribol* 1(3):161–176.

Mansoori, G.A. and Soelaiman, T.A.F. 2005. Nanotechnology—An introduction for the standards community. *J ASTM Int* 2(6):1–22.

Mishra, A.K., Mishra, R.S., Narayan, R., and Raju, K.V.S.N. 2010. Effect of nano ZnO on the phase mixing of polyurethane hybrid dispersions. *Prog Org Coat* 67(4):405–413.

Mittal, K.L. (Ed.). 2006. *Contact Angle, Wettability and Adhesion*. Taylor & Francis Group, Boca Raton, FL, Vol. 4.

Mittal, V., Kim, J.K., and Pal, K. 2011. *Recent Advances in Elastomeric Nanocomposites*, Advanced Structured Materials. Springer-Verlag, Berlin, Germany.

Mody, N., Tekade, R.K., Mehra, N.K., Chopdey, P., and Jain, N.K. 2014. Dendrimer, liposomes, carbon nanotubes and PLGA nanoparticles: One platform assessment of drug delivery potential. *AAPS PharmSciTech* 15(2):388–399.

Monje, A.E. and Reséndiz, J.R.H. 2013. Synthesis of urethane base composite materials with metallic nanoparticles. *Mater Res Soc Symp Proc* 1547:141–147.

Mori, Y., Ono, T., Miyahira, Y., Nguyen, V.Q., Matsui, T., and Ishihara, M. 2013. Antiviral activity of silver nanoparticle/chitosan composites against H1N1 influenza A virus. *Nanoscale Res Lett* 8(1):93.

Morones, J.R., Elechiguerra, J.L., Camacho, A. et al. 2005. The bactericidal effect of silver nanoparticles. *Nanotechnology* 16:2346–2353.

Mothé, C.G. and de Araújo, C.R. 2000. Properties of polyurethane elastomers and composites by thermal analysis. *Thermochim Acta* 357–358:321–325.

Neelgund, G.M. and Oki, A. 2011. Deposition of silver nanoparticles on dendrimer functionalized multiwalled carbon nanotubes: Synthesis, characterization and antimicrobial activity. *J Nanosci Nanotechnol* 11(4):3621–3629.

Pal, A., Shah, S., and Devi, S. 2007. Synthesis of Au, Ag and Au–Ag alloy nanoparticles in aqueous polymer solution. *Colloids Surf A Physicochem Eng Asp* 302(1–3):51–57.

Parisi, C., Vigani, M., and Rodríguez-Cerezo, E. 2015. Agricultural nanotechnologies: What are the current possibilities? *Nanotoday* 10(2):124–127.

Patra, J.K. and Gouda, S. 2013. Application of nanotechnology in textile engineering: An overview. *J Eng Technol Res* 5(5):104–111.

Paul, S., Roohpour, N., Wilks, M., and Vadgama, P. 2013. Antimicrobial, mechanical and thermal studies of silver particle-loaded polyurethane. *J Funct Biomater* 4:358–375.

Prasad, R., Kumar, V., and Prasad, K.S. 2014. Nanotechnology in sustainable agriculture: Present concerns and future aspects. *Afr J Biotechnol* 13(6):705–713.

Premanathan, M., Karthikeyan, K., Jeyasubramanian K., and Manivannan, G. 2011. Selective toxicity of ZnO nanoparticles toward Gram-positive bacteria and cancer cells by apoptosis through lipid peroxidation. *Nanomed Nanotechnol Biol Med* 7(2):184–192.

Qiu, M., Khisamutdinov, E., Zhao, Z. et al. 2000. RNA nanotechnology for computer design and *in vivo* computation. *Philos Trans A Math Phys Eng Sci* 371:20120310, doi: 10.1098/rsta.2012.0310.

Rahimi, A. and Mashak, A. 2013. Review on rubbers in medicine: Natural, silicone and polyurethane rubbers. *J Plast Rubb Compos Macromol Eng* 42(6):223–230.

Rai, M., Yadav, A., and Gade, A. 2009. Silver nanoparticles as a new generation of antimicrobials. *Biotechnol Adv* 27:76–83.

Raimondi, F., Scherer, G.G., Kötz, R., and Wokaun, A. 2005. Nanoparticles in energy technology: Examples from electrochemistry and catalysis. *Angew Chem Int Ed Engl* 44(15):2190–2209.

Salata, O.V. 2004. Applications of nanoparticles in biology and medicine. *J Nanobiotechnol* 2:3–9.

Sawai, J., Shoji, S., Igarashi, H. et al. 1998. Hydrogen peroxide as an antibacterial factor in zinc oxide powder slurry. *J Ferment Bioeng* 86:521–522.

Sawai, J. and Yoshikawa, T. 2004. Quantitative evaluation of antifungal activity of metallic oxide powders (MgO, CaO and ZnO) by an indirect conductimetric assay. *J Appl Microbiol* 96:803–809.

Schroeder, A., Heller, D.A., Winslow, M.M. et al. 2012. Treating metastatic cancer with nanotechnology. *Nat Rev Cancer* 12:39–50.

Silpa, R., Shoma, J., Sumod, U.S., and Sabitha, M. 2012. Nanotechnology in cosmetics: Opportunities and challenges. *J Pharm Bioallied Sci* 4(3):186–193.

Sirelkhatim, A., Mahmud, S., Seeni, A. et al. 2015. Review on zinc oxide nanoparticles: Antibacterial activity and toxicity mechanism. *Nano-Micro Lett* 7:219–242.

Sun, L., Rippon, J.A., Cookson, P.G., and Wang, X. 2008. Nano zinc oxide for UV protection of textiles. *Int J Technol Transfer Commercialisation* 7(2/3):224–235.

Tapmeier, T.T., Moshnikova, A., Beech, J. et al. 2015. The pH low insertion peptide pHLIP Variant 3 as a novel marker of acidic malignant lesions. *Proc Natl Acad Sci USA* 112(31):9710–9715.

Tarafdar, J.C., Sharma, S., and Raliya, R. 2013. Nanotechnology: Interdisciplinary science of applications. *Afr J Biotechnol* 12(3):219–226.

Teo, A.J.T., Mishra, A., Park, I., Kim, Y.J., Park, W.T., and Yoon, Y.J. 2016. Polymeric biomaterials for medical implants and devices. *ACS Biomater Sci Eng* 2(4):454–472.

Thanh, N.T.K. and Green, L.A.W. 2010. Functionalisation of nanoparticles for biomedical applications. *Nano Today* 5:213–230.

van Broekhuizen, P., van Broekhuizen, F., Cornelissen, R., and Reijnders, L. 2011. Use of nanomaterials in the European construction industry and some occupational health aspects thereof. *J Nanopart Res* 13:447–462.

Vigneshwaran, N., Kumar, S., Kathe, A.A., Varadarajan, P.V., and Prasad, V. 2006. Functional finishing of cotton fabrics using zinc oxide-soluble starch nanocomposites. *Nanotechnology* 17:5087–5095.

Vigneshwaran, N., Varadarajan, P.V., and Balasubramanya, R.H. 2010. *Application of Metallic Nanoparticles in Textiles*, Nanotechnologies for the Life Sciences. Wiley-VCH Verlag GmbH, Weinheim, Germany.

Vlad, S. 2005. Influence of the hard segment contents on mechanical behavior of some poly(ether-urethane-urea)s. *Mater Plast* 42(1):63–67.

Vlad, S., Butnaru, M., Filip, D. et al. 2010a. Polyetherurethane membranes modified with renewable resource as a potential candidate for biomedical applications. *Dig J Nanomater Biostruct* 5(4):1089–1100.

Vlad, S., Ciobanu, C., Gradinaru, R.V., Gradinaru, L.M., and Nistor, A. 2011. Antibacterial evaluation of some polyurethane membranes modified by zinc oxide nanoparticles. *Dig J Nanomater Biostruct* 6(3):921–930.

Vlad, S., Cristea, M., Ciobanu, C. et al. 2010b. Characterization of some soft polyesterurethane films. *J Optoelectron Adv Mater* 12(11):2278–2287.

Vlad, S., Filip, D., Macocinschi, D. et al. 2010c. New polyetherurethanes based on cellulose derivative for biomedical applications. *Optoelectron Adv Mater Rapid Commun* 4(3):407–414.

Vlad, S., Gradinaru, L.M., Ciobanu, C. et al. 2015. Polycarbonate urethane-hydroxypropyl cellulose membranes with zinc oxide nanoparticles. *Cellulose Chem Technol* 49(9–10):905–913.

Vlad, S. and Oprea, S. 2007. Effect of polyols on the physico-mechanical properties of some polyurethanes. *J Optoelectron Adv Mater* 9(4):994–999.

Vlad, S., Tanase, C., Macocinschi, D. et al. 2012. Antifungal behaviour of polyurethane membranes with zinc oxide nanoparticles. *Dig J Nanomater Biostruct* 7(1):51–58.

Volkova, E.R., Tereshatov, V.V., Karmanov, V.I., Makarova, M.A., and Slobodinyuk, A.I. 2013. Polyurethane adhesive composition cured at room temperature. *Polym Sci Ser D* 6:120–124.

Volodina, L.A., Zhigach, A.N., Leypunsky, I.O. et al. 2013. The influence of physical-chemical characteristics of surface modified copper nanoparticles on *E. coli* cell population growth suppression and on electrostatic properties of their membranes. *Biophysics* 58(3):394–401.

Weerakkody, D., Moshnikova, A., Thakur, M.S. et al. 2013. Family of pH (low) insertion peptides for tumor targeting. *Proc Natl Acad Sci USA* 110:15834–15839.

Wiechers, J.W. and Musee, N. 2010. Engineered inorganic nanoparticles and cosmetics: Facts, issues, knowledge gaps and challenges. *J Biomed Nanotechnol* 6:408–431.

Wu, W., Wu, Z., Yu, T., Jiang, C., and Kim, W.S. 2015. Recent progress on magnetic iron oxide nanoparticles: Synthesis, surface functional strategies and biomedical applications. *Sci Technol Adv Mater* 16:023501.

Yan, J., Liu, P., Ma, C., Lin, Z., and Yang, G. 2016. Plasmonic near-touching titanium oxide nanoparticles to realize solar energy harvesting and effective local heating. *Nanoscale* 8(16):8826–8888.

Zdrahala, R.J. and Zdrahala, I.J. 1999. Biomedical applications of polyurethanes: A review of past promises, present realities, and a vibrant future. *J Biomater Appl* 14(1):67–90.

Zhang, H., Li, W., Yang, X. et al. 2007. Development of polyurethane elastomer composite materials by addition of milled fiberglass with coupling agent. *Mater Lett* 61(6):1358–1362.

Zhang, L., Gu, F.X., Chan, J.M. et al. 2008. Nanoparticles in medicine: Therapeutic applications and developments. *Clin Pharmacol Ther* 83(5):761–769.

Zhang, Y., Huang, R., Zhu, X.F., Wang, L.Z., and Wu, C.X. 2012. Synthesis, properties, and optical applications of noble metal nanoparticle-biomolecule conjugates. *Chin Sci Bull* 57(2–3):238–246.

4

Smart Materials with Phosphorus and Nitrogen Functionalities Suitable for Biomedical Engineering

Diana Serbezeanu, Tachita Vlad-Bubulac, Maria Butnaru, and Magdalena Aflori

CONTENTS

4.1 Introduction

Today, the field of synthetic and biological polymers is extensively impacting various areas of chemistry, biochemistry, molecular biology, nanotechnology, electronics, medicine, life sciences, materials, etc. Synthetic polymers have played a fascinating role in the successful development of biomedical devices and drug delivery systems. However, until recently, polymers for health care applications were commonly adopted from other industries without their substantial redesign for medical use. In many life science applications, research studies are facing major challenges in creating materials with specific patterns of degradation profiles, biological interactions, release characteristics, and physicochemical and mechanical properties (Langer and Tirrell 2004). One of the ways to obtain new polymers with sophisticated functions is connected with the synthesis of novel monomer units where the required function is linked to the chemical structure of these units. However, the potential of this approach is rather limited, because complicated and diverse functions of polymer materials would then require a very complex structure of monomer units, which normally means that the organic synthesis is more expensive and less robust.

The alternative approach is to use known monomer units or polymer and to try and design a copolymer chain with a given sequence of these units. There are practically infinite possibilities of varying sequences in copolymers: from the variation of some simple characteristics like composition of monomer units, average length of blocks, availability of branching, etc., to more sophisticated features like long-range correlations or gradient structure. Therefore, in this approach, a wide variety of novel functional copolymers could be tailored. The study of materials capable of self-assembling in supramolecular structures with desired functionalities and physical properties, at the nano- and microscopic levels, is actually one of the domains of greatest scientific interest, offering the possibility of designing and preparing new functional advanced materials by building using the so-called bottom-up technique. Phosphorus-containing materials can be employed for a wide range of technological applications. For instance, they are largely used in industry due to their binding ability toward metals (Clearfield 2006). Indeed, organophosphonates exhibited interesting complexing properties and were used as dispersants, as corrosion-inhibiting agents, or for preventing deposit formation. The necessity of new high performance materials based on polymers makes important the scientific research in order to satisfy more important needs: flame retardancy and minimization environmental impacts. Recently, the development of free halogen materials due to the latest legislation gave new opportunities for using phosphorylated polymers in applications that require flame retardant performances (Canadell et al. 2007, Singh and Jain 2009), where phosphorus is known to be highly efficient. Phosphorylated halogen-free flame retardant coatings can lead to the formation of char or a protective coating that avoids the transport of oxygen to the burning area and extinguishes the fire. Human life loss is often the result of advanced toxicity of the atmosphere resulting from the fire. Thus, the use of halogenated flame retardants was drastically minimized in Europe and the United States, while in China they are still produced at a high scale. To date, a universal composition that is highly efficient for all polymers or even for a few of them has not been discovered. Each class of polymers has its own type of flame retardant used to improve the flame resistance. Although halogen-based flame retardants will be banned, there is an increasing need for other efficient materials, which leave open the interest in the development and production of new high-performance systems to improve the flame resistance of polymeric materials (Petreus et al. 2010, Carja et al. 2014, Hamciuc et al. 2016).

Recently, interest in phosphorus-based materials used in biomedical fields has been accelerating because they have proved to be biodegradable and blood compatible and shown reduced protein adsorption and strong interactions with dentin, enamel, or bones. As a consequence, they appear to be an interesting class of materials, which will lead to further developments in this area of application. For instance, phosphonated groups were preferred because they improved hydrolytic stability and were proved to be efficient as calcium sequestrants, inhibiting the crystal growth of calcium phosphate (Francis et al. 1969).

The main goal of this chapter is to make a brief rundown of our interest for the synthesis and characterization of novel compounds containing phosphorus or nitrogen functionalities in the main and/or side chain, which could be recommended for applications in top fields of biomedicine (biosensors, drug controlled release, and tissue engineering). Because the domain of polymers containing phosphorous or nitrogen functionalities in the main and/or side chain is very wide, we have summarized in this chapter only the most recent studies on some polyphosphoesters (PPEs) (polyphosphonates, polyphosphites, and polyphosphoramidates) and polyimide (PI) nanofibers, suitable for biomedical applications.

4.2 Biomedical Applications of Polyphosphoesters

Polymers play a key role in the development of drug delivery systems, medical devices, and biosensors. More than ever, they are facing challenging requirements, as clinical science dictates increasingly sophisticated sets of properties and design parameters. Interaction with specific biological targets, biocompatibility, environmental responsiveness, modulated degradation, and formation of supramolecular assemblies are among the desired features that have to be integrated in next-generation biomedical polymers. Yet, most synthetic macromolecules used in the biomedical area have not been designed originally for these specific applications, and they lack the desired chemical flexibility. PPEs are phosphorus-containing polymers in which the PPE linkages from the backbone are repeated in the structural unit (Figure 4.1).

The pentavalent nature of the phosphorus atom allows the introduction of bioactive molecules, leading to the modification of the physical and chemical properties of the polymers. Depending on the nature of their side groups, PPEs can be categorized as polyphosphates, polyphosphonates, polyphosphites, or polyphosphoramidates. The biodegradable backbone of PPEs, their water solubility, and the possibility of attaching reactive pendant groups make these polymers promising materials for biomedical applications (Zhao et al. 2003, Huang and Zhuo 2008). The most common methods to synthesize PPEs are

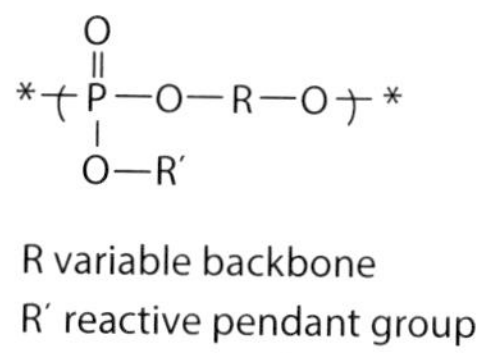

$$*\!-\!\!\left[\begin{matrix}O\\ \|\\ P\\ |\\ O-R'\end{matrix}\!-O-R-O\right]\!\!-*$$

R variable backbone
R′ reactive pendant group

FIGURE 4.1
General structure of PPEs.

polycondensation, ring opening polymerization, and postpolymerization modification. The oldest method for preparing PPEs is the polycondensation reaction between alkyl/aryl phosphoric dichloride and diols (Gefter 1962a,b, Troev 2012a,b). Through polycondensation of ethyl dichlorophosphate with a diol carrying a positive charge and a cholesterol moiety, Wen et al. (2004) synthesized amphiphilic cationic PPEs (poly{[(cholesteryl oxocarbonylamidoethyl) methyl bis(ethylene) ammonium iodide] ethyl phosphate}) for gene delivery applications. The most efficient route in the synthesis of the PPEs is considered to be the ring-opening polymerization (Zhao et al. 2003, Wang et al. 2012, Babu and Muralidharan 2014, Lapienis 2016, Penczek and Pretula 2016). For the first time, Penczek and Klosinski (1990) used the ring-opening polymerization of the five- or six-membered H-phosphonate with subsequent treatment to synthesize poly(alkylene phosphate).

PPEs have found potential applications in drug/gene delivery and cell-responsive tissue engineering. Leong and coauthors (Wen et al. 2003) tested the *in vivo* biocompatibility of poly(D,L-lactide–co-ethyl ethylene phosphate)s in mouse brain. The results showed that there are no significant differences in inflammatory reaction in the brain section between salin and injected poly(D,L-lactide–co-ethyl ethylene phosphate)s microspheres. Also, poly(D,L-lactide–co-ethyl ethylene phosphate)s were used in drug delivery studies by Leong and coauthors (Zhao et al. 2003). In this study, PACLIMER microspheres, containing 10% (W/W) paclitaxel in poly(D,L-lactide–co-ethyl ethylene phosphate)s, have been evaluated for a relevant animal model (OVCAR-3) and a phase I human trial for advanced ovarian cancer. The results confirmed the sustained release of hemotherapeutic agents, and the desired biodegradation kinetics and biocompatibility of PPE carriers.

A series of copolymers of poly(ethyl ethylene phosphate) synthesized by ring opening polymerization were investigated by Wang et al. (2009a) for drug delivery system applications. These copolymers were found to form nanosized vesicles in aqueous solution using a thin-film hydration method. Doxorubicin (DOX) was loaded into these nano-sized vesicles and showed the inhibition of cell proliferation. Also, DOX was loaded into the thermoresponsive triblock copolymer of poly(propylene oxide) and poly(ethyl ethylene phosphate) (Wang et al. 2009b). Wu et al. (2009) synthesized nanoparticles starting from a diacrylate version of triblock copolymers of poly(propylene oxide) and poly(ethyl ethylene phosphate), which were further cross-linked by reacting the diacrylates. The swollen gel was tested for drug delivery of DOX. A series of star-shaped polymers were investigated by Cuong et al. (2011) as potential DOX carriers. Du et al. (2011) synthesized a dual pH-sensitive PPE-based polymer-DOX conjugate nanoparticles.

Another application of PPEs, also of interest is hydrogel-based skin-wound dressing. Armes and coauthors (Madsen et al. 2008) synthesized a series of thermoresponsive ABA triblock copolymer gelators based on poly(2-(methacryloyloxy)ethyl phosphorylcholine) and poly(2-hydroxypropyl methacrylate) with possible application in wound dressing. They observed that these copolymer gels had no significant adverse effects when placed directly on tissue-engineered skin under conditions that mimic those found for the human skin. Iwasaki and coauthors (Wachiralarpphaithoon et al. 2007) have prepared a highly porous, biodegradable hydrogel starting from poly(2-methacryloyloxyethyl phosphorylcholine), which was cross-linked with PPEs using the gas forming technique. The cell viability of the hydrogel was investigated and no dead cells were observed after culturing for 96 h. The authors concluded that this new highly porous hydrogel might be useful for cell- and tissue-engineering applications. Wang and coauthors (Du et al. 2007) have synthesized biodegradable hydrogels based on PPEs and poly(ethyleneglycol) by UV photo-cross-linking with potential applications in tissue engineering.

In our group, phosphorus-modified poly(vinyl alcohol) was prepared from PVA and various phosphonic dichlorides by solution polycondensation at moderate temperature. The phosphorylated PVA was used to prepare new hydrogels. PVA/PPE–chondroitin sulphate (CS) hydrogels have been prepared by the epichlorohydrin-cross-linking of PVA/PPE with CS at different compositions. From SEM data, it was observed that the hydrogels displayed microporous structures, with the pores average diameters ranging from 60.3 to 6.2 μm, depending on the CS content (Figure 4.2).

The obtained hydrogels, which have the advantages of all the components (PVA, PPE, and CS), have been investigated as potential materials for drug delivery systems (Vlad-Bubulac et al. 2013a,b). The mixed PVA/PPE–CS hydrogels have been loaded with metoprolol tartrate, a drug widely used as

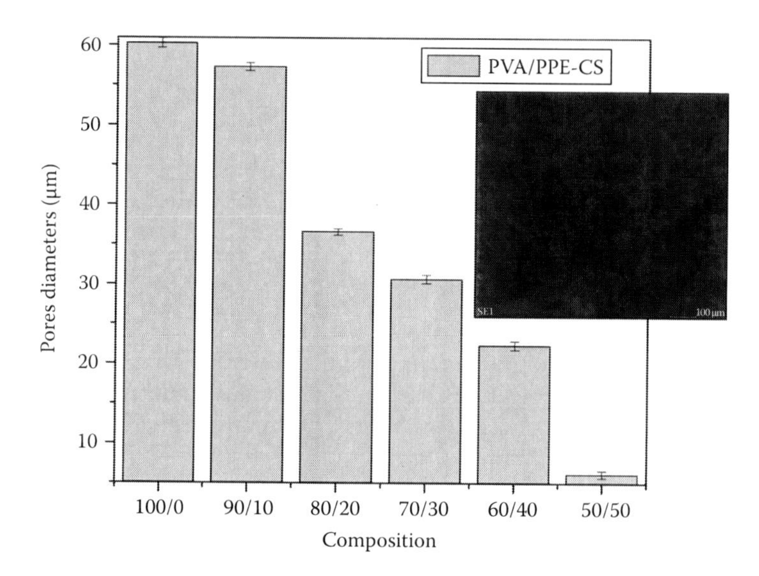

FIGURE 4.2
The average pores diameters measured from SEM versus composition of PVA/PPE-CS. (Data adapted from Vlad-Bubulac, T. et al., *Cent. Eur. J. Chem.*, 11(3), 446, 2013b.)

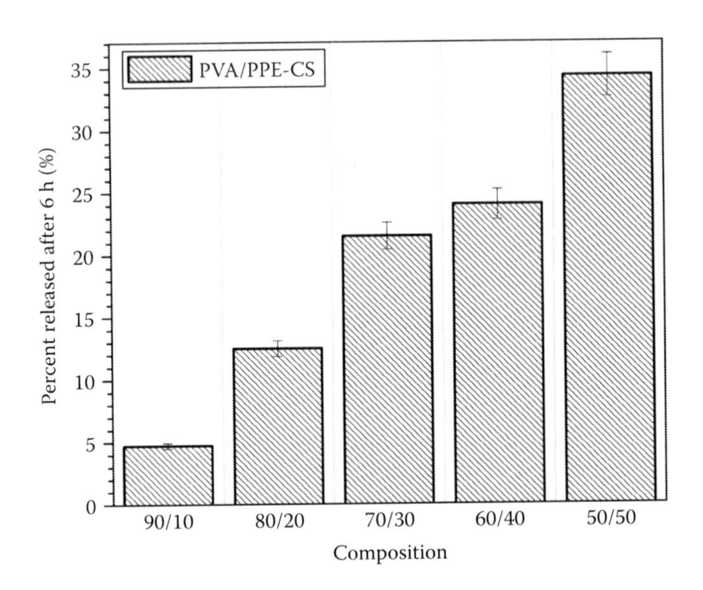

FIGURE 4.3
Cumulative metoprolol release obtained at the end of releasing period (6 h). (Data adapted from Vlad-Bubulac, T. et al., *Rev. Chim.* (*Bucharest*) 64(6), 663, 2013a.)

a choice in the management of hypertension, angina pectoris, and arrhythmias. Swelling and drug delivery studies were conducted in a phosphate buffer solution (pH 7.4) at 37°C. The release profiles of the drug from the hydrogels were strictly dependent on the CS content. From Figure 4.3, an increase in the percentage of released drug with the increasing CS content can be observed. The highest cumulative metoprolol release obtained at the end of releasing period (6 h) was 36% for 50/50 APV/PPE-CS composition.

Also, PPEs and polyphosphoramidates can be used as gene delivery vectors. Leong and coauthors (Wang et al. 2001a) synthesized poly(2-aminoethyl propylene phosphate), a new biodegradable gene carrier, starting from (4-methyl-2-oxo-2-chloro-1,3,2-dioxaphospholane), which was obtained by the ring-opening polymerization of 4-methyl-2-oxo-2-hydro-1,3,2-dioxaphospholane in the presence of triisobutylaluminum as an initiator, followed by chlorination of P–H. This polymer binds DNA effectively and presents the capability for controlled release of plasmids from this system. Poly(2-hydroxyethyl propylene phosphate) (Huang et al. 2004), a nonionic PPE, was synthesized by chlorination of poly(4-methyl-2-oxo-2-hydro-1,3,2-dioxaphospholane), followed by esterification with 2-benzyloxyethanol and deprotection of the hydroxyl group by catalytic hydrogenation in the presence of Pd–C. *In vitro* degradation and biocompatibility of this polymer, and the intramuscular transfection efficiency of naked DNA co-delivered with poly(2-hydroxyethyl propylene phosphate) was investigated. It shows minimal cytotoxicity and good tissue compatibility in the muscle and it was observed that the expression of luciferase in the mouse muscle after intramuscular injection is enhanced up to fourfold by poly(2-hydroxyethyl propylene phosphate) at 0.01%–0.5% concentration in saline, compared with that of naked DNA in saline at the same dose. Leong and coauthors (Wang et al. 2002) synthesized a novel polyphosphoramid with a spermidine residue in the side chain. In this paper, the authors investigated the polymer–DNA complexation and protection ability and cytotoxicity and the parameters that affect DNA transfection efficiencies. This gene carrier offered significant protection to DNA against nuclease degradation, and showed lower cytotoxicity than polyethylenimine in the cell culture. Also, PPEs are attractive candidates in the development of degradable and biocompatible polymers for fabrication of nerve guide conduits (Wan et al. 2001, Wang et al. 2001b). In this respect, poly(bis(hydroxyethyl)terephthalate-ethyl ortho-phosphate/terephthaloylchloride) was investigated as a nerve guide conduit material. The nerve guide conduits obtained show nontoxicity *in vitro* and low inflammatory response after *in vivo* implantation and promote the axonal regeneration. However, these reports appear in isolation and current efforts in the field do not appear to have followed the PPE pathway.

Ishihara and coauthors synthesized a biocompatible polymer with good mechanical properties and feasibility for use in an implantable artificial pancreas (Uchiyama et al. 2002). Also, the biocompatibility of poly(2-methacryloyloxyethyl phosphorylcholine-co-*n*-butyl methacrylate) was investigated by Nowak and coauthors in an *in vivo* rat model (Nowak et al. 2000). Poly(2-methacryloyloxyethyl phosphorylcholine) has been investigated as a biocompatible membrane/coating for the sensor by several groups (Medeiros et al. 2011, Madsen et al. 2013). A pH-sensitive molecularly imprinted nanosphere/hydrogel composite coating, with the hydrogel including a 2-methacryloyloxyethyl phosphorylcholine moiety, has been reported by Wang et al. (2010). Wang et al. (2010) investigated a nanosphere/hydrogel composite poly(2-hydroxyethyl methacrylate-*N*-vinyl-2-pyrrolidinone-2-methacryloyloxyethyl phosphorylcholine) as a coating for implantable glucose biosensors, and they concluded that this new nanosphere/hydrogel composite system can potentially prolong the lifetime of the sensor in vivo.

4.3 Biomedical Applications of Electrospun Polyimide Nanofibers

Aromatic PIs represent one of the well-known classes of polymers that have found extensive applications as fibers, films, coatings, photoresists, and composites due to their properties, such as high thermal stability, chemical resistance, excellent electrical and mechanical properties (Liaw et al. 2012). Additionally, PIs have been used in a various range of applications, including liquid crystal alignments (He et al. 2007), gas separation membranes (White et al. 1995, Sanders et al. 2013), composites (Chen et al. 2015), Langmuir–Blodgett film (Nishikata et al. 1992), electroluminescent devices (Choi et al. 2008), electrochromic materials (Hsiao et al. 2016), polymer electrolytes (Liaw et al. 2012), fuel cells, polymer memory materials (Zhao et al. 2016), fiber optics, blending applications (Tsai et al. 2016), etc. Also, these polymers are used as substrates and insulation layers in flexible microfabricated nerve electrodes (Song et al. 2013).

The electrospinning technique is considered to be a cheap, straightforward method for producing membranes with a very large surface-to-volume ratio that can be used as optical sensors (Urrutia et al. 2013, Camposeo et al. 2015), tissue-engineering scaffolds (Lannutti et al. 2007, Liu et al. 2013, Hasan et al. 2014), as well as barriers for protective clothing (Lee and Obendorf 2007, Raza et al. 2014).

PIs are insoluble and infusible in common organic solvents, leading to the difficulty of being electrospun directly from solution. In the literature are found sporadic reports about the preparation of PI nanofibers and application of electrospun PI nanofibers (Nah et al. 2003, Yang et al. 2003, 2011, Huang et al. 2006a,b, Shuiliang et al. 2008, Chen et al. 2009, Cheng et al. 2010, Chisca et al. 2013, Ding et al. 2013, 2016, Butnaru et al. 2015, Magdalena et al. 2015, Serbezeanu et al. 2015a,b, 2016).

So far, there is a lack of scientific papers investigating the biomedical applications of electrospun PI nanofibers. In this respect, we investigated the successful processing of these solutions into composite nanofibers from gold nanoparticles in a 4,4′-oxydiphthalic anhydride/4,4′-diamino-4″-hydroxy triphenylmethane-based PI matrix having biological activity. Previously, we reported the synthesis and the preparation of PI fibers incorporating gold salt using the electrospinning technique which could be used as catalysts (Magdalena et al. 2015).

In this chapter, we present the biological activity of the electrospun gold–PI nanofibers. In this respect, preosteoblast cell line MC3T3-E1, subclone 4 cells (passage 21) were thawed and multiplied in cell culture flasks with a surface area of 75 cm^2, in α-minimum essential medium (MEM) culture medium, without ascorbic acid, supplemented with 10% fetal bovine serum (BFS) and 1% antibiotic medium. The initial cell density was 2000 cells/cm^2 of culture surface area.

The membranes (PI–Au) were cropped into small pieces of 5 × 5 mm, decontaminated by immersion in a sterile solution of ethylic alcohol 70% for 20 min, and then washed three times in sterile phosphate-buffered saline. The prepared materials were prebalanced in complete culture medium at 37°C for 24 h.

MTT assays were performed by the direct contact method on the samples prebalanced in complete culture medium, at 37°C for 24 h. The MTT test was run in 24-well culture plates populated with the preosteoblast cell line MC3T3-E1, subclone 4 cells. The initial cell density was 104 cells/well, in

0.5 mL of α-MEM culture medium. The contact of the materials with the cells has been carried out when a semi-confluent monolayer of cells was achieved (48 h after culture initiation). Every individual 5 × 5 mm sample of the material was introduced into the well, upon cell culture. The direct contact of the material with the cells was maintained for a period of 72 h, at 37°C, 95% humidity, and 5% CO_2. Each sample was tested in triplicate. All experimentally obtained results were compared with those obtained in control cultures, in the absence of the testing material. The MTT 3-(4,5-dimethylthiazol-2-yl)-2,5-diphenyltetrazolium bromide test was performed according to the techniques described in the literature. The principle of the method consists in the reduction of MTT, a yellow tetrazolium dye, to its insoluble derivative—formazan, a purple compound, under the activity of mitochondrial dehydrogenase in living cells. To complete the MTT test, the culture medium and the treated fragment of material from each well have been removed; then, to the remaining cells, the MTT solution in α-MEM was added without BFS. After 3 h of incubation, the absorbance of formazan solution was measured using a Tecan Plate Reader spectrophotometer, at the wavelength of 570 nm. Absorbance values of formazan from wells containing experimental samples were related to those obtained from control wells and, thus, percentage viability of cells was calculated for culture incubated with the tested material. The MTT test results revealed the better biocompatibility of the gold-coated sample, in comparison with the blank sample (without gold). After 72 h of cell incubation, the cell viability was more than 80% in the presence of PI–Au sample, and only 60% (cytotoxicity) in the case of the contact with the sample without gold (Figure 4.4).

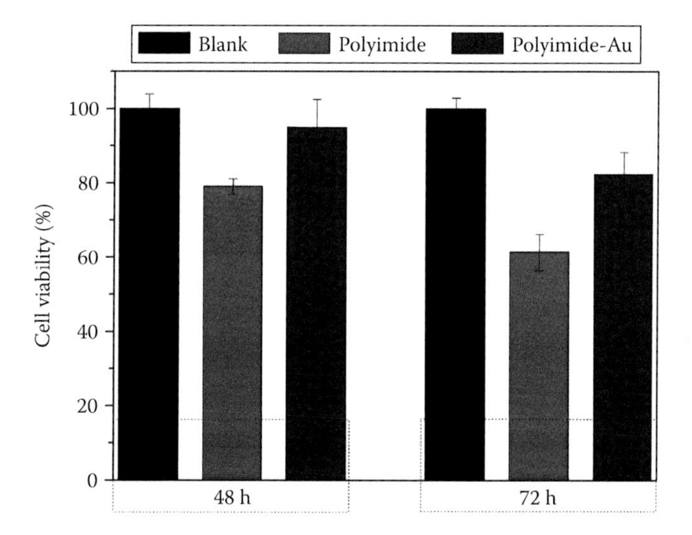

FIGURE 4.4
Effect of polyimide and polyimide-Au on fibroblast viability using the MTT assay.

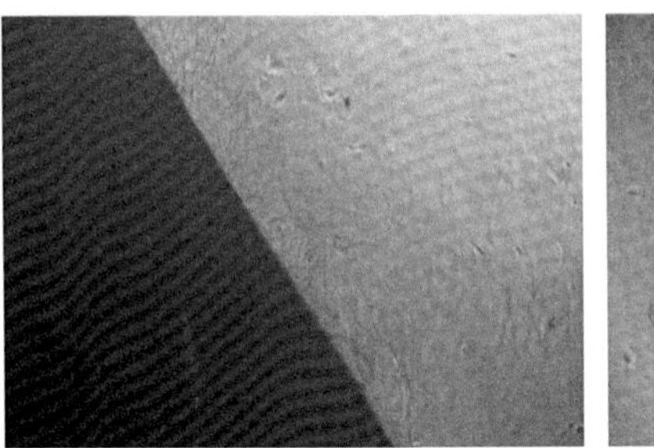 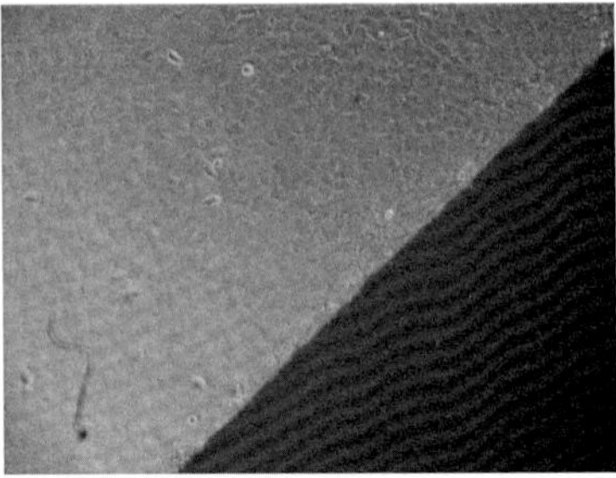

FIGURE 4.5
Photomicrographs of viability of MC3T3-E1 cells in polyimide and polyimide-Au nanofibers after culture of 72 h.

Cytocompatibility of PI–Au sample was demonstrated by microscopy, the photomicrographs revealing the formation of dense agglomeration in proximity of the direct contact between the cell and the material (Figure 4.5).

4.4 Conclusions

This study focused specifically on the recent efforts in the development of the biomedical applications of PPEs (polyphosphonates, polyphosphites, and polyphosphoramidates) and PI electrospun nanofibers. The PPE structure enables a variety of architectures with tunable properties leading to their use in various fields of biomedicine. Another task of this chapter was to investigate the biomedical applications of electrospun PI nanofibers. In this respect, we investigated the biocompatibility of the synthesis of gold nanoparticles in a 4,4′-oxydiphthalic anhydride/4,4′-diamino-4″-hydroxy triphenylmethane-based PI matrix. For the first time, electrospun PI–Au nanocomposites were investigated in terms of biological activity. Finally, in view of their potential biomedical applications, the cytotoxicity of the prepared nanocomposites was evaluated using the preosteoblast cell line MC3T3-E1, subclone 4 cells. These nanocomposites can be used as antimicrobial coatings in the biomedical field.

Acknowledgments

The authors acknowledge the financial support of CNCSIS–UEFISCSU, Project Number PN-II-RU-TE-0123 nr. 28/29.04.2013, and of the European Regional Development Fund, Project POINGBIO, ID P_40_443, Contract no. 86/8.09.2016.

References

Aflori M., Serbezeanu D., Carja I.-D., and Fortunato G. Gold nanoparticles incorporated into electrospun polyimide fibers. *Chem. Lett.* 44(10) (2015): 1440–1442.

Babu H. V. and Muralidharan K. Polyethers with phosphate pendant groups by monomer activated anionic ring opening polymerization: Syntheses, characterization and their lithium-ion conductivities. *Polymer* 55(1) (2014): 83–94.

Butnaru I., Serbezeanu D., Bruma M., Sava I., Gaan S., and Fortunato G. Physical and thermal properties of poly(ethylene terephthalate) fabric coated with electrospun polyimide fibers. *High Perform. Polym.* 27(5) (2015): 616–624.

Camposeo A., Moffa M., and Persano L. (2015) Electrospun fluorescent nanofibers and their application in optical sensing. In: Macagnano A., Zampetti E., and Kny E. (Eds.). *Electrospinning for High Performance Sensors*, Springer International Publishing, Cham, Switzerland, pp. 129–155.

Canadell J., Hunt B. J., Cook A. G., Mantecón A., and Cádiz V. Flame retardance and shrinkage reduction of polystyrene modified with acrylate-containing phosphorus and crosslinkable spiro-orthoester moieties. *Polym. Degrad. Stabil.* 92(8) (2007): 1482–1490.

Carja I.-D., Serbezeanu D., Vlad-Bubulac T. et al. A straightforward, eco-friendly and cost-effective approach towards flame retardant epoxy resins. *J. Mater. Chem. A* 2(38) (2014): 16230–16241.

Chen D., Liu T., Zhou X., Tjiu W. C., and Hou H. Electrospinning fabrication of high strength and toughness polyimide nanofiber membranes containing multiwalled carbon nanotubes. *J. Phys. Chem. B* 113(29) (2009): 9741–9748.

Chen Y., Gao X., Wang J. et al. Properties and application of polyimide-based composites by blending surface functionalized boron nitride nanoplates. *J. Appl. Polym. Sci.* 132(16) (2015): n/a–n/a.

Cheng C., Chen J., Chen F. et al. High-strength and high-toughness polyimide nanofibers: Synthesis and characterization. *J. Appl. Polym. Sci.* 116(3) (2010): 1581–1586.

Chisca S., Musteata V. E., Stoica I., Sava I., and Bruma M. Effect of the chemical structure of aromatic-cycloaliphatic copolyimide films on their surface morphology, relaxation behavior and dielectric properties. *J. Polym. Res.* 20(3) (2013): 1–11.

Choi M.-C., Kim Y., and Ha C.-S. Polymers for flexible displays: From material selection to device applications. *Prog. Polym. Sci.* 33(6) (2008): 581–630.

Clearfield A. Coordination chemistry of phosphonic acids with special relevance to rare earths. *J. Alloys Compd.* 418(1–2) (2006): 128–138.

Cuong N.-V., Hsieh M.-F., Chen Y.-T., and Liau I. Doxorubicin-loaded nanosized micelles of a star-shaped poly(ε-caprolactone)-polyphosphoester block copolymer for treatment of human breast cancer. *J. Biomater. Sci. Polym. Ed.* 22(11) (2011): 1409–1426.

Ding Y., Hou H., Zhao Y., Zhu Z., and Fong H. Electrospun polyimide nanofibers and their applications. *Prog. Polym. Sci.* 61 (2016): 67–103.

Ding Y., Wu Q., Zhao D., Ye W., Hanif M., and Hou H. Flexible PI/$BaTiO_3$ dielectric nanocomposite fabricated by combining electrospinning and electrospraying. *Eur. Polym. J.* 49(9) (2013): 2567–2571.

Du J.-Z., Du X.-J., Mao C.-Q., and Wang J. Tailor-made dual pH-sensitive polymer–doxorubicin nanoparticles for efficient anticancer drug delivery. *J. Am. Chem. Soc.* 133(44) (2011): 17560–17563.

Du J.-Z., Sun T.-M., Weng S.-Q., Chen X.-S., and Wang J. Synthesis and characterization of photo-cross-linked hydrogels based on biodegradable polyphosphoesters and poly(ethylene glycol) copolymers. *Biomacromolecules* 8(11) (2007): 3375–3381.

Francis M. D., Graham R., Russell G., and Fleisch H. Diphosphonates inhibit formation of calcium phosphate crystals in vitro and pathological calcification in vivo. *Science* 165(3899) (1969): 1264–1266.

Gefter Y. L. (1962a) Chapter II—Saturated organophosphorus compounds dihydroxylcompounds. In: Gefter Y. L. (Ed.). *Organophosphorus Monomers and Polymers*, Pergamon Press, Oxford, U.K., pp. 93–140.

Gefter Y. L. (1962b) Chapter V—Heterochain high molecular weight compounds containing phosphorus in main chain. In: Gefter Y. L. (Ed.). *Organophosphorus Monomers and Polymers*, Pergamon Press, Oxford, U.K., pp. 213–253.

Hamciuc C., Vlad-Bubulac T., Serbezeanu D. et al. Environmentally friendly fire-resistant epoxy resins based on a new oligophosphonate with high flame retardant efficiency. *RSC Adv.* 6(27) (2016): 22764–22776.

Hasan A., Memic A., Annabi N. et al. Electrospun scaffolds for tissue engineering of vascular grafts. *Acta Biomater.* 10(1) (2014): 11–25.

He Y., Liu B., Ren H., and Wang X. Polyimide liquid crystal alignment layers prepared by soft-lithography. *Front. Chem. China* 2(3) (2007): 318–321.

Hsiao S.-H., Hsiao Y.-H., and Kung Y.-R. Synthesis and characterization of new redox-active and electrochromic polyimides with (4-morpholinyl)triphenylamine units. *J. Electroanal. Chem.* 764 (2016): 31–37.

Huang C., Chen S., Reneker D. H., Lai C., and Hou H. High-strength mats from electrospun poly(p-phenylene biphenyltetracarboximide) nanofibers. *Adv. Mater.* 18(5) (2006a): 668–671.

Huang C., Wang S., Zhang H. et al. High strength electrospun polymer nanofibers made from BPDA–PDA polyimide. *Eur. Polym. J.* 42(5) (2006b): 1099–1104.

Huang S.-W., Wang J., Zhang P.-C., Mao H.-Q., Zhuo R.-X., and Leong K. W. Water-soluble and nonionic polyphosphoester: Synthesis, degradation, biocompatibility and enhancement of gene expression in mouse muscle. *Biomacromolecules* 5(2) (2004): 306–311.

Huang S.-W. and Zhuo R.-X. Recent advances in polyphosphoester and polyphosphoramidate-based biomaterials. *Phosphorus Sulfur Silicon Relat. Elem.* 183(2–3) (2008): 340–348.

Langer R. and Tirrell D. A. Designing materials for biology and medicine. *Nature* 428(6982) (2004): 487–492.

Lannutti J., Reneker D., Ma T., Tomasko D., and Farson D. Electrospinning for tissue engineering scaffolds. *Mater. Sci. Eng. C* 27(3) (2007): 504–509.

Lapienis G. (2012). Ring-opening polymerization of cyclic phosphorus monomers. In: Matyjaszewski K. and Moller M. (Eds.). *Polymer Science: A Comprehensive Reference*, Vol. 4, Elsevier, Amsterdam, the Netherlands, pp. 477–505.

Lee S. and Obendorf S. K. Use of electrospun nanofiber web for protective textile materials as barriers to liquid penetration. *Text. Res. J.* 77(9) (2007): 696–702.

Liaw D.-J., Wang K.-L., Huang Y.-C., Lee K.-R., Lai J.-Y., and Ha C.-S. Advanced polyimide materials: Syntheses, physical properties and applications. *Prog. Polym. Sci.* 37(7) (2012): 907–974.

Liu H., Ding X., Zhou G., Li P., Wei X., and Fan Y. Electrospinning of nanofibers for tissue engineering applications. *J. Nanomater.* 2013 (2013): 11.

Madsen J., Armes S. P., Bertal K., Lomas H., MacNeil S., and Lewis A. L. Biocompatible wound dressings based on chemically degradable triblock copolymer hydrogels. *Biomacromolecules* 9(8) (2008): 2265–2275.

Madsen J., Canton I., Warren N. J. et al. Nile blue-based nanosized pH sensors for simultaneous far-red and near-infrared live bioimaging. *J. Am. Chem. Soc.* 135(39) (2013): 14863–14870.

Medeiros S. F., Santos A. M., Fessi H., and Elaissari A. Stimuli-responsive magnetic particles for biomedical applications. *Int. J. Pharm.* 403(1–2) (2011): 139–161.

Nah C., Han S. H., Lee M.-H., Kim J. S., and Lee D. S. Characteristics of polyimide ultrafine fibers prepared through electrospinning. *Polym. Int.* 52(3) (2003): 429–432.

Nishikata Y., Fukui S.-I., Kakimoto M.-A., Imai Y., Nishiyama K., and Fujihira M. Preparation of polyimide Langmuir-Blodgett films possessing a triphenylamine unit and their application to photodiodes. *Thin Solid Films* 210 (1992): 296–298.

Nowak T., Nishida K., Shimoda S. et al. Biocompatibility of MPC: In vivo evaluation for clinical application. *J. Artif. Organs* 3(1) (2000): 39–46.

Penczek S. and Klosinski P. (1990) *Models of Biopolymers by Ring-Opening Polymerization*, CRC Press, Boca Raton, FL.

Penczek S. and Pretula J. B. (2016) Ring-opening polymerization. In: Reedijk J. et al. (Eds.). *Reference Module in Chemistry, Molecular Sciences and Chemical Engineering*, Elsevier, Oxford, U.K. ISBN 9780124095472. https://doi.org/10.1016/B978-0-12-409547-2.11351-4.

Petreus O., Avram E., and Serbezeanu D. Synthesis and characterization of phosphorus-containing polysulfone. *Polym. Eng. Sci.* 50(1) (2010): 48–56.

Raza A., Li Y., Sheng J., Yu J., and Ding B. (2014) Protective clothing based on electrospun nanofibrous membranes. In: Ding B. and Yu J. (Eds.). *Electrospun Nanofibers for Energy and Environmental Applications*, Springer, Berlin, Germany, pp. 355–369.

Sanders D. F., Smith Z. P., Guo R. et al. Energy-efficient polymeric gas separation membranes for a sustainable future: A review. *Polymer* 54(18) (2013): 4729–4761.

Serbezeanu D., Butnaru I., Varganici C.-D., Bruma M., Fortunato G., and Gaan S. Phosphorus-containing polyimide fibers and their thermal properties. *RSC Adv.* 6(44) (2016): 38371–38379.

Serbezeanu D., Popa A. M., Sava I. et al. Design and synthesis of polyimide—Gold nanofibers with tunable optical properties. *Eur. Polym. J.* 64(0) (2015a): 10–20.

Serbezeanu D., Popa A. M., Stelzig T., Sava I., Rossi R. M., and Fortunato G. Preparation and characterization of thermally stable polyimide membranes by electrospinning for protective clothing applications. *Text. Res. J.* 85(17) (2015b): 1763–1775.

Shuiliang C., Ping H., Andreas G. et al. Electrospun nanofiber belts made from high performance copolyimide. *Nanotechnology* 19(1) (2008): 015604.

Singh H. and Jain A. K. Ignition, combustion, toxicity, and fire retardancy of polyurethane foams: A comprehensive review. *J. Appl. Polym. Sci.* 111(2) (2009): 1115–1143.

Song Y.-A., Ibrahim A. M. S., Rabie A. N., Han J., and Lin S. J. Microfabricated nerve–electrode interfaces in neural prosthetics and neural engineering. *Biotechnol. Genet. Eng. Rev.* 29(2) (2013): 113–134.

Troev K. D. (2012a) 1—Poly(alkylene H-phosphonate)s. In: Troev K. D. (Ed.) *Polyphosphoesters: Chemistry and Application*, Elsevier, Oxford, U.K., pp. 1–127.

Troev K. D. (2012b) 3—Poly[alkylene(arylene) alkyl or arylphosphonate]s. In: Troev K. D. (Ed.) *Polyphosphoesters: Chemistry and Application*, Elsevier, Oxford, U.K., pp. 263–320.

Tsai C.-L., Yen H.-J., and Liou G.-S. Highly transparent polyimide hybrids for optoelectronic applications. *React. Funct. Polym.* 108 (2016): 2–30.

Uchiyama T., Watanabe J., and Ishihara K. Biocompatible polymer alloy membrane for implantable artificial pancreas. *J. Membr. Sci.* 208(1–2) (2002): 39–48.

Urrutia A., Goicoechea J., Rivero P. J., Matías I. R., and Arregui F. J. Electrospun nanofiber mats for evanescent optical fiber sensors. *Sens. Actuators B Chem.* 176 (2013): 569–576.

Vlad-Bubulac T., Oprea A.-M., Serbezeanu D., Carja I.-D., and Hamciuc C. In vitro release of metoprolol tartrate from poly(vinyl alcohol)/phosphoester—Chondroitin sulfate Semi-IPNs. *Rev. Chim. (Bucharest)* 64(6) (2013a): 663–666.

Vlad-Bubulac T., Serbezeanu D., Oprea A.-M., Carja I.-D., Hamciuc C., and Cazacu M. Preparation and characterization of new hydrogels based on poly(vinyl alcohol)/phosphoester—Chondroitin sulphate. *Cent. Eur. J. Chem.* 11(3) (2013b): 446–456.

Wachiralarpphaithoon C., Iwasaki Y., and Akiyoshi K. Enzyme-degradable phosphorylcholine porous hydrogels cross-linked with polyphosphoesters for cell matrices. *Biomaterials* 28(6) (2007): 984–993.

Wan A. C. A., Mao H.-Q., Wang S., Leong K. W., Ong L. K. L. L., and Yu H. Fabrication of poly(phosphoester) nerve guides by immersion precipitation and the control of porosity. *Biomaterials* 22(10) (2001): 1147–1156.

Wang C., Javadi A., Ghaffari M., and Gong S. A pH-sensitive molecularly imprinted nanospheres/hydrogel composite as a coating for implantable biosensors. *Biomaterials* 31(18) (2010): 4944–4951.

Wang F., Wang Y.-C., Yan L.-F., and Wang J. Biodegradable vesicular nanocarriers based on poly(ε-caprolactone)-block-poly(ethyl ethylene phosphate) for drug delivery. *Polymer* 50(21) (2009a): 5048–5054.

Wang J., Mao H.-Q., and Leong K. W. A Novel Biodegradable gene carrier based on polyphosphoester. *J. Am. Chem. Soc.* 123(38) (2001a): 9480–9481.

Wang J., Yuan Y. Y., and Du J. Z. (2012) 4.29—Polyphosphoesters: Controlled ring-opening polymerization and biological applications. In: Matyjaszewski K. and Möller M. (Eds.). *Polymer Science: A Comprehensive Reference*, Elsevier, Amsterdam, the Netherlands, pp. 719–747.

Wang J., Zhang P.-C., Lu H.-F. et al. New polyphosphoramidate with a spermidine side chain as a gene carrier. *J. Control. Release* 83(1) (2002): 157–168.

Wang S., Wan A. C. A., Xu X. et al. A new nerve guide conduit material composed of a biodegradable poly(phosphoester). *Biomaterials* 22(10) (2001b): 1157–1169.

Wang Y.-C., Xia H., Yang X.-Z., and Wang J. Synthesis and thermoresponsive behaviors of biodegradable Pluronic analogs. *J. Polym. Sci. Part A Polym. Chem.* 47(22) (2009b): 6168–6179.

Wen J., Kim G. J. A., and Leong K. W. Poly(D,L-lactide-co-ethyl ethylene phosphate)s as new drug carriers. *J. Control. Release* 92(1–2) (2003): 39–48.

Wen J., Mao H.-Q., Li W., Lin K. Y., and Leong K. W. Biodegradable polyphosphoester micelles for gene delivery. *J. Pharm. Sci.* 93(8) (2004): 2142–2157.

White L. S., Blinka T. A., Kloczewski H. A., and Wang I. F. Properties of a polyimide gas separation membrane in natural gas streams. *J. Membr. Sci.* 103(1) (1995): 73–82.

Wu J., Liu X.-Q., Wang Y.-C., and Wang J. Template-free synthesis of biodegradable nanogels with tunable sizes as potential carriers for drug delivery. *J. Mater. Chem.* 19(42) (2009): 7856–7863.

Yang K. S., Edie D. D., Lim D. Y., Kim Y. M., and Choi Y. O. Preparation of carbon fiber web from electrostatic spinning of PMDA-ODA poly(amic acid) solution. *Carbon* 41(11) (2003): 2039–2046.

Yang Y., Li X., Cheng L. et al. Core–sheath structured fibers with pDNA polyplex loadings for the optimal release profile and transfection efficiency as potential tissue engineering scaffolds. *Acta Biomater.* 7(6) (2011): 2533–2543.

Zhao J., Peng L., Zhu Y.-L., Song Y.-J., Wang L.-J., and Shen Y.-Z. Synthesis and memory characteristics of novel soluble polyimides based on asymmetrical diamines containing carbazole. *Polymer* 91 (2016): 118–127.

Zhao Z., Wang J., Mao H.-Q., and Leong K. W. Polyphosphoesters in drug and gene delivery. *Adv. Drug Deliv. Rev.* 55(4) (2003): 483–499.

5

Key Considerations in the Design of Polymeric Micro- and Nanoparticles for Drug Delivery Systems

Marieta Constantin and Gheorghe Fundueanu

CONTENTS

5.1 Introduction

The administration of drugs using controlled delivery formulations has represented a great triumph in terms of efficiency of medical treatments.

These remarkable achievements are the result of intense and interdisciplinary efforts involving contributions from chemistry, pharmacology, engineering, and other related sciences. Controlled delivery formulations are usually polymeric supports in which drugs are chemically (covalently or ionically) linked or physically entrapped and are released in a controlled manner over a predetermined period of time. When the polymeric support takes the form of micro- and nanoparticles, the advantages are considerable. Thus, these particulate systems can transport the drug to the desired place and maintain its concentration in the required therapeutic domain. Moreover, the release rate can be controlled by varying the surface/size/weight ratio. The flexibility of the route of administration is another major advantage. Basically, these particles can be administered via any route of access into the organism: oral, inhalation, topical, intra-arterial, and intravenous. In addition, the use of the bioadhesive properties of microparticulate systems gives them the possibility of other routes of administration: ocular, nasal, anal, vaginal, etc.

Micro- and nanoparticles can be synthesized both from synthetic and natural polymers by a large number of methods: emulsion or suspension polymerization, precipitative polymerization, solvent evaporation from simple or double emulsion, suspension cross-linking, coacervation, etc. Despite a large number of advantages of synthetic polymers, natural polymers are preferred because they are biodegradable and the degradation products are nontoxic. Polysaccharides are a class of natural polymers widely used in the production of micro- and nanoparticles since they are the most abundant materials in nature. These polymers are highly stable, biocompatible, biodegradable, and enzymatic, and hydrolytic degradation products (sugars) are nontoxic and easily metabolized in the organism. In their natural state, many polysaccharides contain pH-sensitive functional units such as carboxyl and amino groups. Other polysaccharides that do not contain natively sensitive groups could be chemically modified, thus resulting in either pH- and/or thermosensitive polymers. These polymers are usually called "intelligent" because the solubilization or the swelling of the polymer network is triggered by small changes of physiological parameters (pH/temperature), thus resulting in a controlled delivery of drugs.

Therefore, this chapter will mainly focus on the synthesis, characterization, and biomedical applications of micro- and nanoparticles based on pH- and temperature-sensitive polysaccharides.

5.2 pH-Sensitive Polysaccharides

pH-sensitive polysaccharides contain weakly acidic (carboxyl) or weakly basic (amino) functional groups. The most representative native polysaccharides possessing pH-sensitive properties are alginic acid, pectin, hyaluronic acid (HA) (carboxylic groups), and chitosan (amino groups). Remarkably, polysaccharides that do not contain these groups can become pH sensitive since they are characterized by the presence of abundant hydroxylic groups that can be chemically modified. The solubility of these linear polymers is deeply influenced by the pH of the aqueous media. For example, alginic acid is not soluble below its pK_a, since the acidic groups will be protonated and hence unionized, but quickly solubilizes above it. In contrast, chitosan is soluble below its pK_a, since the ionization of the amino groups will increase at low pH, and precipitates above pK_a. Correspondingly, the hydrogels obtained from alginic acid will be relatively unswollen at low pH. With increasing pH, the hydrogel will swell to a greater degree. The opposite holds for hydrogels obtained from chitosan (Figure 5.1).

5.2.1 Native pH-Sensitive Polysaccharides

5.2.1.1 Alginic Acid

Alginic acid is a pH-sensitive, naturally occurring polymer usually obtained from brown algae. From the chemical point of view, it can be defined as a linear block copolymer composed of sequences with consecutive β-1,4-D-mannuronic acid residues (M-blocks), α-L-guluronic acid residues (G-blocks), and alternating M and G residues (MG-blocks) (Draget et al. 1994). Because of its biocompatibility, low toxicity, and mucoadhesiveness, alginate is also an attractive polymer for biomedical applications (Yoshioka et al. 2003). The pK_a of guluronic acid and mannuronic acid in 0.1 M NaCl are known to be 3.65 and 3.38, respectively. This polymer will be insoluble or in the collapsed state in the stomach (pH = 1.2) while in the intestine (pH = 7.4) it will be either in the soluble or the swollen state. Based on these characteristics, alginic acid was frequently used as a platform for controlled delivery to the small and large intestines.

For example, Işıklan et al. (2011) developed pH-sensitive polymers based on graft copolymers of sodium alginate (NaAlg) with itaconic acid (IA) using cerium ammonium nitrate. These polymers were further crosslinked with glutaraldehyde and transformed into microspheres. The results showed that NaAlg-*g*-IA microspheres are pH responsive; the release of nifedipine from grafted microspheres was slower in simulated gastric

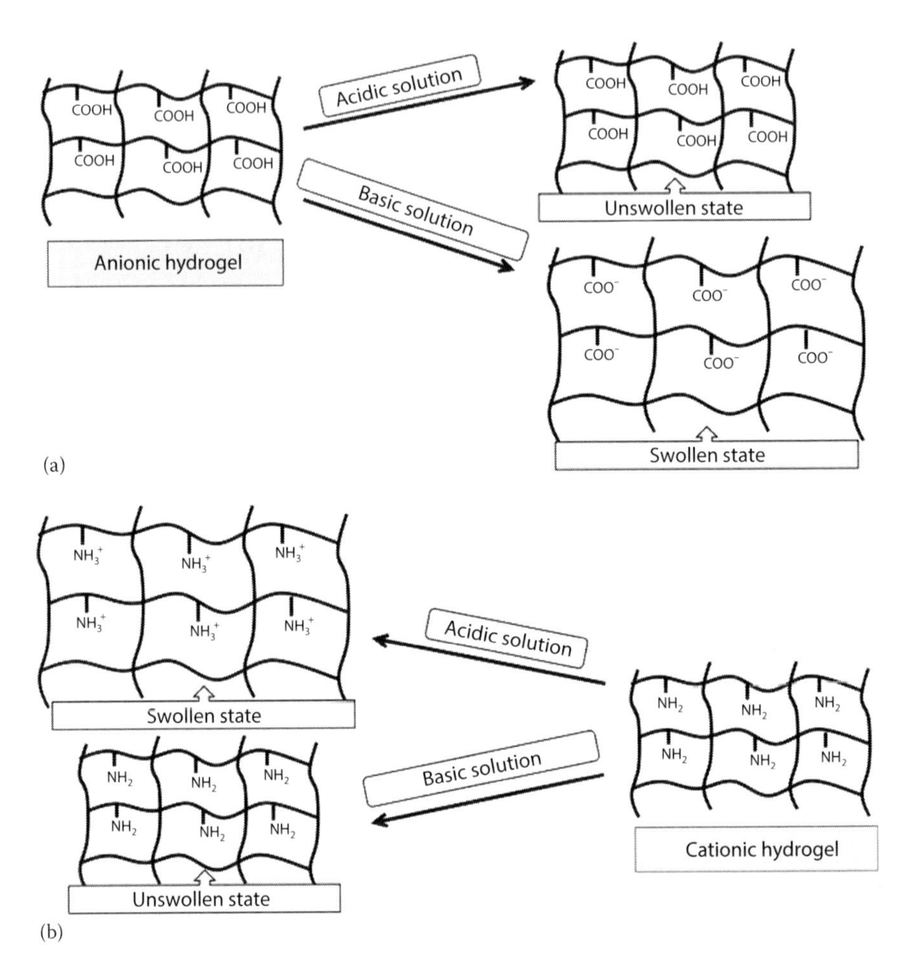

FIGURE 5.1
Swelling behavior of anionic (alginic acid) (a) and cationic (chitosan) hydrogel (b).

fluids (pH = 1.2) than in simulated intestinal fluids (buffer solution at pH 7.4). In another study, Agarwal et al. (2015) described the preparation, characterization, and application of calcium alginate–carboxymethyl cellulose beads for colon-specific oral drug delivery. The microspheres were prepared by ionic gelation method, and the physicochemical characterization was done by SEM, XRD, EDAX, and DSC. The authors exploited the influence of pH on swelling, mucoadhesivity, and colonic microflora-catered biodegradability of the formulations for colon-specific drug delivery. It was demonstrated that the swelling and mucoadhesivity of the microspheres was higher in the simulated colonic environment. The release studies of anticancer drug 5-fluorouracil were performed in simulated intestinal fluids in the presence of colonic enzymes. It was shown that the presence of enzymes significantly increased (>90%) the amount of released drug. Mukhopadhyay et al. (2015) prepared alginate nanoparticles by ionotropic gelation under mild conditions for the entrapment and controlled release of insulin. Then, the nanoparticles were complexed with oppositely charged chitosan to improve insulin stability and to control the moment and rate of drug release. The nanoparticles displayed an almost spherical shape with an average particle size of 100–200 nm determined by light scattering (DLS) and an insulin encapsulation of 85%. The pH sensitivity of the nanoparticles was confirmed since almost the entire amount of insulin was retained in the simulated gastric fluid followed by its sustained release in the simulated intestinal fluid.

Besides medicine, alginic acid microspheres were frequently used for different biotechnological applications. For example, alginate beads were used to enhance the quality and safety of the wine (Bleve et al. 2016; de Andrade Neves et al. 2014). Bleve et al. (2016) carried out the simultaneous immobilization of *Saccharomyces cerevisiae* and *Oenococcus oeni* in alginate beads and used them in microvinification tests to produce Negroamaro wine. Coimmobilization of *S. cerevisiae* and *O. oeni* increases the efficiency of the process, resulting in low volatile acidity levels and ethanol and glycerol concentrations comparable with those obtained by yeast and bacteria cells in the free form. Moreover, the coimmobilization process showed a substantial decrease of the time requested for complete alcoholic and malolactic fermentation. The alginate beads can be considered as small reactors where the immobilized cells could be efficiently reused for the wine fermentation at least three times without any apparent loss of cell metabolic activities.

5.2.1.2 Hyaluronic Acid

HA is a nonsulfated member of glycosaminoglycan family. It is a naturally occurring linear polysaccharide consisting of alternating units of β-1,4-D-glucuronic acid and β-1,3-*N*-acetyl-D-glucosamine. It is degraded in vivo by omnipresent enzymes such as hyaluronidase, the concentration of which is amplified at the tumor site (Choi et al. 2011). HA has a pK_a value of about 3.0. Therefore, below the pK_a, the carboxylic groups are in the protonated state and the polysaccharide gel is collapsed. Above the pK_a, the carboxylic groups are ionized and more hydrophilic, and the hydrogel will be in the swollen state. In recent years, HA has been extensively investigated for use in tumor-targeted delivery because of its ability to specifically bind to various cancer cells (Camci-Unal et al. 2013; Yao et al. 2013). It is well known that the tumor interstitial fluid is, due to hypoxia, more acidic, with a pH of around 6.5, while in the blood plasma the pH is 7.4 (Zhu et al. 2013), and the pH in late endosomes may decrease to 5.0 (Nelson et al. 2013). Therefore,

Qiu et al. (2014) developed a pH-sensitive system based on micelles from HA conjugated with hydrophobic poly(L-histidine) for the acid-triggered rapid release of doxorubicin inside tumor cells. After internalization, both HA and poly(L-histidine) are in the ionized state (the remaining carboxyl groups pass into carboxylate and the imidazole ring is protonated) and induce the rupture of lysosomal membrane, facilitating the release of the entrapped drug into the cytoplasm. The most important advantage of this novel drug delivery system is the possession of smart functions, such as active targeting and pH-triggered doxorubicin release, resulting in a substantial increase in the therapeutic efficacy.

Han et al. (2012) designed and developed HA nanoparticles for oral administration of insulin. The nanoparticles were prepared by the reverse-emulsion freeze-drying method and displayed an average size of 182 nm and high entrapment efficiency (95%). The pH-sensitive HA nanoparticles have several advantages. First, the collapsed polymeric matrix protects the insulin against the harsh gastric fluid of the stomach and does not destroy the junction integrity of epithelial cells allowing long-term safe chronic treatment. Second, the amount of insulin released in the simulated gastric fluid in the first two hours is very low. By changing the pH from 1.2 to 6.8 (simulated intestinal fluid), the HA polymeric network swells extensively and a large amount of insulin was released (Figure 5.2). Therefore, the pH-sensitive HA nanoparticles could be a promising candidate for oral administration of insulin.

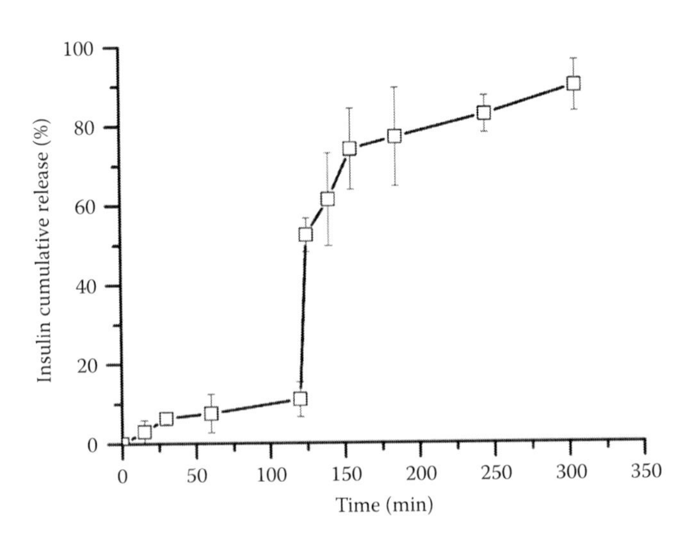

FIGURE 5.2
In vitro release profiles of insulin from HA nanoparticles in the simulated gastric fluid (pH 1.2) and intestinal fluid (pH 6.8). Each value represents mean ± S.D. (n = 3). (From Han, L. et al., *AAPS PharmSciTech*, 13, 836, 2012.)

5.2.1.3 Pectin

Pectin is a heteropolysaccharide present in the primary cell walls of plants consisting of galacturonic acid residues bonded via α-1,4 glycosidic linkage and different amount of neutral sugars as side chains. Galacturonic acid can be found in the methylesterified form at C-6 and/or O-acetylated at O-2 and/or O-3 (Voragen et al. 2009). Pectins are generally classified based on the degree of esterification or degree of methylation (DM) of contained carboxyl groups with methanol. High-methoxyl pectins have a DM of 50% or greater while low-methoxyl pectins have a DM of less than 50%. Therefore, the degree of esterification is an important pectin characteristic in the gelling process. The nonesterified residues can be ionized/protonated resulting in a polyanion with pH-sensitive properties. Accordingly, in the presence of cations, pectin can be cross-linked intra- and/or intermolecularly resulting in weak or strong hydrogel networks. The pH sensitivity and the DM control the gelation of the pectin. Thus, Da Silva and Rao (1995) reported pectin having low DM gels in the presence of Ca^{2+} in a large pH domain and pectin having high DM gels at a low pH (<3.5) in the presence of a cosolute. The binding of Ca^{2+} to pectin is not simple ionic interaction but involves intermolecular chelate binding of the cation, leading to the formation of macromolecular aggregates ("egg-box" cavity) (Figure 5.3).

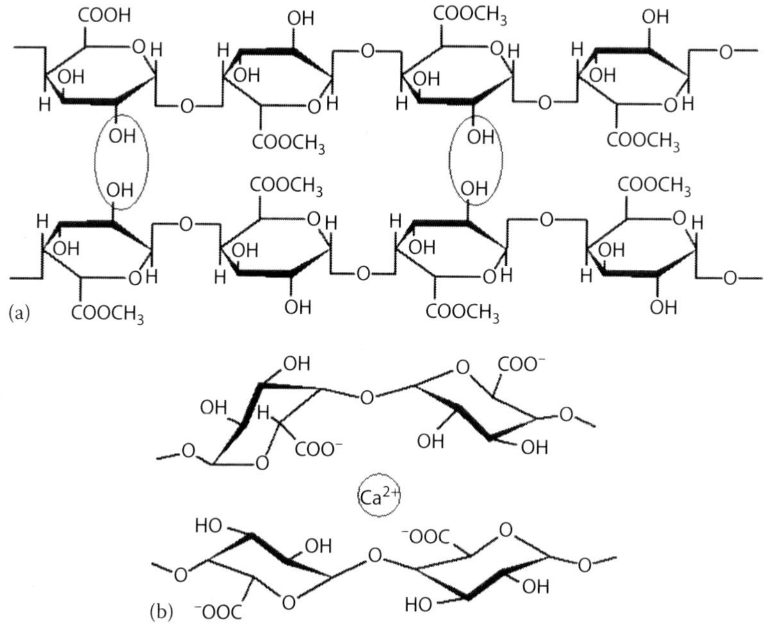

FIGURE 5.3
Mechanism of pectin gelation: (a) HM pectin gelation mechanism and (b) LM pectin gelation mechanism.

The pH sensitivity of pectin was also exploited for the colon release of drugs. Thus, Tan et al. (2016) reported the synthesis of beads based on pectin and carboxymethyl sago pulp cross-linked with calcium and further by electron beam irradiation for oral administration of diclofenac. It was shown that less than 9% of the drug has been released at pH 1.2, because of the low swelling degree of beads at this pH. The protonated anionic groups of pectin determine the hydrogel beads to remain intact. In the simulated intestinal fluid (pH = 6.8), the carboxyl groups are ionized (pK_a of pectin is between 3.5 and 4.5), and the microgels start to swell, releasing almost the entire amount of entrapped drug.

Dutta and Sahu (2012) developed a magnetic nanocarrier of 100–150 nm from pectin and chitosan with a high encapsulation efficiency of diclofenac, taken as the model drug. The in vitro drug release was pH sensitive. Thus, in the simulated gastric fluid (0–2 h), almost no drug was released. In contrast, the amount of drug released in phosphate buffer solution at pH 7.4 was substantially increased and was in good agreement with swelling-controlled mechanism on the basis of the Korsmeyer–Peppas model.

Pectin was also used as coating material with pH-sensitive properties. Thus, Puga et al. (2013) prepared chitosan microgels loaded with 5-fluorouracil for oral and topical chemotherapy. Then, the microgels were coated with pectin layers at the solid–air interface in an efficient way. The size of the microgels changed from 280 μm for chitosan seeds to 557 μm for pectin-coated microgels. Remarkably, the microgels coated with only one layer of calcium cross-linked pectin display a substantial decrease of drug release rate in acidic pH (Figure 5.4).

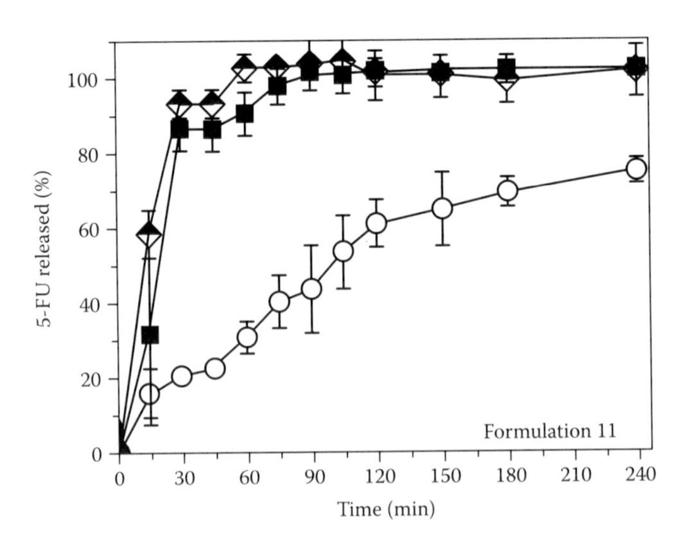

FIGURE 5.4
5-Fluorouracil release profiles in water (squares), HCl 1% (circles), and in phosphate buffer pH 7.4 (diamonds) from apple pectin-coated microgels. (From Puga, A.M. et al., *Carbohydr. Polym.*, 98, 331, 2013.)

In fact, this pectin has a lower methoxy content and therefore a high content of pH-sensitive units that can form multiple interaction points with chitosan or with the cross-linker. In contrast, in phosphate buffer at pH 7.4, a fast release rate occurred. In these conditions, the electrostatic interactions between carboxylic groups of pectin and calcium ions as well as amino groups of chitosan are weakened, favoring the release of drug.

5.2.1.4 Chitosan

Chitosan is considered one of the most valuable polysaccharides for biomedical and pharmaceutical applications due to its biocompatibility, biodegradability, lack of toxicity, and antimicrobial and antitumoral properties. Moreover, chitosan is the most abundant biopolymer obtained by *N*-deacetylation of chitin that is a major component of the shells of crustaceans.

Chitosan is a linear polysaccharide composed of randomly distributed β-(1–4)-linked D-glucosamine (deacetylated unit) and *N*-acetyl-D-glucosamine (acetylated unit). The presence of primary amines in chitosan confers important pH-sensitive properties that could be exploited in the controlled delivery of drugs. The amino group in chitosan has a pK_a value of ~6.5, which leads to protonation in an acidic fluid and deprotonation in neutral and basic media. In fact, protonation is one of the most commonly utilized mechanisms to achieve pH-triggered drug delivery. By exploiting the acidic microenvironments in the tumor (pH = 5.0–6.8) (Kallinowski and Vaupel 1988; Thistlethwaite et al. 1985), pH-responsive assemblies based on chitosan (microgels, micelles) can solubilize (swell) at the tumor site and release the necessary dose of the drug. Therefore, Yu et al. (2016) developed pH-sensitive nanospheres with a diameter of about 100 nm by electrostatic interactions between the positively charged amino group of chitosan grafted with β-cyclodextrin and the negatively charged sodium tripolyphosphate. The nanospheres are characterized by a hollow cavity entrapping doxorubicin with an entrapment efficiency of above 60%. The release rate of the drug from nanospheres increases with the decrease of the pH and the increase of temperature and ionic strength. For example, at pH = 5.2 and 37°C more than 90% of the entrapped drug was released with a continuous release rate. The in vitro cytotoxicity tests reveal that doxorubicin-loaded nanospheres exhibited inhibition against cancer cells.

In another work, Deng et al. (2011) reported a one-step method to prepare monodispersed SiO_2 nanoparticles decorated with pH-sensitive chitosan. First, the monodispersed cationic polystyrene nanospheres were prepared by free emulsion polymerization using α,α′-azodiisobutyramidine dihydrochloride, as the initiator. These nanospheres were further used as a template to prepare SiO_2 nanoparticles using tetraethoxysilane (TEOS) (Figure 5.5). Decoration of SiO_2 nanospheres with chitosan was performed in the presence of (3-glycidyloxypropyl) trimethoxysilane (GPTMS) (Wu and Sailor 2009) (Figure 5.5). The resulting nanospheres with a pH-sensitive chitosan

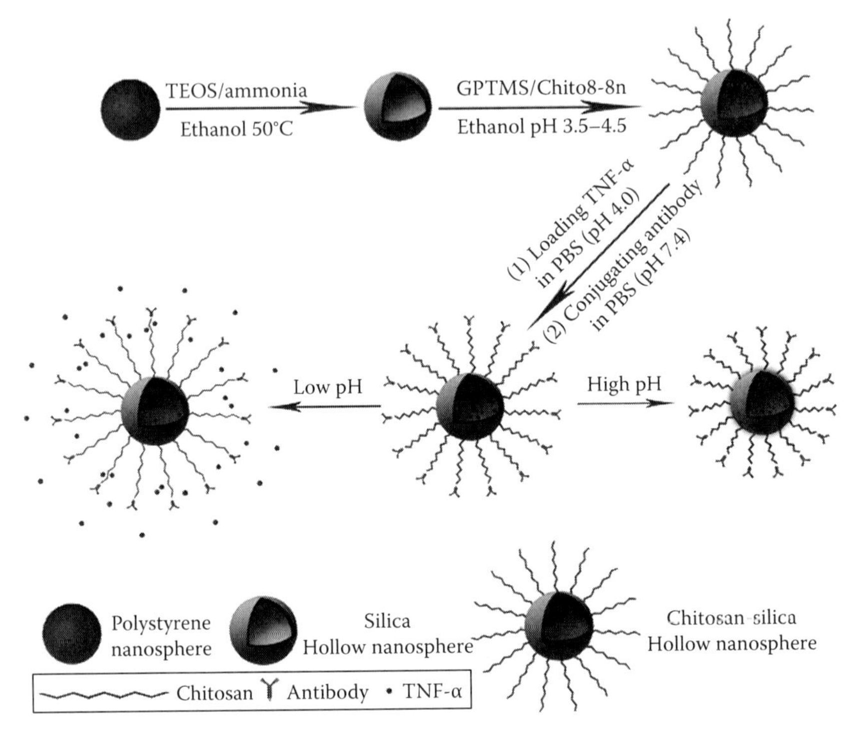

FIGURE 5.5
Schematic diagram illustrating the formation of nanocarriers (CSeSiO$_2$-TNF-α conjugated with antibody) and the drug release behavior at different pH values. (From Deng, Z. et al., *Biomaterials*, 32, 4976, 2011.)

layer are conjugated to the antibody molecule (to ErbB 2), resulting in the preferred nanocarriers for targeted TNF-α drug delivery to tumor cells.

Bovine serum albumin (BSA), taken as the model protein drug, was encapsulated in nanospheres and the release studies were performed in phosphate buffer solutions at different pH values (pH = 7.4 and pH = 4) (Figure 5.6). SiO_2 nanospheres decorated with chitosan released just 17.4% of the BSA at pH = 7.4 in the first 100 h, while in pH = 4.0, a rapid release occurred (83.7% within 24 h). This difference in release rates can be ascribed to the collapse and swelling of the chitosan layers on the surface of SiO_2 nanospheres. Under acidic conditions, the chitosan passes in the protonated form, more hydrophilic. The polymeric chains swell, leading to opening of the pores of nanospheres and favoring the release of BSA. In contrast, at a neutral pH of 7.4, the chitosan chains are in the deprotonated state, are more hydrophobic, and shrink, creating a shield that hampers the release of protein. The results clearly proved that chitosan played an important role in the release mechanism.

When the pH is low, the chitosan polymer chains swell in the medium opening the pores of the nanocarriers so that the loaded drugs can be easily

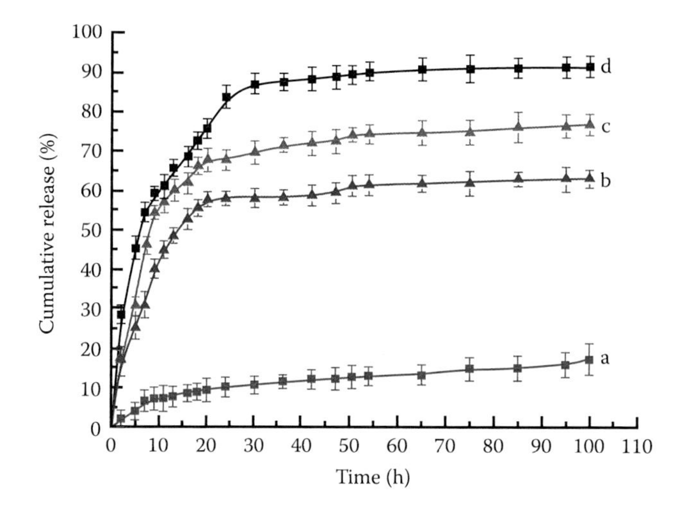

FIGURE 5.6
Release profiles of BSA as one model protein drug from $CSeSiO_2$ and SiO_2 HNPs in the PBS media at different pH values: (a) $CSeSiO_2$ HNPs, pH 7.4, (b) SiO_2 HNPs, pH 7.4, (c) SiO_2 HNPs, pH 4.0, and (d) $CSeSiO_2$ HNPs, pH 4.0. (From Deng, Z. et al., *Biomaterials*, 32, 4976, 2011.)

released from the nanocarriers. In contrast, at a high pH, the chitosan polymer chains are deprotonated and collapse to form a shield layer on the porous surface on the nanocarriers. This blocks and restricts drugs release from the hollow interior.

Unsoy et al. (2014) prepared magnetic nanoparticles coated with chitosan for *in vitro* targeted delivery of doxorubicin on breast cancer cells. The release rate of drug was substantially influenced by the pH. At low pH (4.2), the swelling ratio of chitosan increased, allowing the release of most of the drug while at pH = 7.4, the nanoparticles are stable. The images obtained by fluorescence microscopy have shown that magnetic nanoparticles loaded with doxorubicin were taken up by the cells and accumulated around the nucleus.

5.2.2 Modified Polysaccharides with Acquired pH Sensitivity

Besides native pH-sensitive polysaccharides, neutral polysaccharides are promising candidates because they can be modified to have tailor-made materials with pH-sensitive properties. Neutral polysaccharides have a great number of functional groups susceptible to chemical modifications. Chemical modification is usually performed on the primary hydroxyl group at C-6 of the sugar unit due to the higher reactivity of this position relative to the secondary hydroxyl group. Among neutral polysaccharides, starch, pullulan, and dextran are widely used as supports for the controlled delivery of drugs because they are highly stable, biocompatible, nontoxic, and can be easily acquired at low cost.

5.2.2.1 Starch

Starch is a polysaccharide composed of amylose and amylopectin. Amylose is a linear polymer consisting of α-D-glucopyranose units linked through (1→4) linkages while amylopectin is a branched polymer linked by (1→6) linkages. Starch is biocompatible and biodegradable and has natural abundance and a low cost of production and is therefore widely used as a support for drug delivery systems.

Carboxymethyl starch (CMS) represents one of the most well-studied starch derivatives, is environmentally safe, and is approved for such applications as food, cosmetics, and pharmaceutical products, as well as for a wide range of environmental and technical purposes. The average number of carboxymethyl groups introduced per sugar unit is defined as the degree of substitution (DS). The most common method for the insertion of carboxymethyl groups is based on the reaction between native starch and monochloroacetic acid in isopropanol/water medium (Anirudhan and Parvathy 2014; Zdanowicz et al. 2014) (Figure 5.7).

Lemieux et al. (2015) developed mucoadhesive microspheres using CMS for the oral delivery of small molecules in GIT (acidic and neutral) simulated conditions. In simulated gastric fluid, the carboxylic groups are protonated and form hydrogen bonds with the model drug, furosemide. Moreover, the polymeric network is not expanded. Therefore, the diffusion of the drug is obstructed, leading to a low release rate. By increasing the DS, more protonated carboxylic groups interacted to result in a more compact network. Therefore, the release rate decreased. In a buffer at pH 7.4, the microspheres swell due to the repulsive forces between ionized polymeric chains and determine a rapid release of the drug (less than 5 min). The bioadhesion of carboxymethylated starch microspheres was much higher to gastric than intestinal mucosa, regardless of the DS. In fact, under acidic conditions, strong hydrogen bonding between mucus and carboxylic functional groups occurred.

Besides carboxymethylation, grafting of pH-sensitive polymers onto neutral polysaccharides is an interesting method to induce pH sensitivity. Thus, Shalviri et al. (2013) designed and developed pH-responsive nanoparticles based on starch grafted with poly(methacrylic acid) and polysorbate 80. The loading efficiency of doxorubicin was very high due to the strong electrostatic

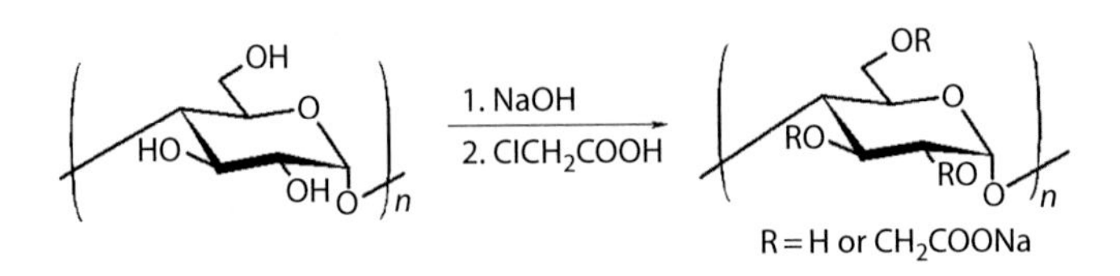

FIGURE 5.7
Schematic representation of carboxymethylation.

interactions between the positively charged drug and the negatively charged nanoparticles. The release rate of the drug was much faster in slightly acidic (pH = 5) than in slightly basic (pH = 7.4) fluid. The higher release rate in acidic pH is the result of the rupture of electrostatic interactions between the drug and polymer as a result of protonation of methacrylic acid. In fact, a rapid release of drug from nanoparticles at a weakly acidic pH is necessary for an effective supply of antitumoral drugs to solid tumors.

5.2.2.2 Pullulan

Pullulan is a water-soluble homopolysaccharide produced by certain strains of the fungus *Aureobasidium pullulans*. From the viewpoint of chemical structure, pullulan is a linear glucan containing α-(1,4) and α-(1,6) linkages in a ratio of 2:1 (Wallenfels et al. 1961). The insertion of pH-sensitive units was also performed by carboxymethylation, as reported previously (Mocanu et al. 2002, 2012). Bruneel and Schacht (1994) proposed an interesting method to insert carboxyl groups by reaction of linear pullulan with succinic anhydride in dimethyl sulfoxide (DMSO) in the presence of dimethyl aminopyridine (DMAP) as the catalyst. Later, Constantin et al. (2007) applied this method to pullulan microspheres and fabricated pH-sensitive microgels. These microspheres with an exchange capacity of around 5.3 meq/g are almost unswollen in simulated gastric fluid (pH = 1.2) but swell extensively (21 times) in simulated intestinal fluid at pH = 7.4. The pH sensitivity of pulluan microgels are exploited in an original manner for the release of diclofenac in the colon. These microgels were coencapsulated with aminated poly(vinyl alcohol) (PVA) loaded with diclofenac in cellulose acetate butyrate (CAB) microcapsules. In the absence of succinoylated pullulan microspheres (SP-Ms), a very low amount of drug was released because the pressure generated by the swelling of PVA microspheres is not sufficient to determine the rupture of CAB coating and to allow the loaded microspheres to escape (Figure 5.8).

With the aim to increase the amount of released drug in the intestine, different amounts of SP-Ms were coencapsulated. These microspheres do not swell in simulated gastric juice but swell extensively (10–20 times) in simulated intestinal fluid causing the rupture of CAB microcapsules and facilitating the escape of loaded microspheres (Figure 5.9). The larger the amount of coencapsulated microspheres, the higher is the drug release rate. In the gastric juice, the amount of released drug is very low (Figure 5.8).

5.2.2.3 Dextran

Dextran is a highly water-soluble polysaccharide consisting mainly of linear chains of α-1,6 linked glucopyranose units and has long been investigated as a blood plasma substitute. Recently, dextran and its derivatives due to its excellent biocompatibility have become of interest as carrier materials for drugs, proteins, and gene delivery (Mai et al. 2015; Mocanu et al. 2015;

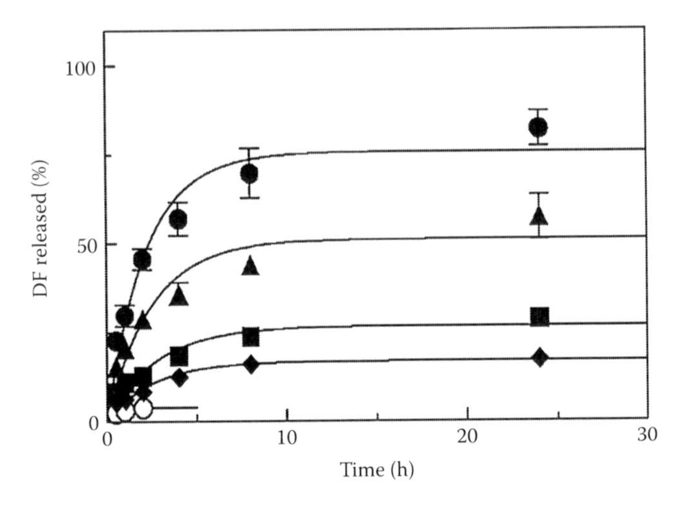

FIGURE 5.8
Release profiles of DF in phosphate buffer at pH 7.4 from encapsulated PVA microspheres in the presence of different percentages of SP-Ms: 0% (●), 5% (■), 15% (▲), and 25% (w/w) (◆). For comparison, the release profile of DF in gastric fluid is depicted, pH 1.2, from encapsulated PVA microspheres in the presence of 25% (w/w) SP-Ms (○). (From Constantin, M. et al., *Int. J. Pharm.*, 330, 129, 2007.)

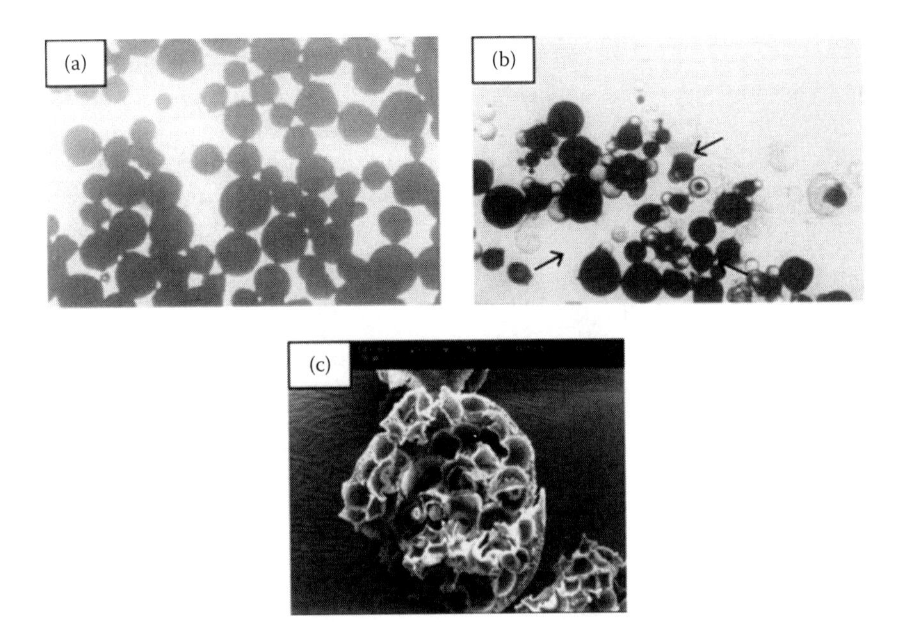

FIGURE 5.9
Optical photomicrographs taken at 1 h (a) after incubation in phosphate buffer, pH = 7.4. (b) The arrows indicate the escape process of SP-Ms. Scanning electron micrograph of the microcapsule after release (c). (From Constantin, M. et al., *Int. J. Pharm.*, 330, 129, 2007.)

Pacelli et al. 2015). Due to the presence of abundant hydroxyl groups, dextran could be chemically modified to obtain pH-sensitive moieties. Thus, Kauffman et al. (2012) synthesized acetalated dextran (Ac-Dex) as a biocompatible polymer that can suffer tunable rapid degradation at slightly acidic conditions present in the phagosome (pH = 5) but slower degradation at extracellular conditions (pH = 7.4) (Broaders et al. 2009). Then, Ac-Dex polymer was transformed in rapamycin-loaded microparticles by oil-in-water solvent evaporation method from single emulsion. Because of the acid sensitivity of Ac-Dex, the microparticles disintegrated and release the loaded drug. Therefore, the amount of released rapamycin was much higher at pH = 5, simulating the phagosomal conditions (50% in 45 h) than at pH = 7.4 (5% in 240 h), which simulate extracellular conditions. It must be noticed that rapamycin does not possess ionizable functional groups, and hence the pH has no influence on its aqueous solubility. In these conditions, it may be concluded that the pH sensitivity of Ac-Dex microparticles is entirely responsible for the different release rates and does not depend on the solubility of the drug at different pH values. The sensitivity of the release rate to pH assumes that drug-loaded microparticles, which passively target phagocytes, would release the drug after phagocytosis and not in the extracellular environment. Suarez et al. (2013) use the same Ac-Dex microparticles as the platform for the delivery of proteins to the heart in postmyocardial infarction. The particles were loaded with a model protein, myoglobin, and a sensitive growth factor, basic fibroblast growth factor (bFGF). The release studies were performed in low-pH environments, as is found in an infarcted heart region. It was found that bFGF preserved its activity after release from the microparticles.

Castiglione et al. (2007) fabricated pH-sensitive dextran microspheres by free radical copolymerization of glycidyl methacrylate dextran and methacrylic acid in the presence of *N,N*-ethylenebisacrylamide used as the cross-linker. Previously, dextran was chemically modified to introduce the polymerizable glycidyl methacrylate unit. The synthesized microparticles displayed a round shape, narrow size distribution, high swelling ratio, and a pH-sensitive swelling behavior. These characteristics recommend the microparticles to be used for controlled delivery of drugs.

5.3 Thermosensitive Polysaccharides

Native polysaccharides show by themselves very limited temperature sensitivity with the exception of gellan and xanthan gums that suffer transitions between an ordered helix structure at low temperature to a disordered coil state at high temperature. To strengthen this temperature sensitivity and to provide other polysaccharide networks with temperature responsiveness, they have to be chemically modified. Therefore, the substitution of the hydroxyl groups of glucose units with more hydrophobic moieties such as methyl (Takahashi et al. 2001), hydroxypropyl (Adrados et al. 2001), or isopropyl groups (Shi and Zhang 2007) confers on them thermosensitive properties. However, the resulting polymers do not show satisfactory thermal characteristics. It follows that the most known method for getting polysaccharide with high thermosensitivity is the insertion of thermosensitive polymers on the main backbone of polysaccharide or ionic cross-linking of chitosan with glycerophosphates. The main polymers that can induce thermosensitivity in polysaccharides are poly(*N*-isopropylacrylamide), poloxamer, polyvinylcaprolactam, and poly(L-lactide).

5.3.1 Poly(*N*-Isopropylacrylamide)

Poly(*N*-isopropylacrylamide) (poly(NIPAAm)) is the most frequently used thermosensitive polymer for biomedical applications (Patrizi et al. 2009; Zhang et al. 2009) because in aqueous solution it possesses a sharp phase transition (lower critical solution temperature, LCST) around the human body temperature (LCST = 32°C) (Heskins and Guillet 1968; Priest et al. 1986). Below the LCST, the polymer is in hydrated state, soluble, and the macromolecular chains are elongated. Above the LCST, the polymer loses the water of hydration, becomes hydrophobic, and collapses. Correspondingly, the poly(NIPAAm)-based hydrogel swells below the LCST and shrinks above it. These temperature-dependent changes of the polymeric chains are exploited for the controlled delivery of drugs or for other biomedical applications. Thus, Fundueanu et al. (2008) prepared thermosensitive pullulan by grafting the copolymer poly(*N*-isopropylacrylamide-*co*-acrylamide) (poly(NIPAAm-*co*-AAm)) on pullulan microspheres (Figure 5.10). First, pullulan microspheres were prepared by cross-linking an aqueous suspension of polymer with epichlorohydrin. Second, the grafting was performed on swollen microspheres in the presence of ceric ions. It is well known that ceric redox catalysts are able to produce radicals on glucopyranosyl units of polysaccharides (McCormick and Park 1981). Then, free radicals initiate the polymerization of comonomers from aqueous solution. In this study, NIPAAm was copolymerized with the hydrophilic AAm to produce a copolymer with a LCST close to the human body temperature (Fundueanu et al. 2009a).

In order to confer double sensitivity, the pH-sensitive functional groups were introduced by chemical reaction of succinic anhydride with the remaining –OH groups of pullulan. It was demonstrated that pullulan microspheres became more hydrophilic after grafting, their swelling degree as well as water uptake increasing substantially. The thermoresponsive properties of modified pullulan microspheres depend on the number and the ionization state (–COOH/–COO–) of carboxylic groups. At a low content of carboxylic groups (0.35 mmol/g), microspheres are thermoresponsive both in the protonated and in the ionized form of carboxylic groups. At an increased number of carboxylic groups (2.25 mmol/g), microspheres are almost unswellable in

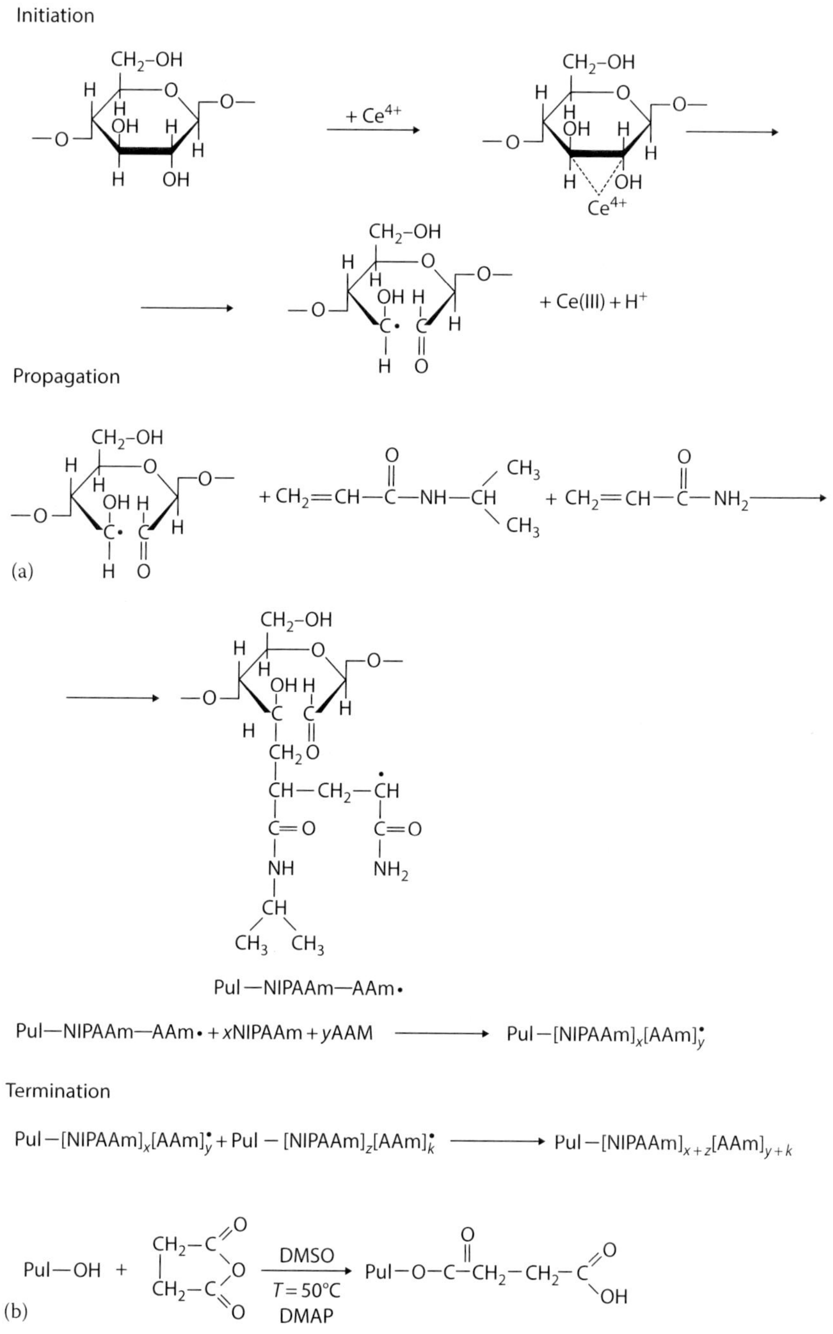

Initiation

$+ Ce^{4+}$

$+ Ce(III) + H^+$

Propagation

(a)

$+ CH_2{=}CH{-}C({=}O){-}NH{-}CH(CH_3)_2 + CH_2{=}CH{-}C({=}O){-}NH_2 \longrightarrow$

Pul—NIPAAm—AAm•

$\text{Pul—NIPAAm—AAm}\bullet + x\text{NIPAAm} + y\text{AAM} \longrightarrow \text{Pul}-[\text{NIPAAm}]_x[\text{AAm}]_y^\bullet$

Termination

$\text{Pul}-[\text{NIPAAm}]_x[\text{AAm}]_y^\bullet + \text{Pul}-[\text{NIPAAm}]_z[\text{AAm}]_k^\bullet \longrightarrow \text{Pul}-[\text{NIPAAm}]_{x+z}[\text{AAm}]_{y+k}$

(b)

$\text{Pul—OH} + \text{succinic anhydride} \xrightarrow[T=50°C,\ \text{DMAP}]{\text{DMSO}} \text{Pul}-O-C(=O)-CH_2-CH_2-C(=O)OH$

FIGURE 5.10
Reaction mechanism of poly(NIPAAm-*co*-AAm) grafting (a) and succinoylation of pullulan microspheres (b). (From Fundueanu, G. et al., *Biomaterials*, 29, 2767, 2008.)

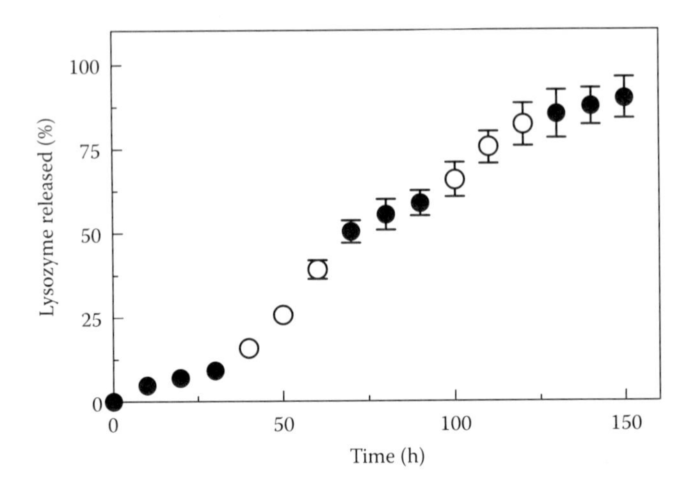

FIGURE 5.11
Effect of temperature cycling (42°C [●] and 22°C [○]) on lysozyme release from graft pullulan microspheres. (From Fundueanu, G. et al., *Biomaterials*, 29, 2767, 2008.)

the protonated state but swell dramatically after ionization losing the thermosensitive properties.

The thermoresponsive microspheres were able to release lysozyme (taken as a molecular model system) by a pulsatile mechanism since a significant amount enzyme is pushed out during the collapse of the polymeric network (Figure 5.11).

In another work, Fundueanu et al. (2010) designed and developed pullulan microspheres with pendant thermosensitive arms able to entrap and release drugs by a strict "on–off" mechanism. First, the authors synthesized pullulan microspheres by suspension cross-linking procedure (Figure 5.12a). Even if the hydroxyl groups of pullulan are susceptible to chemical modifications, they are not reactive enough, and therefore a great number was chloroacetylated (Figure 5.12b). The thermosensitive arms (semitelechelic oligomers with NH_2 end groups) were prepared by free radical polymerization of NIPAAm with AAm using cysteamine as the chain transfer agent (Fundueanu et al. 2009b). Then, the functionalized pullulan microspheres were coupled with semitelechelic oligomers by reaction between the amino-end groups of oligomers and the chlorine present on modified pullulan (Figure 5.12c).

Inverse size exclusion chromatography was used to predict the size of the drug molecule that could be loaded/released by an "on–off" mechanism. It was found that FITC-Dextran 4000 is the perfect molecule for such a purpose. Release studies were conducted under simulated physiological conditions (phosphate buffer at pH = 7.4) below and above the LCST of the semitelechelic thermoresponsive oligomer. Above the LCST, pendant thermosensitive arms are in the collapsed state and no steric obstructions occur;

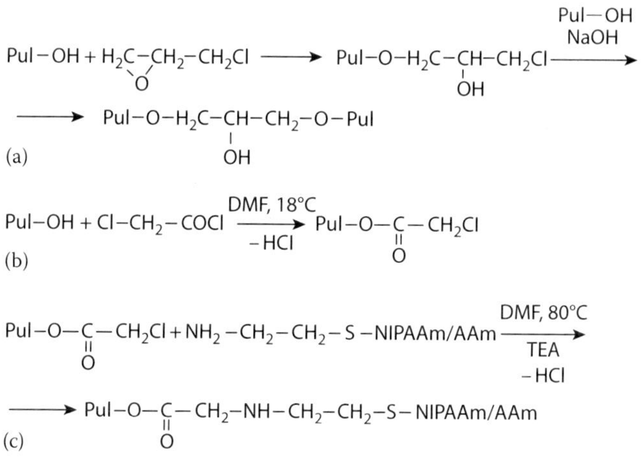

$$\text{Pul-OH} + H_2C\text{-}CH\text{-}CH_2\text{-}CH_2Cl \ (\text{epoxide, O}) \longrightarrow \text{Pul-O-}H_2C\text{-}CH(OH)\text{-}CH_2Cl \xrightarrow{\text{Pul-OH, NaOH}}$$

$$\longrightarrow \text{Pul-O-}H_2C\text{-}CH(OH)\text{-}CH_2\text{-O-Pul}$$

(a)

$$\text{Pul-OH} + Cl\text{-}CH_2\text{-}COCl \xrightarrow[\text{-HCl}]{\text{DMF, 18°C}} \text{Pul-O-}C(=O)\text{-}CH_2Cl$$

(b)

$$\text{Pul-O-}C(=O)\text{-}CH_2Cl + NH_2\text{-}CH_2\text{-}CH_2\text{-S-NIPAAm/AAm} \xrightarrow[\text{TEA, -HCl}]{\text{DMF, 80°C}}$$

$$\longrightarrow \text{Pul-O-}C(=O)\text{-}CH_2\text{-NH-}CH_2\text{-}CH_2\text{-S-NIPAAm/AAm}$$

(c)

FIGURE 5.12
Synthesis of thermosensitive pullulan microspheres: cross-linking (a), acetylation (b), and coupling (c) reactions. (From Fundueanu, G. et al., *Biomaterials*, 31, 9544, 2010.)

therefore, the FITC-Dextran 4000 is rapidly released. In contrast, when the temperature is decreased below the LCST, the thermosensitive arms expand and steric interactions block the diffusion of the model molecule.

Çakmak et al. (2013) developed thermosensitive dextran microspheres by grafting poly(NIPAAm) onto the surface of the microbeads by surface-initiated atom transfer radical polymerization (SI-ATRP) (Figure 5.13). Previously, hydroxyl groups of dextran microspheres were activated with 2-bromopropionyl bromide to obtain ATRP macroinitiator. Then, NIPAAm was polymerized on the microspheres by ATRP in the presence of CuBr/2,2′-dipyridyl used as a catalyst complex.

The resulting poly(NIPAAm)-grafted dextran microcarriers displayed thermoresponsive properties and could be used as an interesting matrix for cell culture and tissue engineering applications.

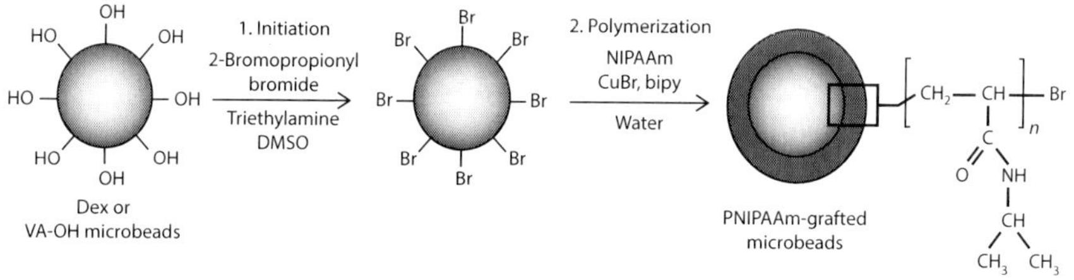

FIGURE 5.13
Schematic representation of the PNIPAAm grafting process through surface-initiated ATRP. (From Çakmak, S. et al., *Mater. Sci. Eng. C: Mater. Biol. Appl.*, 33, 3033, 2013.)

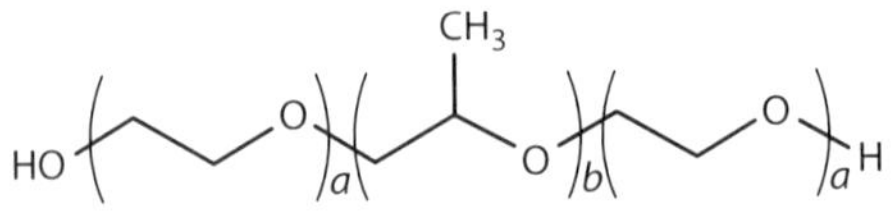

FIGURE 5.14
Chemical structure of poloxamer.

5.3.2 Poloxamers

Besides poly(NIPAAm), poloxamers are largely used to confer thermosensitivity to polysaccharides (Jung et al. 2017; Mayol et al. 2008; Yu et al. 2017). Poloxamers are nonionic triblock copolymers possessing a central hydrophobic chain of polyoxypropylene and two hydrophilic chains of polyoxyethylene (Figure 5.14).

Thus, Mocanu et al. (2011) prepared carboxymethyl pullulan microspheres by suspension cross-linking procedure; then various amounts of poloxamer were inserted by reaction between carboxylic groups of polysaccharide and the terminal hydroxyl groups of polyoxyethylene in the presence of the coupling agent, dicyclohexyl carbodiimide. These microparticles have both pH and temperature sensitivity and have been used for the loading of biologically active proteins through ionic or hydrophobic interactions. It was proved that the release of proteins depends on the pH, temperature, and duration.

Poloxamers also have the capacity to form temperature-dependent micellar aggregates and, after further temperature increase, gel due to micelle aggregation. Aqueous poloxamer solutions are thermosensitive: at low temperatures, they are in the liquid state, whereas at body temperature they form stable gels. This property of reverse thermal gelation and the low toxicity (FDA approval) render these copolymers attractive as in situ gel-forming matrix materials for controlled drug delivery systems.

In situ gel formation is widely used in ophthalmic therapy because it ensures an increased ocular bioavailability and a prolonged delivery of drugs (Cho et al. 2016; Gratieri et al. 2011). Thus, Cho et al. (2003) developed an ophthalmic drug delivery system by grafting the poloxamer onto the HA. The grafting reaction was performed by coupling mono amine-terminated poloxamer with an HA backbone using 1-ethyl-3-(3-dimethylaminopropyl)-carbodiimide and *N*-hydroxylsuccinimide as coupling agents. The authors demonstrated that the gelation temperature of graft copolymers is deeply influenced by the percentage of the HA and concentration of poloxamer. In vitro release studies have proven that the ophthalmic formulation is able to control the release of the entrapped ciprofloxacin in a prolonged period of time due to in situ gel formation and viscous properties of HA.

5.3.3 Glycerophosphates

Besides poloxamers, polyol salts, such as α- and β-glycerophosphate (Figure 5.15), are the most common compounds that induce thermogelling in chitosan aqueous solution (Kim et al. 2010; Niranjan et al. 2013).

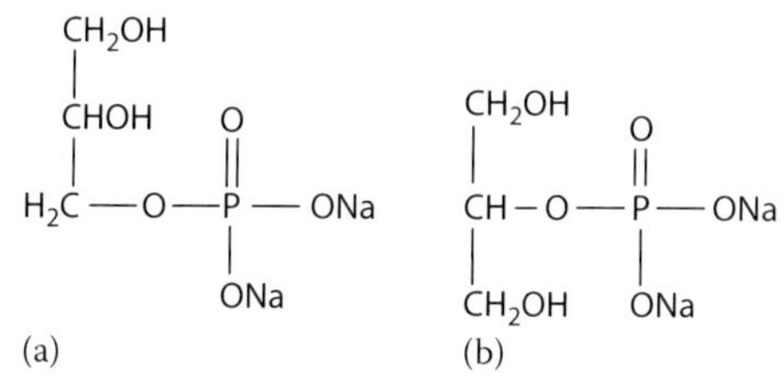

CH_2OH
CHOH O
H_2C—O—P— ONa
ONa
(a)

CH_2OH O
CH–O—P— ONa
CH_2OH ONa
(b)

FIGURE 5.15
Chemical structure of α- (a) and β-glycerophosphate (b).

Chitosan solution remains a liquid below room temperature at physiologically acceptable pH values (6.8–7.4) in the presence of glycerophosphate salts but gels when the temperature reaches the physiological value. The effective interactions responsible for the sol/gel transition are multiple: (1) the intermolecular hydrogen bonds are reconstructed due to the reduction of electrostatic interactions between the unprotonated amines groups in neutral conditions, (2) ionic interactions between chitosan and glycerophosphate via the ammonium and the phosphate groups, respectively, and (3) hydrophobic interactions between the chitosan chains enhanced by the structuring action of glycerol in water (Chenite et al. 2000).

Most of the hydrogels are used as macroscopic devices, the synthesis of thermogelling micro- and nanogels being a difficult task. Thus, Wu et al. (2008) developed uniformly sized pH-sensitive chitosan microspheres by combining the Shirasu porous glass (SPG) membrane emulsification technique and the thermal gelation method. First, the aqueous phase consisting of quaternized chitosan and α-β-glycerophosphate was dispersed in the oil phase using the SPG membrane emulsification technique to form uniform W/O emulsion. Then, the aqueous microdroplets hardened into microspheres at 37°C by thermal gelation method. The resulting microspheres had a variation coefficient of diameters below 15% and display a porous structure. Very interestingly, the microspheres solubilized rapidly in acidified solution (pH = 5) but were stable in neutral solution (pH = 7.4). The release rates of BSA, taken as the model drug, were high in acidic solution and low in neutral fluid. Due to this pH sensitivity, the chitosan microspheres can be used for the delivery of drugs to the tumor sites.

Hsiao et al. (2012) developed thermogelling injectable nanogels by combining self-assembled nanocapsules of chitosan with amphiphilic moieties and glycerophosphate disodium salt and glycerol. Native chitosan was first chemically modified by partial substitution with carboxymethyl moieties to increase the solubility of the polysaccharide in water and by partial substitution with hydrophobic hexanoyl moieties to increase their amphiphilic character (Liu et al. 2006).

Carboxymethyl hexanoyl chitosan self-assembled into nanocapsules in aqueous media.

Both in acidic and neutral pH, the amine groups of chitosan are protonated and nanocapsules have positive charges. Therefore, β-glycerophosphate was used to neutralize the positive charges and diminish repulsive forces between chitosan nanocapsules at higher temperatures, giving rise to a sol–gel transition with increased temperature. Additionally, glycerol was added to produce a supplementary increase of the gel strength. *In vitro* drug release studies using ethosuximide demonstrated that nanogels released the drug in a prolonged period of time with no burst release. Moreover, all investigated formulations have no cytotoxic effect on human retinal pigmented epithelium cells.

5.3.4 Poly(*N*-Vinylcaprolactam)

Poly(*N*-vinylcaprolactam) (poly(NVCL)) is the most popular temperature-responsive polymer after poly(NIPAAm). This polymer displays a sharp phase transition (LCST) in aqueous solution between 32°C and 34°C (Tager et al. 1993). The phase transition is reversible similar to poly(NIPAAm) and the corresponding hydrogel undergoes swelling/collapsing processes at the same temperature as that for linear polymer (Cortez-Lemus and Licea-Claverie 2016). The fact that this polymer is less known in the last few years, compared to poly(NIPAAm), has likely been due to the difficulty in polymerizing NVCL in a controlled fashion.

Thus, Rejinold et al. (2011) developed nanoparticles from thermoresponsive chitosan-*g*-poly(*N*-vinylcaprolactam) copolymer as carrier for 5-fluorouracil to cancer cells. First, carboxyl-terminated poly(*N*-vinylcaprolactam) was prepared by free radical polymerization in the presence of mercaptopropionic acid as the chain transfer agent. Then, the poly(NVCL)–COOH was grafted onto chitosan using (1-ethyl-3-(3-dimethylaminopropyl)carbodiimide/*N*-hydroxy succinimide) as the condensing agent. Finally, thermoresponsive nanoparticles were fabricated using the ionic cross-linking method with sodium tripoly phosphate. The nanoparticles displayed a phase transition at 38°C. The 5-FU drug was incorporated into the carrier during the cross-linking reaction. The release rate of the drug was controlled mainly by the swelling and diffusion and was much higher above than below LCST. Cytotoxicity tests demonstrated that nanoparticles in the concentration range of 0.1–1 g/mL are nontoxic to an array of cell lines. Also, nanoparticles loaded with the drug have a comparatively high toxicity to cancer cells but they have a less toxic effect on normal cells. The uptake by the cells of nanoparticles loaded with 5-fluorouracil was confirmed from the green fluorescence inside cells due to the rhodamine-123 conjugation. The obtained results showed that these thermo-responsive nanoparticles have great potential for cancer therapy.

Previously, Prabaharan et al. (2008) synthesized pH- and/or thermo-sensitive beads starting from the thermo-responsive chitosan-*g*-poly(*N*-vinylcaprolactam) copolymer obtained by a coupling reaction between carboxyl end groups of poly(vinylcaprolactam) and amino groups of chitosan (Figure 5.16).

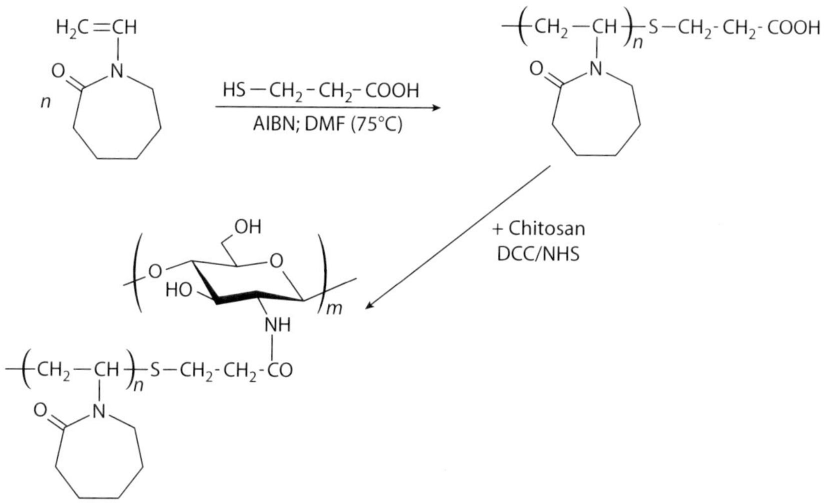

FIGURE 5.16
Synthesis of chitosan-*g*-poly(vinylcaprolactam).

The beads loaded with ketoprofen were obtained by dropping an aqueous copolymer solution with the drug into 100 mL of 10% sodium tripolyphosphate through a syringe. During the gelation process, the pH of the sodium tripolyphosphate solution was maintained at pH = 4.4 with dilute HCl. As expected, the swelling degree of the obtained beads depended on the pH and temperature, being higher at pH = 2.2 than at pH = 7.4, and decreasing with the increase of temperature. The release rates of ketoprofen from pH/sensitive beads were deeply influenced by pH and temperature. The amount of released drug was higher in simulated physiological fluids with low pH and at low temperature below the LCST. The cytotoxic effect of chitosan-*g*-poly(vinylcaprolactam) beads against human endothelial cell line was insignificant in the concentration range of 0–400 μg/mL.

5.3.5 Poly(L-Lactide)

Seo et al. (2012) developed thermo-responsive nanogels from pullulan-*g*-poly(L-lactide) copolymers (Figure 5.17) with different lactide contents as an anticancer drug (doxorubicin) delivery carrier. First, water-insoluble pullulan-*g*-poly(L-lactide) was synthesized via a one-pot method using triethylamine as catalyst and pullulan as macroinitiator (Cho et al. 2009). The thermo-responsive properties of the copolymers are the result of the disruption of polymer–water hydrogen bonding in controlling the contraction of the chains followed by the polymer collapse as a result of changes in the hydrophobic interactions (Inomata et al. 1990). The resulting copolymer was then transformed in nanogels via the dialysis method. In the micelle

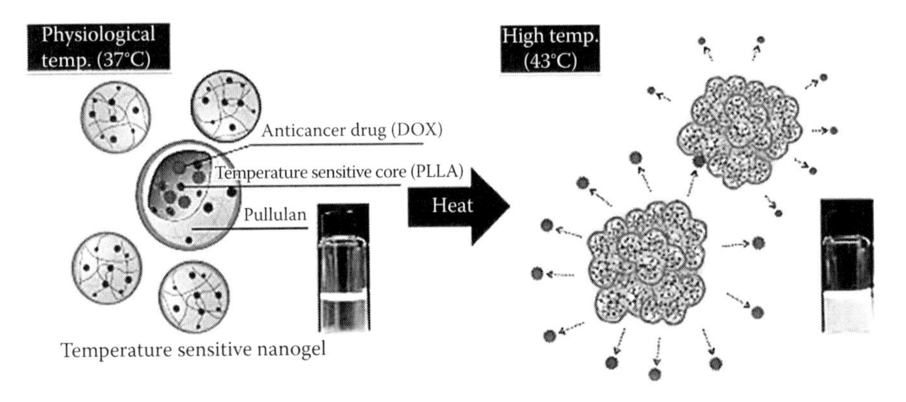

FIGURE 5.17
Molecular structure of the pullulan-*g*-poly(L-lactide) copolymer and the schematic representation of drug release from thermosensitive nanogels triggered by temperature. (From Seo, S. et al., *Carbohydr. Polym.*, 87, 1105, 2012.)

structure, poly(L-lactide) is supposed to form the hydrophobic inner core and pullulan acts as hydrophilic outer shell. The hydrophobic core plays an important role in loading and release of doxorubicin. The authors observed that a large amount of the drug was released by increasing the temperature from 37°C to 43°C because the stronger hydrophobic interactions between the lactide units caused the shrinkage of the nanogels and the expulsion of the drug (Figure 5.17). Also, the loaded nanogels were effective for killing cancer cells at higher temperatures.

5.4 Conclusions

Polysaccharides represent an important class of natural polymers that can be used as support in the development of pH- and/or temperature-sensitive carriers for controlled delivery of drugs or other biologically active compounds. Most of them have native pH sensitivity, and the others can acquire this property by being chemically modified with appropriate functionalities. Native polysaccharides have not or have very limited temperature sensitivity but the insertion of thermosensitive polymers such as poly(*N*-isopropylacrylamide), poloxamer, polyvinylcaprolactam, or poly(L-lactide) induces a dramatic increase of their thermosensitivity.

Also, chitosan obtains temperature-dependent gelling properties in the presence of glycerophosphates.

Native and modified polysaccharides could be transformed in micro- or nanoparticles by numerous methods such as suspension cross-linking, ionic gelation, self-assembly, dialysis, and nanoprecipitation, solvent evaporation/removal, etc. These microparticulate carriers are capable of transporting high amounts of drugs to the desired place and release it at the appropriate rates when the pH and/or temperature changes.

Acknowledgments

The authors acknowledge the financial support for this research through the European Regional Development Fund, Project POINGBIO, ID P_40_443, Contract no. 86/8.09.2016.

References

Adrados, B. P., Galaev, I. K., Nilsson, K., and Mattiasson, B. 2001. Size exclusion behavior of hydroxypropylcellulose beads with temperature-dependent porosity. *J Chromatogr A* 930:73–78.

Agarwal, T., Narayana, S. N., Pal, K., Pramanik, K., Giri, S., and Banerjee, I. 2015. Calcium alginate-carboxymethyl cellulose beads for colon-targeted drug delivery. *Int J Biol Macromol* 75:409–417.

Anirudhan, T. S. and Parvathy, J. 2014. Novel semi-IPN based on crosslinked carboxymethyl starch and clay for the in vitro release of theophylline. *Int J Biol Macromol* 67:238–245.

Bleve, G., Tufariello, M., Vetrano, C., Mita, G., and Grieco, F. 2016. Simultaneous alcoholic and malolactic fermentations by *Saccharomyces cerevisiae* and *Oenococcus oeni* cells co-immobilized in alginate beads. *Front Microbiol* 7:943.

Broaders, K. E., Cohen, J. A., Beaudette, T. T., Bachelder, E. M., and Fréchet, J. M. 2009. Acetalated dextran is a chemically and biologically tunable material for particulate immunotherapy. *Proc Natl Acad Sci USA* 106:5497–5502.

Bruneel, D. and Schacht, E. 1994. Chemical modification of pullulan: 3. Succinoylation. *Polymer* 35:2656–2658.

Çakmak, S., Çakmak, A. S., and Gümüşderelioğlu, M. 2013. PNIPAAm-grafted thermoresponsive microcarriers: Surface-initiated ATRP synthesis and characterization. *Mater Sci Eng C Mater Biol Appl* 33:3033–3040.

Camci-Unal, G., Cuttica, D., Annabi, N., Demarchi, D., and Khademhosseini, A. 2013. Synthesis and characterization of hybrid hyaluronic acid-gelatin hydrogels. *Biomacromolecules* 14:1085–1092.

Castiglione, M., Puoci, F., Iemna, F. et al. 2007. pH-sensitive microspheres obtained by derivatized dextran. *Chim Oggi* 25:9–11.

Chenite, A., Chaput, C., Wang, D. et al. 2000. Novel injectable neutral solutions of chitosan form biodegradable gels in situ. *Biomaterials* 21:2155–2161.

Cho, I. S., Park, C. G., Huh, B. K. et al. 2016. Thermosensitive hexanoyl glycol chitosan-based ocular delivery system for glaucoma therapy. *Acta Biomater* 39:124–132.

Cho, J. K., Park, W., and Na, K. 2009. Self organized nanogels from pullulan-*g*-poly(L-lactide) synthesized by one-pot method: Physicochemical characterization and in vitro doxorubicin release. *J Appl Polym Sci* 113:2209–2216.

Cho, K. Y., Chung, T. W., Kim, B. C. et al. 2003. Release of ciprofloxacin from poloxamer-graft-hyaluronic acid hydrogels in vitro. *Int J Pharm* 260:83–91.

Choi, K. Y., Yoon, H. Y., Kim, J. H. et al. 2011. Smart nanocarrier based on PEGylated hyaluronic acid for cancer therapy. *ACS Nano* 5:8591–8599.

Constantin, M., Fundueanu, G., Bortolotti, F., Cortesi, R., Ascenzi, P., and Menegatti, E. 2007. A novel multicompartimental system based on aminated poly(vinyl alcohol) microspheres/succinoylated pullulan microspheres for oral delivery of anionic drugs. *Int J Pharm* 330:129–137.

Cortez-Lemus, N. A. and Licea-Claverie, A. 2016. Poly(*N*-vinylcaprolactam), a comprehensive review on a thermoresponsive polymer becoming popular. *Prog Polym Sci* 53:1–51.

Da Silva, J. A. L. and Rao, M. A. 1995. Rheology of structure development in high methoxyl pectin/sugar systems. *Food Technol* 10:70–73.

De Andrade Neves, N., de Araujo Pantoja, L., and dos Santos, A. S. 2014. Thermovinification of grapes from the Cabernet Sauvignon and Pinot Noir varieties using immobilized yeasts. *Eur Food Res Technol* 238:79–84.

Deng, Z., Zhen, Z., Hu, X., Wu, S., Xu, Z., and Chu, P. K. 2011. Hollow chitosan–silica nanospheres as pH-sensitive targeted delivery carriers in breast cancer therapy. *Biomaterials* 32:4976–4986.

Draget, K. I., Skjåk Bræk, G., and Smidsrød, O. 1994. Alginic acid gels: The effect of alginate chemical composition and molecular weight. *Carbohydr Polym* 25:31–38.

Dutta, R. K. and Sahu S. 2012. Development of diclofenac sodium loaded magnetic nanocarriers of pectin interacted with chitosan for targeted and sustained drug delivery. *Colloids Surf B Biointerfaces* 97:19–26.

Fundueanu, G., Constantin, M., and Ascenzi, P. 2008. Preparation and characterization of pH- and temperature-sensitive pullulan microspheres for controlled release of drugs. *Biomaterials* 29:2767–2775.

Fundueanu, G., Constantin, M., and Ascenzi, P. 2009a. Poly(*N*-isopropylacrylamide-*co*-acrylamide) cross-linked thermoresponsive microspheres obtained from preformed polymers: Influence of the physico-chemical characteristics of drugs on their release profiles. *Acta Biomater* 5:363–373.

Fundueanu, G., Constantin, M., and Ascenzi, P. 2009b. Fast-responsive porous thermoresponsive microspheres for controlled delivery of macromolecules. *Int J Pharm* 379:9–17.

Fundueanu, G., Constantin, M., Oanea, I., Harabagiu, V., Ascenzi, P., and Simionescu, B. C. 2010. Entrapment and release of drugs by a strict "on-off" mechanism in pullulan microspheres with pendant thermosensitive groups. *Biomaterials* 31:9544–9553.

Gratieri, T., Gelfuso, G. M., de Freitas, O., Rocha, E. M., and Lopez, R. F. 2011. Enhancing and sustaining the topical ocular delivery of fluconazole using chitosan solution and poloxamer/chitosan in situ forming gel. *Eur J Pharm Biopharm* 79:320–327.

Han, L., Zhao, Y., Yin, L. et al. 2012. Insulin-loaded pH-sensitive hyaluronic acid nanoparticles enhance transcellular delivery. *AAPS PharmSciTech* 13:836–845.

Heskins, M. and Guillet, J. E. 1968. Solution properties of poly(*N*-isopropylacrylamide). *J Macromol Sci Chem* 2:1441–1455.

Hsiao, M. H., Larsson, M., Larsson, A. et al. 2012. Design and characterization of a novel amphiphilic chitosan nanocapsule-based thermo-gelling biogel with sustained in vivo release of the hydrophilic anti-epilepsy drug ethosuximide. *J Control Release* 161:942–948.

Inomata, H., Goto, S., and Saito, S. 1990. Phase transition of N-substituted acrylamide gels. *Macromolecules* 23:4887–4888.

Işıklan, N., İnal, M., Kurşun, F., and Ercan, G. 2011. pH responsive itaconic acid grafted alginate microspheres for the controlled release of nifedipine. *Carbohydr Polym* 84:933–943.

Jung, Y., Park, W., Park, H., Lee, D. K., and Na, K. 2017. Thermo-sensitive injectable hydrogel based on the physical mixing of hyaluronic acid and Pluronic F-127 for sustained NSAID delivery. *Carbohydr Polym* 156:403–408.

Kallinowski, F. and Vaupel, P. 1988. pH distributions in spontaneous and isotransplanted rat tumours. *Br J Cancer* 58:314–321.

Kauffman, K. J., Kanthamneni, N., Meenach, S. A., Pierson, B. C., Bachelder, E. M., and Ainslie, K. M. 2012. Optimization of rapamycin-loaded acetalated dextran microparticles for immunosuppression. *Int J Pharm* 422:356–363.

Kim, S., Nishimoto, S. K., Bumgardner, J. D., Haggard, W. O., Gaber, M. W., and Yang, Y. 2010. A chitosan/beta-glycerophosphate thermo-sensitive gel for the delivery of ellagic acid for the treatment of brain cancer. *Biomaterials* 31:4157–4166.

Lemieux, M., Gosselin, P., and Mateescu, M. A. 2015. Carboxymethyl starch mucoadhesive microspheres as gastroretentive dosage form. *Int J Pharm* 496:497–508.

Liu, T. Y., Chen, S. Y., Lin, Y. L., and Liu, D. M. 2006. Synthesis and characterization of amphiphatic carboxymethyl-hexanoyl chitosan hydrogel: Water-retention ability and drug encapsulation. *Langmuir* 22:9740–9745.

Mai, K., Zhang, S., Liang, B., Gao, C., Du, W., and Zhang, L. M. 2015. Water soluble cationic dextran derivatives containing poly(amidoamine) dendrons for efficient gene delivery. *Carbohydr Polym* 123:237–245.

Mayol, L., Quaglia, F., Borzacchiello, A., Ambrosio, L., and La Rotonda, M. I. 2008. A novel poloxamers/hyaluronic acid in situ forming hydrogel for drug delivery: Rheological, mucoadhesive and in vitro release properties. *Eur J Pharm Biopharm* 70:199–206.

McCormick, C. L. and Park, L. S. 1981. Water-soluble copolymers. III. Dextran-*g*-poly-(acrylamides) control of grafting sites and molecular weight by Ce(IV)-induced initiation in homogeneous solutions. *J Polym Sci Polym Chem Ed* 19:2229–2241.

Mocanu, G., Mihai, D., Dulong, V., Picton, L., Le Cerf, D., and Moscovici, M. 2011. Anionic polysaccharide hydrogels with thermosensitive properties. *Carbohydr Polym* 83:52–59.

Mocanu, G., Mihai, D., Picton, L., LeCerf, D., and Muller, G. 2002. Associative pullulan gels and their interaction with biological active substances. *J Control Release* 83:41–51.

Mocanu, G., Nichifor, M., and Stanciu, M. C. 2015. New shell crosslinked micelles from dextran with hydrophobic end groups and their interaction with bioactive molecules. *Carbohydr Polym* 119:228–235.

Mocanu, G., Souguir, Z., Picton, L., and Le Cerf, D. 2012. Multi-responsive carboxymethyl polysaccharide crosslinked hydrogels containing Jeffamine side-chains. *Carbohydr Polym* 89:578–585.

Mukhopadhyay, P., Chakraborty, S., Bhattacharya, S., Mishra, R., and Kundu, P. P. 2015. pH-sensitive chitosan/alginate core-shell nanoparticles for efficient and safe oral insulin delivery. *Int J Biol Macromol* 72:640–648.

Nelson, C. E., Kintzing, J. R., Hanna, A., Shannon, J. M., Gupta, M. K., and Duvall, C. L. 2013. Balancing cationic and hydrophobic content of PEGylated siRNA polyplexes enhances endosome escape, stability, blood circulation time, and bioactivity in vivo. *ACS Nano* 7:8870–8880.

Niranjan, R., Koushik, C., Saravanan, S., Moorthi, A., Vairamani, M., and Selvamurugan, N. 2013. A novel injectable temperature-sensitive zinc doped chitosan/β-glycerophosphate hydrogel for bone tissue engineering. *Int J Biol Macromol* 54:24–29.

Pacelli, S., Paolicelli, P., and Casadei, M. A. 2015. New biodegradable dextran-based hydrogels for protein delivery: Synthesis and characterization. *Carbohydr Polym* 126:208–214.

Patrizi, M. L., Piantanida, G., Coluzza, C., and Masci, G. 2009. ATRP synthesis and association properties of temperature responsive dextran copolymers grafted with poly(*N*-isopropylacrylamide). *Eur Polym J* 45:2779–2787.

Prabaharan, M., Grailer, J. J., Steeber, D. A., and Gong, S. 2008. Stimuli-responsive chitosan-graft-poly(*N*-vinylcaprolactam) as a promising material for controlled hydrophobic drug delivery. *Macromol Biosci* 8:843–851.

Priest, J. H., Murray, S. L., Nelson, R. J., and Hoffman, A. S. 1986. Lower critical solution temperatures of aqueous copolymers of *N*-isopropylacrylamide and other N-substituted acrylamides. *ACS Symp Ser* 350:255–264.

Puga, A. M., Lima, A. C., Mano, J. F., Concheiro, A., and Alvarez-Lorenzo, C. 2013. Pectin-coated chitosan microgels crosslinked on superhydrophobic surfaces for 5-fluorouracil encapsulation. *Carbohydr Polym* 98:331–340.

Qiu, L., Li, Z., Qiao, M. et al. 2014. Self-assembled pH-responsive hyaluronic acid–*g*-poly((L)-histidine) copolymer micelles for targeted intracellular delivery of doxorubicin. *Acta Biomater* 10:2024–2035.

Rejinold, N. S., Chennazhi, K. P., Nair, S. V., Tamura, H., and Jayakumar, R. 2011. Biodegradable and thermo-sensitive chitosan-*g*-poly(*N*-vinylcaprolactam) nanoparticles as a 5-fluorouracil carrier. *Carbohydr Polym* 83:776–786.

Seo, S., Lee, C. S., Jung, Y. S., and Na, K. 2012. Thermo-sensitivity and triggered drug release of polysaccharide nanogels derived from pullulan-*g*-poly(L-lactide) copolymers. *Carbohydr Polym* 87:1105–1111.

Shalviri, A., Chan, H. K., Raval, G. et al. 2013. Design of pH-responsive nanoparticles of terpolymer of poly(methacrylic acid), polysorbate 80 and starch for delivery of doxorubicin. *Colloids Surf B Biointerfaces* 101:405–413.

Shi, H. Y. and Zhang, L. M. 2007. New grafted polysaccharides based on *O*-carboxymethyl-*O*-hydroxypropyl guar gum and *N*-isopropylacrylamide: Synthesis and phase transition behavior in aqueous media. *Carbohydr Polym* 67:337–342.

Suarez, S., Grover, G. N., Braden, R. L., Christman, K. L., and Almutairi, A. 2013. Tunable protein release from acetalated dextran microparticles: A platform for delivery of protein therapeutics to the heart post-MI. *Biomacromolecules* 14:3927–3935.

Tager, A. A., Safronov, A. P., Sharina, S. V., and Galaev, I. Y. 1993. Thermodynamic study of poly(*N*-vinylcaprolactam) hydration at temperatures close to lower critical solution temperature. *Colloid Polym Sci* 271:868–872.

Takahashi, M., Shimazaki, M., and Yamamoto, J. 2001. Thermoreversible gelation and phase separation in aqueous methyl cellulose solutions. *J Polym Sci B Polym Phys Ed* 39:91–100.

Tan, H. L., Tan, L. S., Wong, Y. Y., Muniyandy, S., Hashim, K., and Pushpamalar, J. 2016. Dual crosslinked carboxymethyl sago pulp/pectin hydrogel beads as potential carrier for colon-targeted drug delivery. *J Appl Polym Sci* 133, doi: 10.1002/app.43416.

Thistlethwaite, A. J., Leeper, D. B., Moylan, D. J. 3rd, and Nerlinger, R. E. 1985. pH distribution in human tumors. *Int J Radiat Oncol Biol Phys* 11:1647–1652.

Unsoy, G., Khodadust, R., Yalcin, S., Mutlu, P., and Gunduz, U. 2014. Synthesis of doxorubicin loaded magnetic chitosan nanoparticles for pH responsive targeted drug delivery. *Eur J Pharm Sci* 62:243–250.

Voragen, A. G. J., Coenen, G. J., Verhoef, R. P., and Schols, H. A. 2009. Pectin, a versatile polysaccharide present in plant cell walls. *Struct Chem* 20:263–275.

Wallenfels, K., Bender, H., Keilich, G., and Bechtler, G. 1961. On pullulan, the glucan of the slime coat of *Pullularia pullulans*. *Angew Chem* 73:245–246.

Wu, J. and Sailor, M. 2009. Chitosan hydrogel-capped porous SiO_2 as a pH responsive nano-valve for triggered release of insulin. *Adv Funct Mater* 19:733–741.

Wu, J., Wei, W., Wang, L. Y., Su, Z. G., and Ma, G. H. 2008. Preparation of uniform-sized pH-sensitive quaternized chitosan microsphere by combining membrane emulsification technique and thermal-gelation method. *Colloids Surf B Biointerfaces* 63:164–175.

Zdanowicz, M., Spychaj, T., and Lendzion-Bieluń, Z. 2014. Crosslinked carboxymethyl starch: One step synthesis and sorption characteristics. *Int J Biol Macromol* 71:87–93.

Zhang, H. F., Zhong, H., Zhang, L. L., Chen, S. B., Zhao, Y. J., and Zhu, Y. L. 2009. Synthesis and characterization of thermosensitive graft copolymer of *N*-isopropylacrylamide with biodegradable carboxymethylchitosan. *Carbohydr Polym* 77:785–790.

Zhu, L., Smith, P. P., and Boyes, S. G. 2013. pH-responsive polymers for imaging acidic biological environments in tumors. *J Polym Sci Part B Polym Phys* 51:1062–1067.

Yao, J., Zhang, L., Zhou, J., Liu, H., and Zhang, Q. 2013. Efficient simultaneous tumor targeting delivery of all-trans retinoid acid and paclitaxel based on hyaluronic acid-based multifunctional nanocarrier. *Mol Pharm* 10:1080–1091.

Yoshioka, T., Tsuru, K., Hayakawa, S., and Osaka, A. 2003. Preparation of alginic acid layers on stainless-steel substrates for biomedical applications. *Biomaterials* 24:2889–2894.

Yu, N., Li, G., Gao, Y., Liu, X., and Ma, S. 2016. Stimuli-sensitive hollow spheres from chitosan-*graft*-β-cyclodextrin for controlled drug release. *Int J Biol Macromol* 93:971–977.

Yu, S., Zhang, X., Tan, G. et al. 2017. A novel pH-induced thermosensitive hydrogel composed of carboxymethyl chitosan and poloxamer cross-linked by glutaraldehyde for ophthalmic drug delivery. *Carbohydr Polym* 155:208–217.

6

Guided Bone Repair Using Synthetic Apatites–Biopolymer Composites

Irina M. Pelin and Dana M. Suflet

CONTENTS

6.1 Introduction

The bone is a complex living tissue and can be briefly described from four synergistic points of view: biological, chemical, mechanical, and engineering. From a *biological* viewpoint, bone is a hard tissue that accomplishes essential functions such as locomotion, support for muscle insertion, and protection of vital organs (Oyen 2008). From a *chemical* standpoint, bone is an active tissue involved in the mineral metabolism of some ions, among which calcium and phosphate have an important role in physiological mineralization of bone matrix and remodeling (Chai et al. 2012), and at the same time being involved in the formation of blood cells. From a *mechanical* point of view, bone is a dynamic, highly mineralized, and vascularized tissue able to respond and adapt to the mechanical loads in a remarkable way, so that the stable equilibrium between bone shape and function is ensured (Hing 2004). Finally, not in the least, from a *materials engineering* perspective, bone is considered an anisotropic composite with open micropores (Currey 1996).

A *restitutio ad integrum* of bone biology and functionality after a trauma or pathological injury requires artificial materials having properties similar or close to normal bone and still represents a target for scientists, even if a wide range of materials have been developed and commercialized. From these, a promising category of materials designed to repair damaged bone are composites based on biopolymers and synthetic apatites, which takes into account that bone is a natural composite containing 70% inorganic components (mainly carbonated and substituted hydroxyapatite [HAP]), about 22% organic components that comprise macromolecules (90% type I collagen and 10% mucopolysaccharides and noncollagenous proteins), and 8% water (Cullinane and Einhorn 2002). Consequently, the synthetic apatite–biopolymer composites will contain synthetic apatites, which are substituted calcium phosphates with the general formula $Ca_{10-x}(PO_4)_{6-x}(HPO_4$ or $CO_3)_x(OH$ or $\frac{1}{2}CO_3)_{2-x}$, $0 \leq x \leq 2$ (Eichert et al. 2009), which will imitate bioapatites and biopolymers—natural polymers—produced by living organisms (as proteins and polysaccharides) that could chemically mimic the structure and functions of the bone's organic matrix.

The development of the composite materials started with scientific insights into complex mineralized composite systems existing in nature. For example, Li and Kaplan affirmed that the formation of natural inorganic–organic composites, such as bone and seashell, is a multistep process, including the assembly of the extracellular matrix, the selective transportation of inorganic ions to discrete organized compartments, subsequent mineral nucleation, and, finally, mineral growth delineated by the preorganized cellular compartments (Li and Kaplan 2003). The need to understand the ability of natural macromolecules to induce mineralization arises from the desire to get detailed information that could be useful to develop new biomaterials able to replace the "gold standard" of bone grafts (autografts). Even if the autograft, a piece of bone harvested from the patient's own body, displays better the most important characteristic of an ideal bone graft substitute, i.e. biocompatibility, the fact that it must be harvested from the patient during (or in an additional) surgical procedure can lead to acute postoperative pain or morbidity of the donor site. An alternative is to use allografts (pieces of bone harvested from fresh dead body), but sometimes this can be unsafe, if no guarantee of healthy donor tissue is given. Therefore, an ideal bone substitute able to guide the bone growth into the graft in order to induce bone repair is a major clinical requirement. The following features are essential for the development of the best bone graft: biocompatibility, bioresorbability, osteoconductivity, osteoinductivity, similarity with bone, ability to be manipulated during surgery, and, not in the least, affordability. Moreover, the composite designed for bone repair should possess a proper balance between physicochemical and mechanical properties, so that its charge, hydrophilicity, porosity, permeability, strength, or stiffness ensures the biodegradability, biocompatibility, and angiogenesis potential of the material.

Taking these requirements into account, this chapter is an overview of the composites developed in world laboratories, intended for future use in orthopedic or dental fields as guided materials for bone repair. Materials shaped in various forms such as membranes/films/multilayer sheets, fibers, sponges, gel/paste, microspheres/irregular particles, and disks/cylinders should be well integrated into the fracture site and facilitate bone healing by their physico-chemical properties. The composites can also be used as drug delivery systems capable of treating bone infections or slowing down bone resorption in some types of pathology. The composites can be made not only by controlling the size and morphology of the components but also by influencing the physicochemical properties, ultimately being able to incorporate specific elements as bioactive principles or growth factors to guide bone repair.

6.2 Basic Bone Biology and Repair

Bone is a dynamic, highly vascularized, and mineralized tissue, having the ability to remodel and repair itself (Hing 2004). Bone is a dense multiphase natural composite made up of cells embedded in a matrix composed of both organic (collagen fibers, lipids, peptides, proteins, glycoproteins, polysaccharides, and citrates) and inorganic (calcium–phosphates, carbonates, sodium, magnesium, and fluoride salts) elements (Cameron 1972). The highly ordered collagen fibers are reinforced by submicroscopic inorganic apatite crystals in such a manner that biochemical, physicochemical, and biomechanical events insure normal function. The type I collagen macromolecule is a heterotrimeric triple helix. The individual triple helices (tropocollagen macromolecules) are 300 nm long and 1.5 nm in diameter and self-assemble into a quarter-staggered array with periodic banding every 67 nm due to regions of overlap (Oyen 2008). This regular arrangement of tropocollagen macromolecules forms larger collagen fibrils, which are in turn grouped to form large collagen fibers. Collagen has both intermolecular and intramolecular cross-links that make bone highly insoluble. The main inorganic phase within bone is somehow incorrectly referred to as hydroxyapatite, a hydrated calcium phosphate ceramic, with a similar (but not identical) crystallographic structure to natural bone apatite. Bone apatite is characterized by calcium, phosphate, and hydroxyl deficiency, internal crystal disorder, and ionic substitution within the apatite lattice resulting in the presence of significant levels of additional trace elements within bone mineral (Hing 2004). Biological apatite rather resembles the A–B-type carbonate-substituted apatite, even if the term HAP is commonly used. So, the apatite is insoluble enough for stability, yet sufficiently reactive to allow the in vivo submicroscopic (5–100 nm) crystallites to be constantly resorbed and reformed as required by the body (Hing 2004).

The organic matrix of bone includes a number of sulfated and acid mucopolysaccharides, of which osteocalcin, bone sialoprotein, osteopontin, and osteonectin are of particular interest, forming so-called noncollagenous proteins. They are produced by bone cells and are believed to regulate bone mineralization and remodeling. Furthermore, in the bone matrix structure, there are some peptides known as growth factors that have an important role in the proliferation of osteoblasts and in their function and motility, resulting in the formation of new bone. The organic matrix of the bone contains cells with various shapes and functions (Figure 6.1).

Healthy bone undergoes remodeling in a cycle of osteoclastic resorption and osteoblastic formation modulated by external mechanical solicitations through a very complex process. In broad lines, mechanical loads cause deformation of the bone matrix that is detected by osteocytes, which in turn send paracrine signals to osteoblasts and osteoclasts. Osteocytes form a functional network that passes intracellular calcium signals from cell to cell, either intracellularly through gap junctions or extracellularly by paracrines like adenosine triphosphate (Robling and Turner 2009).

The pathology of bone is substantial and various and includes osteoporosis, osteogenesis imperfecta, osteomyelitis, osteomalacia, osteosarcoma, and so on, as a function of the following causative agents: perturbation in bone metabolism, genetic defect that determines abnormal production of collagen, bacterial infection, inadequate mineralization of the bone, genetic factors, or radiation therapy.

Bone defects often result from trauma and tumor resection or as a consequence of periodontal disease. In the case of bone traumatism, bone heals

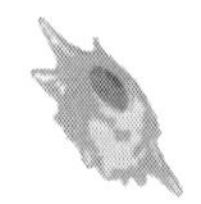

Osteogenic cell
(localized in the inner layer of the periosteum; evolves into osteoblast)

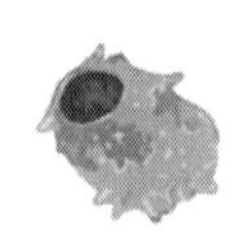

Osteoblast
(synthesizes and secretes collagen matrix and calcium salts; when the area from its surrounding calcifies, it turns into osteocyte)

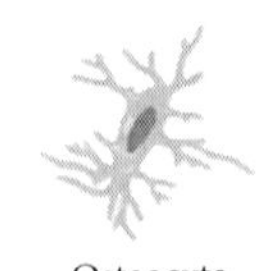

Osteocyte
(mature bone cell; has cytoplasmic processes that extend into canaliculi and make contact with the processes of other osteocytes)

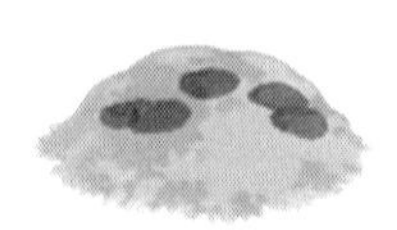

Osteoclast
(large cell with abundant acidophilic cytoplasm, that breaks down and resorbs bone)

FIGURE 6.1
Bone cells and their functions.

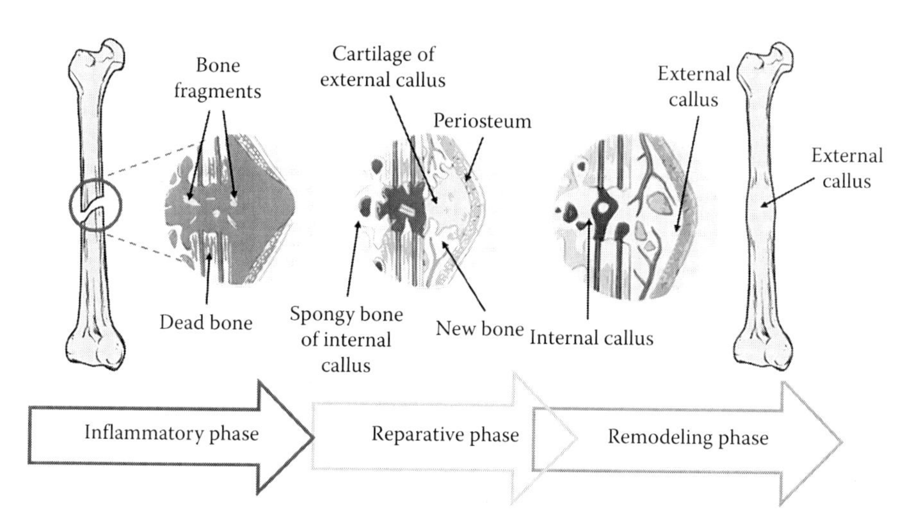

FIGURE 6.2
The bone self-repair process.

by itself, and the process of repair goes through three distinct but overlapping phases: inflammatory, reparative, and remodeling phases (Figure 6.2). Briefly, in the inflammatory phase, a hematoma develops within the fracture site in the first few hours and lasts up to several days. In the reparative phase, fibroblasts begin to form a stroma that supports vascular ingrowth. Fracture healing is completed during the remodeling phase in which the healing bone is restored to its original shape, structure, and mechanical strength. Remodeling of the bone occurs slowly over months to years and is facilitated by mechanical stress exercised on the bone (Kalfas 2001).

To shorten the healing time of injured bone in case of small or large fractures using minimal or normal invasive surgery, an increased interest is in inserting a bone substitute that can be regarded as a part of a system of gears, which together with cells and signaling molecules will guide bone repair (Figure 6.3). Therefore, a complete understanding of the mechanisms of interaction between the three components could offer valuable information for new biomaterials to be considered as treatment indication in the case of bone defects.

6.3 Synthetic Apatites–Biopolymer Composites

A modern approach that could support bone repair involves using resorbable porous composite obtained via biomimetic route, which can provide a temporary matrix with proper features that will allow the osteoblasts' insertion and activity (Figure 6.4).

Signaling molecules: cytokines, growth factors, molecules involved in cell adhesion
Cells: stem cells, marrow, stromal cells, osteoblasts
Matrix/scaffold: membrane/film/ multilayer sheet, fibers, sponge, gel/paste, microspheres, disk/cylinder

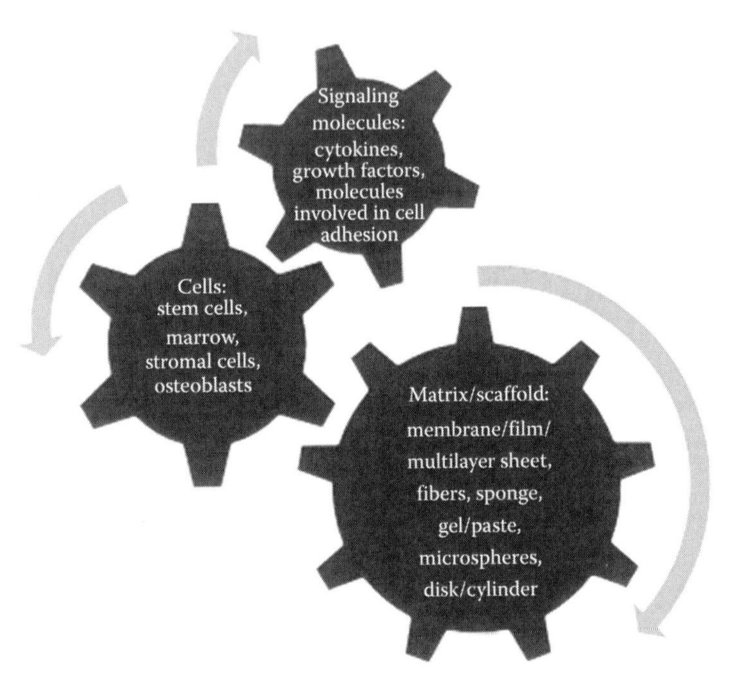

FIGURE 6.3
A gear system representation of the main components necessary to guide bone repair.

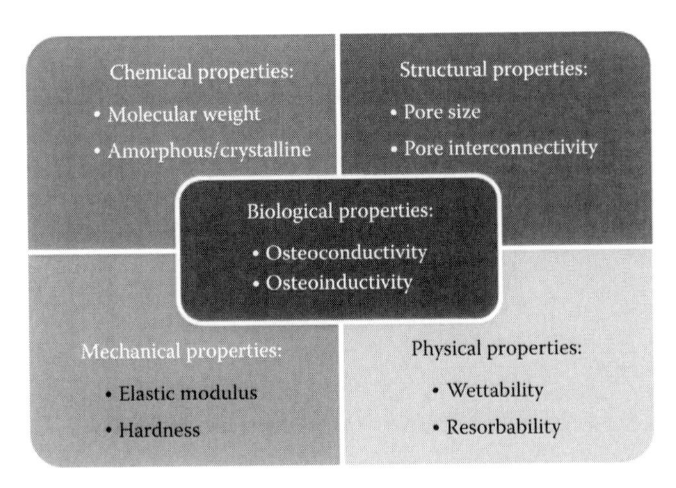

FIGURE 6.4
Interrelation between properties required for a composite useful in bone regeneration.

The term "composite" in materials science refers to a solid that contains two or more distinct constituent materials or phases, on a scale larger than the atomic one, and in which properties are significantly modified in comparison with those of a homogeneous material (Lakes 2007).

Given the fact that bone is a natural composite with two major components, apatite and collagen, many papers describe various combinations between natural polymers and synthetic apatite and try to prove that new bone substitutes capable of guiding bone repair can be fabricated.

6.3.1 Synthetic Apatites

The inorganic part of bones or teeth contains a type of calcium orthophosphate—hydroxyapatite—that is similar in composition and structure with hydroxylapatite, an OH^--containing mineral. Apatite is more flexible than most other minerals, meaning that it is very accommodating to chemical substitutions that will slightly modify the structure of a mineral but will have a major impact on solubility, hardness, brittleness, strain, thermal stability, and optical properties. Ionic substitutions, F^-, Cl^-, Na^+, K^+, Fe^{2+}, Zn^{2+}, Sr^{2+}, Mg^{2+}, citrate, and carbonate, are found in bone apatite lattice, bone apatite containing approximately 7 wt% carbonate, and tooth enamel about 3.5 wt% carbonate. Carbonate ions can substitute in the apatite structure either in the OH^- site ("A-type" substitution) or in the PO_4^- site ("B-type" substitution), but in biological apatite, it is generally accepted that CO_3^{2-} dominantly replaces PO_4^{3-} (Wopenka and Pasteris 2005).

Some of the calcium phosphates used in the composite formulations for bone repair do not have an apatitic crystalline structure. Table 6.1 presents different apatitic and nonapatitic calcium phosphates from Wopenka and Pasteris (2005).

From the crystallographic viewpoint, the HAP, $Ca_{10}(PO_4)_6(OH)_2$, is the most apatitic form of calcium phosphates, belongs to space group P63/m, and has the unit cell parameters: $a = b = 0.943$ nm and $c = 0.688$ nm. Hydroxyapatite (HAP) has two different binding sites on the particle surface (Figure 6.5), which are able to interact with functional groups of proteins: the C sites, rich in calcium ions that bind to acidic groups of proteins and are arranged rectangularly with the interdistances of 0.943 nm and 0.344 nm ($c/2$) for the a (or b) and c directions, respectively, and the P sites, which are attached to basic groups of proteins and are arranged hexagonally on the *ab* particle face at a distance of 0.943 nm (Kandori et al. 2007).

The results obtained by Kandori et al. concerning the adsorption characteristics of some proteins (like bovine serum albumin) onto HAP modified with pyrophosphoric acid could offer useful information when composites with natural polymer are envisaged as bone substitutes. Taking into account that the bioceramics for bone repair composed only of HAP provide high strength to loading but are not resorbed and could lead in

TABLE 6.1

Apatitic and Nonapatitic Calcium Phosphates

Typical Acronym	Chemical Name	Chemical Formula	Mineral Name	Structure	Ca/P Ratio
HAP, HA	Tribasic calcium phosphate	$Ca_5(PO_4)_3(OH)$	Hydroxylapatite	Apatitic	1.67
ACP	Amorphous calcium phosphate	?	N.A.	N.A.	?
PCHA, PCA	Poorly crystalline hydroxyapatite	$Ca_5(PO_4)_3(OH)$	Hydroxylapatite	Apatitic	1.67
CAP	Carbonated apatite, other names used: carbonate apatite, carbonated hydroxy(l)apatite	Variable[a]	No accepted mineral name; in the past, geologic carbonated fluorapatite was called "francolite," and geologic carbonated hydroxylapatite was called "dahllite" or "dahlite"	Apatitic	1.6–2.0
TCP	Tricalcium phosphate	$Ca_9(PO_4)_6$	"Whitlockite"	Nonapatitic	1.5
β-TCMP	Magnesium-substituted tricalcium phosphate	$(Ca,Mg)_9(PO_4)_6$	"Whitlockite"	Nonapatitic	≤1.50
?	"Tricalcium phosphate"	$Ca_9(Mg,Fe^{2+})(PO_4)_6(HPO_4)$	Geologically occurring Whitlockite	Nonapatitic	1.28
CPPD	Calcium pyrophosphate dihydrate	$Ca_2P_2O_7 \cdot 2H_2O$	Does not exist as geologic mineral	Nonapatitic	1
γ-CPP	γ-Calcium pyrophosphate	$Ca_2P_2O_7$	Does not exist as geologic mineral	Nonapatitic	1
OCP	Octacalcium phosphate	$Ca_8H_2(PO_4)_6 \cdot 5H_2O$	Does not exist as geologic mineral	Nonapatitic	1.33
MON	Dibasic calcium phosphate	$Ca(HPO_4)$	Monetite	Nonapatitic	1
DCPD	Dicalcium phosphate dihydrate	$Ca(HPO_4) \cdot 2H_2O$	Brushite	Nonapatitic	1

Source: Reprinted from Wopenka, B. and Pasteris, J.D., *Mater. Sci. Eng. C*, 25, 131, 2005. With permission.

[a] Can have different stoichiometry.

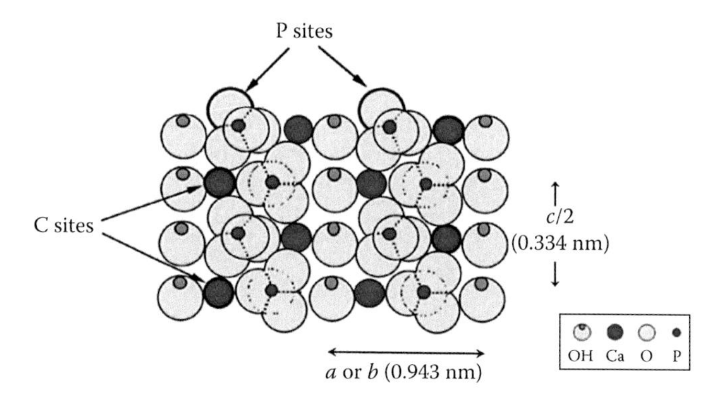

FIGURE 6.5
Crystal structure of hydroxyapatite with active sites. (Reprinted from Kandori, K. et al., *Colloids Surface B*, 58, 98, 2007. With permission.)

time to the injury of the bone after callus formation, the matrices for bone reconstruction containing the organic reinforcement will improve the resorbability of the substitute, permitting the new bone to replace the lost bone effectively.

To obtain composites for bone repair, another aspect concerning the structure of the apatite is that the apatite nanocrystals are covered with a fragile but structured surface hydrated layer (Cazalbou et al. 2004) containing relatively mobile ions (mainly bivalent anions and cations: Ca^{2+}, HPO_4^{2-}, CO_3^{2}) in "nonapatitic" sites that are responsible for most of the properties of the apatites (Dorozhkin 2009a).

The methods used to obtain HAP can be divided into solid-state reactions and wet methods, which include precipitation, hydrothermal synthesis, and hydrolysis of other calcium orthophosphates (Dorozhkin 2009b). The precipitates are generally nonstoichiometric, suggesting the formation of intermediate precursor phases, even under ideal stoichiometric conditions. HAP can be prepared in aqueous solutions by mixing stoichiometric quantities of Ca- and PO_4-containing solutions at pH > 9, followed by boiling for several days in CO_2-free atmosphere (the aging or maturation stage), filtration, drying, and sintering at about 1000°C. The first precipitates are rich in nonapatitic environments (amorphous calcium phosphate and calcium-deficient HAP), and in order to obtain HAP, a maturation stage is very important. The Ca/P molar ratio of 1.67 was found to be attained in less than 5 h after the completion of the reaction at 90°C (Rodriguez-Lorenzo and Vallet-Regi 2000). The aging time may vary from a few hours to a few months (depending on the reactants' purity, pH, and temperature), and the longer the aging period, the better improved are the quality and characteristics of the crystals (Koutsopoulos 2002).

6.3.2 Biopolymers

Biopolymers are generally considered natural polymers from bioresources, and in this chapter, only a few proteins or polysaccharides will be evoked as organic component in the fabrication of composites with applicability in bone reconstruction. It has been demonstrated that biopolymers such as collagen, gelatin, fibroin, cellulose, chitosan, curdlan, xanthan, pullulan, dextran, hyaluronan, starch, alginate, and agarose are able to interact with synthetic apatites to form temporary substitutes for hard tissue repair or can be used as scaffolds in bone tissue engineering. Natural polymers have attractive properties for the fabrication of biocompatible and bioresorbable composites, and their structural, physicochemical, or mechanical properties can be tailored by changing the concentrations or by introducing various functional groups. In the following section, biopolymers that are frequently used in the fabrication of composites with synthetic apatites such as collagen, gelatin, fibroin, cellulose, and chitosan will be briefly presented.

6.3.2.1 Collagen

Collagen is the major protein of all connective tissues, including skin, bone, tendon, and cartilage, and is a generic term that covers a large family of distinct proteins, each having specific structures, functions, and distributions in the extracellular matrix. There are at least 28 genetically distinct types, which have in common a characteristic triple-helical sequence: (Gly-X-Y)$_n$, where glycine is found in every third position (Ramshaw et al. 2009).

Composites containing collagen and HAP are desirable biomaterials since the bone is a natural composite primarily composed of apatite crystals and collagen. The HAP–collagen complex has attracted considerable attention as an artificial bone substitute in the treatment of bone defects in odontology and orthopedics (Wahl and Czernuszka 2006). Due to the immunogenic reactions, careful attention was paid, especially if the source of collagen was calfskin, knowing that the major antigenic determinants are located in the telopeptides at both ends of the collagen macromolecules. Therefore, atelocollagen, from which the antigenic telopeptides have been removed, is recommended due to its low antigenicity (Miyamoto et al. 1998).

A common way to obtain a composite was by directly mixing HAP nanoparticles with collagen solution, but Cui and coworkers (2007) stated that by direct blending of two components, it is difficult to control the homogeneity and the uniform distribution of HAP particles, and HAP is often aggregated and randomly distributed in the fibrous matrix. This means that there is only a compositional similarity with natural bone but not a structural one. Moreover, the weak binding between HAP and collagen results in a no cooperation effect in vivo for bone defect repair. The collagen degrades fast, while HAP remains in the original form and does not attend the remodeling progress of bone. To overcome this problem, a mimetic method was applied in order to prepare nano-HAP-collagen composite that could favor bone repair. This method consists in the immersion of a collagen membrane in a simulated body fluid (SBF), a solution in which the ionic concentration is the same as in human blood plasma. It has been observed that no nucleation of apatite crystals takes place on the surface of the membrane when it is soaked in SBF without citric acid. On the other hand, when the membrane is soaked in SBF containing citric acid, the nucleation of HAP crystals is gradually stimulated, but the mineralization of the collagen takes place only at the surface, and due to this barrier formation, the subsequent calcification inside the matrix is impeded (Cui et al. 2007). Relatively recent approaches that allow the fabrication of bone substitutes via the biomimetic route imply the inducing of the direct nucleation of HAP nanocrystals onto collagen fibers (TenHuisen et al. 1995; Miyamoto et al. 1998; Kikuchi et al. 2001, 2003, 2004a,b,c; Itoh et al. 2002b; Lickorish et al. 2004; Yunoki et al. 2006; Gelinsky et al. 2008; Pelin et al. 2009; Wang and Liu 2014), or the combination of the mineralized collagen fibers, which are generated using a simple one-step coprecipitation method that involves collagen self-assembly, with an in situ apatite precipitation in a collagen-containing modified SBF (Xia et al. 2013).

6.3.2.2 Gelatin

Gelatin shows a chemical similarity with collagen and consists of a mixture of helical fibril fragments resulted from the hydrolysis of collagen, and constitutes a few amino acids joined by peptide linkages (Hillig et al. 2008). It is less expensive to use gelatin as an organic component in composites, and taking into account its gel-like mechanical consistency, excellent adhesiveness, and body resorbability, it could be a better alternative to collagen. For example, a nanocomposite of gelatin–HAP was prepared via biomimetic process, by precipitation of HAP in an aqueous solution of gelatin at pH 8 and 38°C by Chang et al. (2003). They observed that HAP nanocrystals were obtained at higher concentration of gelatin, when a large number of carboxylic groups are able to bind ionic calcium and form HAP nuclei through a heterogeneous reaction. The coprecipitated nanocomposites showed chemical bond formation between HAP nanocrystals and gelatin macromolecules. Composites with HAP and gelatin were obtained by solvent-casting method combined with freeze-drying (Narbat et al. 2006), mixing an aqueous slurry of HAP into a gelatin hydrosol (Hillig et al. 2008), coprecipitation method (Chiu et al. 2012), wet-chemical method (Chao et al. 2015), solvent-casting combined with freeze-drying and lamination techniques (Samadikuchaksaraei et al. 2016), and using embedded HAP nanoparticles with gelatin and adding tannic acid, a polyphenol used as cross-linking agent (Sartuqui et al. 2016). From the mentioned researches, only few were finalized by evaluation of their biocompatibility in cell culture or implantation into defect bone model.

6.3.2.3 Fibroin

Fibroin is a natural polymer that has been extensively used for tissue engineering applications due to its mechanical properties, but also for its environmental stability, biocompatibility, controlled biodegradability, and morphologic flexibility (Polo-Corrales et al. 2014). For example, composites with fibroin and HAP were prepared by alternating lamination of untreated fibroin and HAP deposited on fibroin films (Kino et al. 2007), by precipitation via biomimetic synthesis (Niu et al. 2010), by electrospinning (Kim et al. 2014), by ion diffusion method (Jin et al. 2015), or by innovative method using ethanol as gelling agent (Ribeiro et al. 2015).

6.3.2.4 Cellulose

Cellulose is the most abundant natural polysaccharide in the world, being traditionally extracted from plants or their wastes. The pure product has significant features, such as biodegradability, nontoxicity, and biocompatibility, which make it valuable as an organic part in composite materials for bone repair. Natural cellulose is a semicrystalline polysaccharide with alternating crystalline and amorphous regions, and once exposed to strong acid medium, amorphous regions hydrolyze faster than crystalline regions due to the higher permeability, leading to the obtaining of cellulose nanocrystals with higher mechanical and chemical stability (Fragal et al. 2016). Composites containing HAP and cellulose were developed by the electrospinning technique (Gouma et al. 2012) or by immersion of modified cellulose nanowhiskers in SBF medium (Fragal et al. 2016).

Although plants are the major contributors of cellulose, various bacteria are able to produce cellulose as an alternative source. Bacterial cellulose has a chemically equivalent structure as plant cellulose. Due to its structure, which consists of only glucose monomer, it possesses remarkable properties such as unique nanostructure, high water holding capacity, high degree of polymerization, high mechanical strength, and high crystallinity, making it a promising material in the biomedical field (Esa et al. 2014). Moreover, bacterial cellulose is an attractive alternative to mimic collagen fibers because of its biocompatibility, high tensile strength in dry and wet states, fine fibril network, high crystallinity, and moldability (Zimmermann et al. 2011). Bacterial cellulose–HAP nanocomposites were obtained by biomineralization method (Zimmermann et al. 2011) or biomimetic pathway (Fang et al. 2009), either by alternative incubation cycles of bacterial cellulose membranes in solution containing calcium and phosphorus or by mixing bacterial cellulose solution with HAP powder (Tazi et al. 2012), by using negatively charged nanofibers on which HAP particles can adsorb, followed by cross-link with gelatin and glutaraldehyde (Park et al. 2015).

6.3.2.5 Chitosan

Chitosan is a biopolymer obtained by partial deacetylation of chitin, a natural polymer present in shells of crustaceans, arthropods, and some fungi. Chitosan is a copolymer of glucosamine and N-acetylglucosamine connected by a β(1–4) linkage and is widely used as a biomaterial due to excellent properties such as biocompatibility, biodegradability, low toxicity, wound healing ability, hemostatic property, and antimicrobial activity (Madhumathi et al. 2009). One of the drawbacks is that chitosan has poor mechanical strength, limiting its applicability as a bone tissue supporting material. However, the advantage of chitosan over other polysaccharides (cellulose, starch, etc.) is that its chemical structure allows specific modifications at the C-2 position, and specific groups can be introduced to design polymers for selected applications (Rinaudo 2006). Moreover, to improve their mechanical properties and osteoconductivity, the association of chitosan or chitosan derivatives with HAP to form composites will lead to materials capable of being used in bone regeneration (LogithKumar et al. 2016).

Composite for bone repair containing chitosan and synthetic apatites can be prepared by a simple mixture of the components (Mukherjee et al. 2003), double diffusion technique (Manjubala et al. 2006), alternative soaking of chitosan membranes in solutions containing calcium and phosphate ions (Madhumathi et al. 2009), or a precipitation method and freeze-gelation technique (Rogina et al. 2016). Nanocomposite gels containing chitosan, collagen, and HAP can be prepared by incorporating HAP into a dual system of collagen/chitosan in situ synthesis (Wang et al. 2009) or by loading a thermosensitive chitosan-β-glycerophosphate solution into a nano-HAP-collagen hydrogel (Huang et al. 2009). Thermosensitive gel with chitosan, nano-HAP, and collagen can be also obtained by a biomimetic approach (Huang et al. 2011). Chitosan can be used as carboxymethyl chitosan for the preparation of injectable gel composites containing gelatin and HAP (Mishra et al. 2011).

6.3.3 Composites in Final Form and Their Biological Testing

Composites containing biopolymers and synthetic apatites can be shaped and biologically tested in various forms (membranes, films, multilayer sheets, fibers, gels, pastes, microspheres or irregular particles, disks, or cylinders) so as to demonstrate their capabilities to be used as bone substitutes or scaffolds for bone tissue engineering, which will accomplish the final goal: to achieve bone structure and functionality as was before injury.

In this section, some examples of composites that were proved to be potential materials for bone tissue repair are briefly presented.

6.3.3.1 Membrane/Film/Multilayer Sheet

Composites developed in the shape of membrane or film or multilayer sheet were intended for clinical procedures (like guided bone regeneration [GBR] or guided tissue regeneration), bone substitute, drug delivery system, or tissue engineering applications. The benefits of using membranes consist in a good biocompatibility, initial mechanical stability, and adhesion without mobility and, depending on the treatment recommendation, with or without resorbability.

- *Membranes with collagen and HAP with and without hyaluronic acid* were made by Bakos and coworkers (1999). They assumed that the combination of excellent biological properties of collagen and hyaluronic acid in a composite with HAP will reduce enzymatic degradation and improve mechanical properties in the wet state, leading to a valuable bone substitute. The aim of their study was to develop a hybrid-type composite that should adhere to both hard and soft tissues, with good cohesion strength, and without disintegrating when immersed in body fluids. They obtained a composite with a higher bend strength compared to the composite without hyaluronic acid. The cytotoxicity test revealed that cell culture was not influenced by the biomaterial and cells retained their epithelial-like character and viability. Higher cohesivity of the new biomaterial could offer new possibilities for application as bone implant material.
- An *apatite-like calcium phosphate–gelatin composite* was developed by Yaylaoglu et al. in order to fill the voids or gaps of bone defects and to be able to release bioactive compounds like drugs and growth hormones and to assist/guide bone repair (Yaylaoglu et al. 1999). They made membranes containing gelatin and calcium-rich apatite, with or without gentamicin–sulfate, which were then implanted in the back limbs of rabbits and it was observed that both implants allow new bone formation. Moreover, drug release from the implant was sufficiently long (more than 6 weeks) for use in the local administration of an antibiotic for treating bone infections like osteomyelitis.
- *Composite collagen–HAP in multilayer sheet form* was prepared by Yamauchi et al. and consisted of, alternately, collagen and calcium phosphate layers with each layer of 6–8 mm thickness. The inorganic layer was mineralized by an alkaline phosphatase (ALP) catalyzed hydrolysis of water-soluble phosphate esters in the presence of calcium ions. A mixture of HAP and ACP was formed in the collagen. The multilayer sheet was flexible, mechanically strong, and water tolerant. The sheets having a HAP layer on top allowed the fibroblast cells to attach and grow (Yamauchi et al. 2004).
- *Composite sheets of nano-HAP and silk fibroin* were synthesized by Tanaka and coworkers (2007). The composite sheet consisted of nanoscaled sintered HAP particles coupled with poly(γ-methacryloxypropyl

trimethoxysilane)-grafted silk fibroin through a covalent linkage. They tested the efficiency of this composite for bone tissue engineering by detecting the capability of osteogenic differentiation of cultured rat marrow mesenchymal cells. The experiments demonstrated that the obtained sheets showed good cell attachment and supported cell proliferation. The results also confirmed that the differentiation of cells was well supported on the crystal surface of the sheets. Their results led to the conclusion that the novel composite is clinically applicable as a bone-bonding biomaterial and can be used for hard tissue regeneration in the fields of orthopedic, maxillofacial, and cranial surgery.

- *Nano-HAP-gelatin composite layers laminated* by gelatin were fabricated by Samadikuchaksaraei et al. (2016). A laminated scaffold was obtained through solvent-casting and freeze-drying methods; then the composite layers were laminated using 10% w/v gelatin as the bonding material and cross-linked by 1% (w/v) glutaraldehyde. Nano-HAP-gelatin/osteoblast-conditioned scaffolds were prepared by culture of human osteoblast cells (G292 cell line). The purpose was to achieve a conditioning of this type of scaffold with the main cellular components of the injured tissue, in order to optimize the reparative potential of the graft. The in vivo results showed a notably increased biocompatibility, osteoinduction, and biodegradation of the conditioned HAP-gelatin scaffold with osteoblasts.
- *Multilayered films consisting of silk fibroin and HAP* were prepared by Kino et al. by alternating lamination using untreated silk fibroin and HAP-deposited onto silk fibroin films (Kino et al. 2007). Silk films with HAP on the surface were prepared by soaking methanol-treated films containing >5 wt% $CaCl_2$ in an SBF solution with the ion concentration 1.5-fold higher than the standard. The multilayered HAP–silk fibroin films had HAP layers with thicknesses of about 3–5 μm and silk fibroin layers with thicknesses of 40–70 μm. The cross-sectional morphology of the multilayered composite films showed macroscopic uniformity of HAP in fibroin. The temperature and compression time of the lamination method markedly influenced the bonding strength between the silk fibroin and HAP layers. The osteocompatibility of the final structure was tested using MC3T3-E1 osteoblasts, and the results, together with those of mechanical testing, suggest that this type of composite can be a good candidate for bioresorbable GBR membrane.
- *Composite membranes with bacterial cellulose and HAP* were obtained by Tazi and coworkers in two ways: by mineralization of the bacterial cellulose membranes through alternative incubation cycles in calcium and phosphorous solutions or by adding 0.33% HAP in bacterial cellulose solution and then casting (Tazi et al. 2012). To study

their potential in adhesion and proliferation of osteoblasts, and also in bone nodule formation, the osteoblasts were cultured in bacterial cellulose–HAP membranes for a few days to 4 weeks. Even the bacterial cellulose membranes supported cell adhesion and had no adverse effect on cell morphology, the osteoblasts adhere and proliferate better on the bacterial cellulose membranes with HAP. They concluded that the osteogenic potential of bacterial cellulose membranes can be optimized by using HAP in order to obtain available scaffolds for bone tissue engineering.

- A *composite membrane containing modified bacterial cellulose and HAP* was developed by Park and coworkers through a complex method that involved the following steps: the obtaining of a nanofibrous 2,2,6,6-tetramethylpiperidine-1-oxyl-oxidized bacterial cellulose (TOBC), the use of a TOBC as a dispersant of HAP nanoparticles in aqueous solution in order to favor the HAP adsorption on TOBC nanofibers, and the addition of gelatin and glutaraldehyde into the colloidal solution to ensure mechanical properties (Park et al. 2015). The well-dispersed HAP particles generated a denser scaffold structure resulting in the increase of the Young's modulus and maximum tensile stress. The porous structures of the HAP–TOBC–gelatin composites were incubated with calvarial osteoblasts, and it was observed that the cell proliferation and differentiation was significantly improved, confirming that this type of material could be used in bone tissue engineering.
- *Composite membranes with chitosan hydrogel and HAP* were prepared by Madhumathi et al. using the wet synthesis method, by alternate soaking of chitosan membranes in $CaCl_2$ (pH 7.4) and Na_2HPO_4 solutions for one, three, and five cycles (Madhumathi et al. 2009). The results showed that HAP deposition occurred on the surface of chitosan hydrogel membranes in about 20 h. Due to the excellent biocompatibility results, these membranes may have potential applications in the tissue engineering field.

6.3.3.2 Fibers

Fibers are used to enhance the strength and fracture resistance of materials, and for this purpose, the reinforcement can be achieved using resorbable or nonresorbable fibers, being either short fibers, randomly distributed in the matrix and forming composites with relatively isotropic properties, or long fibers, aligned in the matrix in certain directions (Xu and Quinn 2002).

- *Composites with fluoro-HAP and collagen fibers* were obtained by Litvinov et al. using directed diffusion of ions from precursors' solutions on collagen fibers (Litvinov and Sudakova 2007). The properties of the prepared materials, high porosity, the nanometer sizes of fluoro-HAP crystals, and their relatively uniform distribution between collagen fibers, ensure a good matrix for bone regeneration when implanted in a mandibular defect. The reason for using fluoride ions in the apatite structure was to suppress osteoclast activity and to provide a combined more positive clinical effect compared to other commercial materials when the implant was inserted at the bone defect site.

- A *composite with collagen nanofibers and nano-HAP* that mimics the extracellular matrix of natural bone was obtained by Ribeiro et al. through simultaneous type I collagen electrospinning and nano-HAP electrospraying using non-denaturing conditions and nontoxic reagents (Ribeiro et al. 2014). The morphological results showed a mesh of collagen fibers with fiber diameters within the nano-meter range embedded with crystals of HAP. They observed that the inclusion of nano-HAP agglomerates by electrospraying in type I collagen nano-fibers improved the adhesion and metabolic activity of MC3T3-E1 osteoblasts. This new nano-structured collagen–nano-HAP composite has great potential for bone healing and can be used as bone repair material.
- A *composite with silk fibroin nanofibers and HAP nanoparticles* was obtained by the electrospinning method by Kim and coworkers (2014). They aimed to enhance the mechanical properties of electrospun fibroin scaffolds by uniformly dispersing HAP nanoparticles inside silk fibroin nanofibers. To improve the uniformity and interfacial bonding between HAP and fibroin fibers, HAP nanoparticles were previously modified with a coupling agent, γ-glycidoxypropyltrimethoxysilane. To investigate the effect of HAP content on the morphology, mechanical properties, and biocompatibility of the composite scaffolds, the ratio fibroin/HAP was varied. The surface of nanofibers became rougher with the increase of HAP content, and it was observed that at content higher than 20%, the HAP particles disrupted the fibroin chains, which resulted in a decrease of the mechanical properties. Osteoblast cultivation and MTT assay demonstrated that the composite scaffolds were biocompatible and can be considered a potential material for bone repair.
- *Nano-HAP–cellulose acetate composite* was fabricated by Gouma and coworkers through the electrospinning technique using two solutions: acetic acid solution in which nano-HAP powder was added and acetone in which cellulose acetate powder was dissolved (Gouma et al. 2012). The obtained composite fibers had a diameter of about 300 nm and a uniform distribution of discrete n-HAP clusters with the average size of 35 nm throughout them. This type of composite was seeded with human osteoblast-like cells (SaOS-2) and cultured for up to 14 days, and it was observed that the composite promoted

favorable adhesion and growth of osteoblasts. Both the morphology and structure composite scaffold played important roles in facilitating cell spreading and differentiation and enhanced apatite mineralization. The authors concluded that this natural, open, hybrid 3D nanoscaffold appears to be a promising bone repair material.

6.3.3.3 **Sponge-Like Material**

Because in many research papers there is no clear distinction between the different forms that the scaffold can have, in this section, some composite scaffolds will be considered as sponge in final form, useful for applications in bone defect therapy. As a function of size, number, distribution, and type of pores, the sponge-like materials possess very good structural and physicochemical properties.

- *Composite sponge with HAP and collagen* was obtained by Kikuchi et al., by control of both HAP and collagen fibrillogenesis via management of the starting concentration (Kikuchi et al. 2003). They obtained a maximum length of the composite fibril of about 20 mm at a starting concentration of 100 mM calcium and a HAP-collagen mass ratio of 80:20. The HAP-collagen composite can be utilized as the scaffold in bone tissue engineering due to its shape easily obtained as sponge, net, or sheet, as well as due to its osteoactivity that enhances the bone remodeling process. In another study, Kikuchi et al. revealed that elastic porous bodies fabricated from the self-organized HAP-collagen nanocomposites by lyophilization demonstrate excellent mechanical and biological properties, providing easier handling to operators and better cell invasiveness both in vitro and in vivo examinations (Kikuchi et al. 2004b).
- *HAP-collagen composites* were prepared by Yunoki et al. by mixing the self-organized HAP-collagen nanocomposite and sodium phosphate buffer at neutral pH and subsequent freeze-drying (Yunoki et al. 2006). They demonstrated that the porous composite exposed to the dehydrothermal treatment showed a rubber-like elasticity in the cyclic compression and an excellent flexibility in the bending test with a high shape-recover property. These features can contribute to easy handling of the composite in clinical treatments for repairing bone defects. The implantation of the porous composite in bone holes showed that the new bone formation occurred without inflammatory response. The in vitro and in vivo bioresorbability of the porous composites clearly indicated that collagen fibril improved their mechanical property and reduced bioresorbability (Yunoki et al. 2007).
- A *porous matrix* was fabricated by Cui et al. by *loading self-assembled lamellar-structured nano-HAP–collagen* composite powders into a collagen–chitosan gel and then cross-linking (Cui et al. 2004).

Three-dimensional scaffolds with acceptable porosity, mechanical properties, and composition similar to natural bone were constructed. The biocompatibility of the scaffold was demonstrated by in vitro cell cultures. The MTT assay and the ALP activity indicate that the presence of nano-HAP–collagen in the collagen–chitosan matrix improved the performance of cocultured osteoblasts on the scaffolds, making this composite a valid biomaterial for bone tissue repair.

- *A collagenous scaffold coated with HAP* was obtained by Lickorish et al. via the biomimetic approach using SBF solution (Lickorish et al. 2004). The scaffold had a porosity of approximately 85%, with pore sizes between 30 and 100 μm. A thin layer (<10 μm) of crystalline HAP was deposited onto the stabilized collagenous scaffold by soaking the collagenous construct in SBF in the presence of calcium silicate glass, as the initiator of HAP deposition on the collagen substrate. In vitro cytotoxicity testing of the composite using L929 fibroblasts and rabbit periosteal cells revealed a cytocompatible material that supported cellular attachment and proliferation. Their results showed that the SBF method provides an effective and rapid path by which bioactive HAP can be deposited onto porous collagen scaffold to obtain composite materials useful in the healing of bone defects.
- *Collagen–HAP composite scaffolds* were fabricated by Sachlos et al. by interfacing a 3D printing and critical point drying technique in order to create a network of microchannels inside the scaffold that may permit the flow of nutrient-rich media and maintain cell survival deep within the scaffold (Sachlos et al. 2008). Microstructural characterization of the composites showed that HAP particles were mechanically interlocked in the collagen matrix. Moreover, the collagen retained its characteristic 67 nm banding pattern representative of native collagen after critical point drying. The in vitro biological response of MG63 osteogenic cells to the composite scaffolds was evaluated using the Alamar Blue™, PicoGreen™, ALP, and Live/Dead™ assays and revealed that the critical point dried scaffolds were noncytotoxic.
- *Collagen–HAP nanocomposite scaffold* was obtained by in situ precipitation and freeze-drying approach by Chen et al. (2016). They demonstrated that the inorganic phase in the nanocomposite was carbonate-substituted HAP with low crystallinity, and the scaffolds presented a well-developed macropore structure with a pore size ranging from 100 to 200 μm. The pore size of the scaffold can be modulated by changing the organic/inorganic weight ratio. The scaffolds promoted the proliferation of MG63 cells, indicating that this composite could be a potential candidate for bone engineering applications.

- *3D open-cell composite scaffolds with gelatin and HAP* were obtained by Narbat et al. through a technique that involved the solvent-casting method combined with the freeze-drying process (Narbat et al. 2006). The scaffolds had porosity higher than 70% and pores ranging from 80 to 400 μm. The values of the mechanical properties for the scaffold with 50 wt% HAP (compressive Young's modulus of 10.2 GPa, compressive strength of 32.1 MPa, and apparent density of 1.17 g/cm^3) were comparable to that of trabecular bone. Concerning the biocompatibility, the scaffolds exhibited good tissue compatibility in L929 fibroblast cell culture.
- *Bacterial cellulose–HAP nanocomposites* were synthetized by Zimmermann and coworkers using an automated pump system to ensure a continuous flow and a constant supply of bacterial cellulose samples with fresh SBF ions (Zimmermann et al. 2011). Previously, bacterial cellulose was negatively charged using a solution containing carboxymethyl cellulose and $CaCl_2$ to favor the nucleation of calcium-deficient HAP. Then, the charged bacterial cellulose samples were immersed in SBF at 37°C to allow the growth of apatite crystals at the nucleation sites. Fluorescence microscopy analysis demonstrated that osteoprogenitor cells preferred adhesion to mineralized bacterial cellulose over pure scaffolds. ALP gene expression showed that the bacterial cellulose–calcium-deficient HAP scaffolds increased the ALP activity of bone cells. A preliminary conclusion was that this type of scaffold is feasible as bone repair material.
- A *3D composite consisting of porous chitosan with oriented nano-HAP crystals* was prepared by Manjubala et al. (2006). The authors attempted to mimic the formation of HAP crystals as in natural bone, and they used a double diffusion technique, which permitted nucleating the inorganic crystals onto three-dimensional porous chitosan scaffolds. These were obtained from chitosan by a thermally induced lyophilization technique that yields highly porous, well-controlled anisotropic open pore architecture. The nucleation of HAP crystals was initiated at ambient conditions on the surface of the chitosan scaffold that was in contact with a calcium solution, and by diffusion of phosphate ions through the scaffold the HAP nuclei were formed. The morphology investigation showed that apatite crystals were formed not only on the surface of the scaffold but also in the pore channels and attached to the pore walls. The in vitro cytocompatibility tests with osteoblast-like cells demonstrated that the biomineralized composite is a suitable substrate for bone regeneration.
- *Highly porous chitosan-HAP scaffolds* were prepared by precipitation reactions and freeze-gelation method by Rogina and coworkers (2016). They demonstrated that various ratios of HAP have different

impact on physicochemical and biological properties of composite scaffolds. The cell culture test showed the cell viability of preosteoblast MC3T3-E1 during 14 days of culture, and based on the detection of osteogenic marker expression, they concluded that chitosan-HAP porous scaffolds with higher content of HAP would ensure proper environment for improving the osteogenesis of MC3T3-E1 preosteoblasts, and this type of scaffold can be a potential candidate for repair of bone tissue defects.

6.3.3.4 Gel/Paste

Sometimes, a low tissue integration of the bone substitute can occur due to improper apposition at the site of implantation, and in this case, an in situ forming three-dimensional matrix is more beneficial. To ensure a better physical contact between the scaffold and the surrounding tissue, these materials (gel/paste) are introduced at the defect site in a minimally invasive manner with a special syringe.

- A *composite paste consisting of HAP and atelocollagen,* with seven parts of HAP by weight and three parts of atelocollagen, including a mixture of atelocollagen (93%) and nerve growth factor (NGF β) in different doses, was obtained and tested in in vitro and in vivo experiments by Letic-Gavrilovic and coworkers (2003). The collagen–HAP–NGF β composites have good chemical and physical properties and satisfactory bone tissue tolerance when implanted, favoring the osseointegration. The delivered osteogenic–neurogenic factor (NGF β) stimulates bone ingrowth in situ. They concluded that this system can contribute to the development of new surgical techniques for craniofacial reconstruction, and it could be a new drug delivery device for sustaining the release of growth factors to improve fracture healing.
- *Nanocomposite gels with HAP, collagen, and chitosan* were prepared by Wang et al. by incorporating HAP into a dual system of collagen-chitosan (5:4) by in situ synthesis as a feasible route for bone substitutes (Wang et al. 2009). To obtain nanocomposites with various amounts of HAP (25%, 40%, 55%, and 70%), calcium and phosphate-containing solutions were added dropwise to the neutral collagen-chitosan system for in situ HAP synthesis. Both nanocomposite and collagen-chitosan mixture had good cytocompatibility and could allow adherence and proliferation of rat Ros 17/2.8 osteoblasts. This observation was further validated by using the MTT technique. These nanocomposites with HAP and pure collagen-chitosan mixture had good cytocompatibility and are expected to be a promising material for bone repair.

- A *3D mineralized silk fibroin hydrogel* was obtained by Jin and coworkers via a simple ion diffusion method, based on the idea that silk fibroin hydrogels containing calcium ions can be used as 3D architecture template for nucleation and growth of HAP crystals (Jin et al. 2015). The obtained 3D HAP–fibroin composites exhibit improved compressive strength. The mineralized hydrogel promoted the viability, proliferation, and differentiation of MG63 osteoblasts. The authors concluded that the template-driven mineralization technique can be an efficient approach to fabricate 3D bone-like biomaterial to repair bone defects.
- A bone-like *nano-HAP-collagen injectable hydrogel loaded with thermosensitive chitosan-β-glycerophosphate* solution was developed by Huang et al. (2009). At low temperature, the system forms an aqueous solution with low viscosity in order to achieve the injection but forms a gel at body temperature. By changing the amount of nano-HAP-collagen, the transition time can be modified. The in vitro cell proliferation assay showed that cells (bone-marrow-derived mesenchymal stem cells) grew normally on the hydrogel. This type of composite can be a suitable biomaterial for bone tissue repair.
- *Injectable composites containing gelatin, carboxymethyl-chitosan, and HAP* were prepared by Mishra et al. (2011). The enzymatically cross-linked injectable gels were obtained in the presence of tyrosinase, p-Cresol, and nano-HAP at physiological pH and temperature. The degree of cross-linking and consequently the gel strength vary with the polymer ratios. All formulations were found to favor murine osteoblast proliferation, but one formulation was found to be the most osteoinductive. The stability study in mice revealed that few formulations are able to lead to stable gels in vivo. The results indicate that this type of gel can be used as injectable hydrogel matrix for bone tissue engineering.
- *A thermosensitive gel with chitosan, nano-HAP, and collagen* was obtained through a biomimetic route by Huang and coworkers (2011). The composite system showed a temperature-dependent phase transition with a physiologically acceptable pH modification. After gelation, the composite gel showed good mechanical stability, which might be due to the association between HAP-collagen and chitosan. Furthermore, the gel showed good cytocompatibility with rat bone marrow stem cells (rBMSCs). It was observed that when rBMSCs and composite were co-injected into the subcutaneous dorsum of rats, rBMSCs survived inside the gel, at the injection site, for at least 28 days, and they improved the biocompatibility of the composite gels. The biocompatibility, cytocompatibility, phase transition process, and rheological property recommend this type of composite to be used as a delivery vehicle for rBMSCs. The great

advantage of this system is that it can be injected into the body in a minimally invasive manner to ensure the scaffold in bone defect repair. At the same time, it provides a promising scaffold in bone tissue engineering.

- *A composite paste containing chitosan glutamate and HAP* was prepared by Mukherjee et al. by mixing HAP from Calcitek (Carlsbad, CA) with chitosan glutamate from Pronova Biomedical (Oslo, Norway) in a ratio of 4:1 (Mukherjee et al. 2003). Their study evaluated the efficiency of the paste used as a delivery vehicle for different biomolecules such as autologous bone marrow aspirate, bone morphogenetic protein, and osteoblasts. The bone mineral density and histological data indicated that the paste containing osteoblasts cultured from bone marrow aspirate induces the formation of the mineralized bone. The mechanical data did not show any difference between the groups, indicating that the bone ingrowth is at too early a stage to reach any significant increase in interfacial strength. No unfavorable reaction was seen and so the paste of chitosan glutamate and HAP could be an effective vehicle to deliver biomolecules for bone ingrowth.

6.3.3.5 Microspheres/Irregular Particles

Microspheres can be used either as carriers for bioactive drugs, growth factors, and genes, which will promote the bone cell proliferation and differentiation, or to enhance the mechanical strength of a scaffold when added into a hydrogel (Shen et al. 2013).

- *Microspheres based on collagen and HAP* were obtained by Hsu and coworkers in order to be applied as bone cavity filling material (Hsu et al. 1999). Bovine collagen in phosphate-buffered saline (PBS) was mixed with HAP powders in a ratio of 35:65 (w/w, collagen-HAP) at 4°C, and the mixture was added into olive oil while stirring at 400 rpm at 37°C for 2 h to allow the reconstitution of collagen. Glutaraldehyde was added to the emulsion at a final concentration of 2.5% in the aqueous droplets, and the mixture was incubated for 1 h. After centrifugation, collagen–HAP microspheres were collected from the lower portion of the tube and washed repeatedly with 0.1 m PBS. The osteoblasts reached confluence on the surface of the gel beads after 7 days of cell culture. The activity of ALP increased with incubation time, as cell density increased and reached a maximum after 7 days. They concluded that gel beads of various densities can be prepared by changing the weight ratio of HAP to collagen and are able to be used as bone filling material. Another research of the group observed by using confocal microscopy that osteoblasts grew confluent on the microspheres and displayed prominent adhesion (Wu et al. 2004). DNA staining demonstrated the presence of cellular mitosis of the osteoblasts grown on microspheres. Furthermore, cellular mitosis of the attached cells could be seen after staining with YOYO-1 iodide. Together these results indicate that osteoblast cells are capable of proliferating, differentiating, and mineralizing in the matrix of the microspheres. This type of microspheres is an excellent carrier for osteoblast cells and is a promising bone filling material.

- *Nanocomposite microspheres based on apatite and gelatin* were developed by Kim and coworkers using the water-in-oil emulsion technique (Kim et al. 2005). The apatite–gelatin viscous nanocomposite solution was successfully formulated into microspheres with an average diameter of ~110 μm by precipitation of HAP nanocrystallites into gelatin matrix. This nanocomposite structure contrasted markedly with that of the conventional composite microspheres that were obtained by directly mixing gelatin with apatite powder. The preliminary cellular responses showed that the microspheres maintained the adhesion and proliferation of the osteoblast cells, suggesting that this type of composite can be used in the bone regeneration field.
- *Gelatin–HAP composite microspheres* composed of 21% gelatin and 79% HAP with uniform morphology and controllable size were synthesized by Chao and coworkers (2015). Through the wet-chemical method, they obtained nano-rods of HAP along gelatin fibers, which tangled into porous microspheres after blending. The cell culture indicates that composite microspheres had no toxicity and the proliferation and differentiation of osteoblast-like cells take place. A greater osteoconductivity and bioactivity were observed 4 weeks postimplantation in a rat calvarial defect model and materialized in a new bone and blood vessel area in the composite scaffolds.
- *Nanocomposite particles of HAP and silk fibroin* were developed by Niu et al. via biomimetic synthesis using a solution of $Ca(OH)_2$ and H_3PO_4 with silk fibroin (Niu et al. 2010). By a precipitation method, HAP nanocrystals were obtained on fibroin surface. The newly obtained composite showed in vitro osteoblast proliferation. By filling the femur bone defects in rabbits, the nanocomposite particles promoted the formation of new bone, proving that it could be a promising material for bone replacement and regeneration.
- *Chitosan-based microspheres with and without biomimetic apatite coatings* were prepared and compared as potential injectable scaffolds for bone regeneration by Shen and coworkers (2013). The microspheres were obtained by emulsion cross-linking and coacervate precipitation, respectively. The apatite coating was successfully prepared, and it was found that, after biomimetic deposition, both coated chitosan microspheres presented better cell attachment and proliferation rates

of MC3T3-E1 cells and higher ALP activity and collagen content. The preparation method and the biomimetic apatite coating contribute to the biological properties of the chitosan microspheres, and consequently, it can be a promising alternative as injectable scaffolds in three-dimensional bone tissue regeneration.

6.3.3.6 Disk/Cylinder

Composites shaped in the disk or cylindrical form are frequently used in clinical practice due to the fact that they can be easily prepared, sterilized, and stored.

- *Self-organized nanocomposites of HAP and atelocollagen* were prepared by Kikuchi et al. through a coprecipitation method, using $Ca(OH)_2$ and H_3PO_4 with controlled pH and temperature, proving that the c-axes of HAP nanocrystals were aligned along collagen fibers as in normal bone (Kikuchi et al. 2001). They demonstrated that the composite shaped in cylindrical form with $2r = 15$ mm and height of 20 mm and implanted in 20 mm bone defects in the beagle tibiae had excellent biocompatibility, being able to be covered with a newly formed bone after 3 months. In another research paper, they argued that the cross-linkage of the composite enhanced its mechanical strength by both inter- and intrafibril cross-linkages among collagen fibrils with the increase of glutaraldehyde concentration (Kikuchi et al. 2004a). The resorption rate in vivo was reduced without any toxic reactions. From the clinical viewpoint, the introduction of cross-linkage into the composite is useful for controlling both the mechanical strength and the bioresorbability so that the replacement with new bone takes place in a reasonable time.
- *A composite with HAP and collagen* loaded with bioactive macromolecule, having bone-like nanostructure, and shaped into cylindrical form was prepared by Itoh et al. in order to develop an artificial vertebra system (Itoh et al. 2002a). To complete the rigid bone union after implantation, they used recombinant human bone morphogenetic proteins (rhBMPs) loaded in the appropriate composite carrier. This carrier is a novel nanocomposite with structure, mechanical strength, and osteoconductive property, which is finally replaced with autogenous bone through self-organization processes. The bone mineral density of the HAP-collagen composite increased after 12 weeks postoperatively. In the rhBMP-treated group, the percentage of bone area increased with time, suggesting that this type of HAP-collagen implant is an effective carrier of rhBMP-2 and it may be effective in weight-bearing bone site. Histological and radiographical analyses suggested that the larger part of the composite material was absorbed

within 13 weeks, and the enhancement of callus formation and bone bridging by rhBMP treatment was effective in preventing collapse of the implant (Itoh et al. 2002b). They concluded that HAP-collagen implant adsorbing rhBMP-2 may be a suitable replacement for the existing ceramics in anterior interbody fusion of the cervical spine.

- *A composite with HAP and collagen* in which an extracellular matrix protein (human recombinant osteocalcin) was added to evaluate the effect on bone healing around the composite was developed by Rammelt et al. (2005). They used a commercially available calcium phosphate cement (Calcibon, BIOMET Merck Biomaterials, Darmstadt, Germany), containing 58 wt% $Ca_3(PO_4)_2$, 24 wt% $CaHPO_4$, 8.5 wt% $CaCO_3$, and 8.5 wt% precipitated HAP, which sets under formation of nanocrystalline HAP, mixed with 2.5 wt% biomimetically mineralized freeze-dried bovine type I collagen to obtain a fiber-reinforced material in which they added human recombinant osteocalcin. Cylinders were prepared and implanted in a rat tibia model. They detected that bone resorption and bone formation take place around the implants, suggesting that the addition of osteocalcin leads to an accelerated onset and increases the rate of bone remodeling around composites. In addition, transformation from woven bone into lamellar bone was accelerated around the implants with osteocalcin. The addition of noncollagenous bone matrix proteins to HAP-collagen composites could be a further step to design a bone-like implant with a high osteogenic potential to enhance bone defect healing.
- *HAP-collagen composites containing model substances* with active functional phosphate and carboxyl groups, such as sodium citrate, phosphoserine, phosphoserine/RGD-peptide, and calcium carbonate, were prepared by Schneiders et al., in order to develop bone replacement materials with improved osteoconductivity (Schneiders et al. 2007). They added sodium citrate, calcium carbonate, phosphoserine, and phosphoserine plus RGD peptide in a nanocrystalline HAP cement containing type I collagen, and the results showed bone remodeling at the early stages of bone healing. The formation of new bone was significantly increased after about a month with respect to total bone contact around these composites. They concluded that the mechanism by which these "model substances" mimic the function of recombinant matrix proteins or growth factors remains a subject for further investigation, and longer-lasting in vivo experiments comprising the impact of mechanical loading must be performed.
- *A nanocomposite cylinder with HAP–gelatin modified siloxane* (GEMOSIL) was obtained by Chiu and coworkers by mixing aqueous slurry of HAP into a gelatin hydrosol to obtain a scaffold for alloplastic graft applications (Chiu et al. 2012). Starting with a buffer solution,

a formable paste was obtained that leads to a hardened composite after the sol–gel reaction. The cohesiveness of the HAP–gelatin powders was modified using 11–19 wt% aminosilane. They showed that by using TiO_2, the osteoconductivity of MC3T3-E1 preosteoblasts was improved. Moreover, titania additives revealed good bone formation in rat calvarial defects. The authors argued that the plastic property of GEMOSIL would be ideal for making complicated scaffold geometries like disks or cylinders as well as injectable scaffolds.

- *A composite hydrogel consisting of silk fibroin and nano-HAP* shaped into sections with 7 mm diameter and 5 mm thickness, with the inorganic particles uniformly dispersed into fibroin matrix, was developed by Ribeiro and coworkers (2015). Macro-/microporous structures with interconnected pores were obtained and influenced the composite properties. The incorporation of nano-HAP in hydrogels was associated with the decrease in the swelling property, while the compression modulus increased with the increase of the nano-HAP concentration. In contact with osteoblast-like cells (MG63 cell line), the new composites showed enhanced cellular metabolic and ALP activities. They concluded that composite hydrogels with nano-HAP were found to be more promising materials for bone tissue engineering purposes.
- *An anisotropic spiral-cylindrical scaffold containing chitosan, sodium carboxymethyl cellulose, and nano-HAP* was obtained by Jiang et al. through synergistic functionalization and curled in a concentric manner, in order to develop a new biomimetic scaffold for bone integration and regeneration (Jiang et al. 2013). The in vivo osteogenesis assessment revealed that the spiral–cylindrical architecture played a dominant role in osseointegration. Newly formed bone tissue grew through the longitudinal direction of the cylinder-shaped scaffold, and the bone marrow penetrated the entire scaffold and formed a medullary cavity in the center of the spiral cylinder. This study demonstrates for the first time that such a type of architecture close to the healthy bone structure can promote complete infiltration of bone tissues in vivo, being a promising candidate for bone repair applications.

6.4 Conclusions

This chapter represents a short overview of bone and some composites based on synthetic apatites and biopolymers that have the potential of being used in bone defect healing. Even if there are on the market many bone graft substitutes used in clinical practice, containing HAP, tricalcium phosphate, carbonate apatite, calcium sulfate, and calcium carbonate, alone or in various ratios, for example, ApaPore, Bio-Oss, BoneSave, CELLPLEX, Endobon, Norian, OsteoGraf, OsSatura, Osteoset, Pro Osteon, Pro Osteon-R, Vitoss, and so forth, and also materials that contain synthetic apatites and biopolymers, for example, Arthrex Quickset, Bio-Oss Collagen, Biostite, Collagraft, Healos, PepGen P-15, OssiMend, Tricos, and so on, the presented examples indicate that there have been numerous endeavors to find the best alternative in bone graft substitutes and the optimal way to ensure bone repair such that excessive blood loss, surgical scars, and infection can be minimized.

Acknowledgments

The authors acknowledge the financial support of this research through the European Regional Development Fund, Project POINGBIO, ID P_40_443, Contract No. 86/8.09.2016.

References

Bakos, D., Soldan, M., and Hernandez-Fuentes, I. 1999. Hydroxyapatite-collagen-hyaluronic acid composite. *Biomaterials* 20:191–195.

Cameron, D.A. 1972. The ultrastructure of bone. In *The Biochemistry and Physiology of Bone*, ed. G.H. Bourne, 2nd edition, Vol. 1, pp. 191–236. New York: Academic Press.

Cazalbou, S., Combes, C., Eichert, D., and Rey, C. 2004. Adaptive physico-chemistry of bio-related calcium phosphates. *J Mater Chem* 14:2148–2153.

Chai, Y.C., Carlier, A., Bolander, J. et al. 2012. Current views on calcium phosphate osteogenicity and the translation into effective bone regeneration strategies. *Acta Biomater* 8:3876–3887.

Chang, M.C., Ko, C.C., and Douglas, W.H. 2003. Preparation of hydroxyapatite-gelatin nanocomposite. *Biomaterials* 24:2853–2862.

Chao, S.C., Wang, M.-J., Pai, N.-S., and Yen, S.-K. 2015. Preparation and characterization of gelatin–hydroxyapatite composite microspheres for hard tissue repair. *Mater Sci Eng C: Mater Biol Appl* 57:113–122.

Chen, L., Hu, J., Ran, J., Shen, X., and Tong, H. 2016. Synthesis and cytocompatibility of collagen/hydroxyapatite nanocomposite scaffold for bone tissue engineering. *Polym Compos* 37:81–90.

Chiu, C.-K., Ferreira, J., Luo, T.-J.M., Geng, H., Lin, F.-C., and Ko, C.-C. 2012. Direct scaffolding of biomimetic hydroxyapatite-gelatin nanocomposites using aminosilane cross-linker for bone regeneration. *J Mater Sci Mater Med* 23:2115–2126.

Cui, F.-Z., Li, Y., and Ge, J. 2007. Self-assembly of mineralized collagen composites, *Mater Sci Eng R* 57:1–27.

Cui, K., Zhu, Y., Wang, X.H., Feng, Q.L., and Cui, F.-Z. 2004. A porous scaffold from bone-like powder loaded in a collagen–chitosan matrix. *J Bioact Compat Pol* 19:17–31.

Cullinane, D.M. and Einhorn, T.A. 2002. Biomechanics of bone. In *Principles of Bone Biology*, eds. J.P. Bilezikian, L.G. Raisz, and G.A. Rodan, pp. 17–32. San Diego, CA: Academic Press.

Currey, J.D. 1996. Biocomposites: Micromechanics of biological hard tissues. *Curr Opin Solid State Mater Sci* 1:440–445.

Dorozhkin, S.V. 2009a. Nanodimensional and nanocrystalline apatites and other calcium orthophosphates in biomedical engineering, biology and medicine. *Materials* 2:1975–2045.

Dorozhkin, S.V. 2009b. Calcium orthophosphates in nature, biology and medicine. *Materials* 2:399–498.

Eichert, D., Drouet, C., Sfihia, H., Rey, C., and Combes, C. 2009. Early works and the way bone mineral was conceived. In *Nanocrystalline Apatite-Based Biomaterials*, eds. D. Eichert, C. Drouet, H. Sfihia, C. Rey, and C. Combes, pp. 3–8. New York: Nova Science Publishers, Inc.

Esa, F., Tasirin, S.M., and Rahman, N.A. 2014. Overview of bacterial cellulose production and application. *Agric Agric Sci Procedia* 2:113–119.

Fang, B., Wan, Y.-Z., Tang, T.-T., Gao, C., and Dai, K.-R. 2009. Proliferation and osteoblastic differentiation of human bone marrow stromal cells on hydroxyapatite/bacterial cellulose nanocomposite scaffolds. *Tissue Eng Pt A* 15(5):1091–1098.

Fragal, E.H., Cellet, T.S.P., Fragal, V.H. et al. 2016. Hybrid materials for bone tissue engineering from biomimetic growth of hydroxiapatite on cellulose nanowhiskers. *Carbohydr Polym* 152:734–746.

Gelinsky, M., Welzel, P.B., Simon, P., Bernhardt, A., and Konig, U. 2008. Porous three-dimensional scaffolds made of mineralized collagen: Preparation and properties of a biomimetic nanocomposite material for tissue engineering of bone. *Chem Eng J* 137:84–96.

Gouma, P., Xue, R., Goldbeck, C.P., Perrotta, P., and Balázsi, C. 2012. Nano-hydroxyapatite—Cellulose acetate composites for growing of bone cells. *Mater Sci Eng C: Biomim* 32:607–612.

Hillig, W.B., Choi, Y., Murtha, S., Natravali, N., and Ajayan, P. 2008. An open-pored gelatin/hydroxyapatite composite as a potential bone substitute. *J Mater Sci Mater Med* 19:11–17.

Hing, K.A. 2004. Bone repair in the twenty-first century: Biology, chemistry or engineering? *Philos Trans R Soc Lond A* 362:2821–2850.

Hsu, F., Chueh, S.-C., and Wang, Y.J. 1999. Microspheres of hydroxyapatite/reconstituted collagen as supports for osteoblast cell growth. *Biomaterials* 20:1931–1936.

Huang, Z., Tian, J., Yu, B., Xu, Y., and Feng, Q. 2009. A bone-like nano-hydroxyapatite/collagen loaded injectable scaffold. *Biomed Mater* 4(5):055005, doi: 10.1088/1748-6041/4/5/055005.

Huang, Z., Yu, B., Feng, Q., Li, S., Chen, Y., and Luo, L. 2011. In situ-forming chitosan/nano-hydroxyapatite/collagen gel for the delivery of bone marrow mesenchymal stem cells. *Carbohydr Polym* 85:261–267.

Itoh, S., Kikuchi, M., Koyama, Y., Takakuda, K., Shinomiya, K., and Tanaka, J. 2002b. Development of an artificial vertebral body using a novel biomaterial, hydroxyapatite/collagen composite. *Biomaterials* 23:3919–3926.

Itoh, S., Kikuchi, M., Takakuda, K. et al. 2002a. Implantation study of a novel hydroxyapatite/collagen (HAp/Col) composite into weight-bearing sites of dogs. *J Biomed Mater Res (Appl Biomater)* 63:507–515.

Jiang, H., Zuo, Y., Zou, Q. et al. 2013. Biomimetic spiral-cylindrical scaffold based on hybrid chitosan/cellulose/nano-hydroxyapatite membrane for bone regeneration. *ACS Appl Mater Interfaces* 5(22):12036–12044.

Jin, Y., Kundu, B., Cai, Y., Kundu, S.C., and Yao, J. 2015. Bio-inspired mineralization of hydroxyapatite in 3D silk fibroin hydrogel for bone tissue engineering. *Colloids Surfaces B* 134:339–345.

Kalfas, I.H. 2001. Principles of bone healing. *J Neurosurg* 10:1–4.

Kandori, K., Tsuyama, S., Tanaka, H., and Ishikawa, T. 2007. Protein adsorption characteristics of calcium hydroxyapatites modified with pyrophosphoric acids. *Colloids Surface B* 58:98–104.

Kikuchi, M., Ikoma, T., Itoh, S. et al. 2004c. Biomimetic synthesis of bone-like nanocomposites using the self-organization mechanism of hydroxyapatite and collagen. *Compos Sci Technol* 64:819–825.

Kikuchi, M., Ikoma, T., Syoji, D. et al. 2004b. Porous body preparation of hydroxyapatite/collagen nanocomposites for bone tissue regeneration. *Key Eng Mater* 254–256:561–564.

Kikuchi, M., Itoh, S., Ichinose, S., Shinomiya, K., and Tanaka, J. 2001. Self-organization mechanism in a bone-like hydroxyapatite/collagen nanocomposite synthesized in vitro and its biological reaction in vivo. *Biomaterials* 22:1705–1711.

Kikuchi, M., Itoh, S., Matsumoto, H.N., Koyama, Y., Takakuda, K., and Tanaka, J. 2003. Fibrillogenesis of hydroxyapatite/collagen self-organized composites. *Key Eng Mater* 240–242:567–570.

Kikuchi, M., Matsumoto, H.N., Yamada, T., Koyama, Y., Takakuda, K., and Tanaka, J. 2004a. Fibrillogenesis of hydroxyapatite/collagen self-organized composites. *Biomaterials* 25:63–69.

Kim, H., Che, L., Ha, Y., and Ryu, W. 2014. Mechanically-reinforced electrospun composite silk fibroin nanofibers. *Mater Sci Eng C* 40:324–335.

Kim, H., Yoon, B.-H., and Kim, H.-E. 2005. Microsphere of apatite-gelatin nanocomposite as bone regenerative filler. *J Mater Sci Mater Med* 16:1105–1109.

Kino, R., Ikoma, T., Yunoki, S. et al. 2007. Preparation and characterization of multilayered hydroxyapatite/silk fibroin film. *J Biosci Bioeng* 103:514–520.

Koutsopoulos, S. 2002. Synthesis and characterization of hydroxyapatite crystals: A review study on the analytical methods. *J Biomed Mater Res* 62:600–612.

Lakes, R.S. 2007. Composite biomaterials. In *Biomaterials*, eds. J.Y. Wong and J.D. Bronzino, pp. 4-1–4-14. Boca Raton, FL: CRC Press/Taylor & Francis.

Letic-Gavrilovic, A., Piattelli, A., and Abe, K. 2003. Nerve growth factor β (NGF β) delivery via a collagen/hydroxyapatite (Col/HAp) composite and its effects on new bone ingrowth. *J Mater Sci Mater Med* 14:95–102.

Li, C. and Kaplan, D.L. 2003. Biomimetic composites via molecular scale self-assembly and biomineralization. *Curr Opin Solid State Mater Sci* 7:265–271.

Lickorish, D., Ramshaw, J.A.M., Werkmeister, J.A., Glattauer, V., and Howlett, C.R. 2004. Collagen–hydroxyapatite composite prepared by biomimetic process. *J Biomed Mater Res* 68A:19–27.

Litvinov, S.D. and Sudakova, T.V. 2007. A polymer–salt composite for replacement of bone defects. *Glass Phys Chem+* 33(4):432–437.

LogithKumar, R., KeshavNarayan, A., Dhivya, S., Chawla, A., Saravanan, S., and Selvamurugan, N. 2016. A review of chitosan and its derivatives in bone tissue engineering. *Carbohydr Polym* 151:172–188.

Madhumathi, K., Shalumon, K.T., Divya Rani, V.V. et al. 2009. Wet chemical synthesis of chitosan hydrogel–hydroxyapatite composite membranes for tissue engineering applications. *Int J Biol Macromol* 45:12–15.

Manjubala, I., Scheler, S., Bossert, J., and Jandt, K.D. 2006. Mineralisation of chitosan scaffolds with nano-apatite formation by double diffusion technique. *Acta Biomater* 2:75–84.

Mishra, D., Bhunia, B., Banerjee, I., Datta, P., Dhara, S., and Maiti, T.K. 2011. Enzymatically crosslinked carboxymethyl–chitosan/gelatin/nano-hydroxyapatite injectable gels for in situ bone tissue engineering application. *Mater Sci Eng C* 31:1295–1304.

Miyamoto, Y., Ishikawa, K., Tatechi, M. et al. 1998. Basic properties of calcium phosphate cement containing atelocollagen in its liquid or powder phases. *Biomaterials* 19:707–715.

Mukherjee, D.P., Tunkle, A.S., Roberts, R.A., Clavenna, A., Rogers, S., and Smith, D. 2003. An animal evaluation of a paste of chitosan glutamate and hydroxyapatite as a synthetic bone graft material. *J Biomed Mater Res B* 67B:603–609.

Narbat, M.K., Orang, F., Hashtjin, M.S., and Goudarzi, A. 2006. Fabrication of porous hydroxyapatite-gelatin composite scaffolds for bone tissue engineering. *Iran Biomed J* 10(4):215–223.

Niu, L., Zou, R., Liu, Q., Li, Q., Chen, X., and Chen, Z. 2010. A novel nanocomposite particle of hydroxyapatite and silk fibroin: biomimetic synthesis and its biocompatibility. *J Nanomater* 2010:1–7. Article ID 729457, https://www.hindawi.com/journals/jnm/2010/729457/.

Oyen, M.L. 2008. The materials science of bone: Lessons from nature for biomimetic materials synthesis. *MRS Bull* 33:49–55.

Park, M., Lee, D., Shin, S., and Hyun, J. 2015. Effect of negatively charged cellulose nanofibers on the dispersion of hydroxyapatite nanoparticles for scaffolds in bone tissue engineering. *Colloids Surfaces B* 130:222–228.

Pelin, I.M., Maier, S.S., Chitanu, G.C., and Bulacovschi, V. 2009. Preparation and characterization of a hydroxyapatite–collagen composite as component for injectable bone substitute. *Mater Sci Eng C* 29:2188–2194.

Polo-Corrales, L., Latorre-Esteves, M., and Ramirez-Vick, J.E. 2014. Scaffold design for bone regeneration. *J Nanosci Nanotechnol* 14(1):15–56.

Rammelt, S., Neumann, M., Hanisch, U. et al. 2005. Osteocalcin enhances bone remodeling around hydroxyapatite/collagen composites. *J Biomed Mater Res* 73A:284–294.

Ramshaw, J.A.M., Peng, Y.Y., Glattauer, V., and Werkmeister, J.A. 2009. Collagens as biomaterials. *J Mater Sci Mater Med* 20:S3–S8.

Rogina, A., Rico, P., Gallego Ferrer, G., Ivankovic, M., and Ivankovic, H. 2016. In situ hydroxyapatite content affects the cell differentiation on porous chitosan/hydroxyapatite scaffolds. *Ann Biomed Eng* 44:1107–1119.

Ribeiro, M., de Moraes, M.A., Beppu, M.M. et al. 2015. Development of silk fibroin/nanohydroxyapatite composite hydrogels for bone tissue engineering. *Eur Polym J* 67:66–77.

Ribeiro, N., Sousa, S.R., van Blitterswijk, C.A., Moroni, L., and Monteiro, F.J. 2014. A biocomposite of collagen nanofibers and nanohydroxyapatite for bone regeneration. *Biofabrication* 6(3):035015, doi: 10.1088/1758-5082/6/3/035015.

Rinaudo, M. 2006. Chitin and chitosan: Properties and applications. *Prog Polym Sci* 31: 603–632.

Robling, A.G. and Turner, C.H. 2009. Mechanical signaling for bone modeling and remodeling. *Crit Rev Eukaryot Gene Expr* 19:319–338.

Rodriguez-Lorenzo, L.M. and Vallet-Regi, M. 2000. Controlled crystallization of calcium phosphate apatites. *Chem Mater* 12:2460–2465.

Sachlos, E., Wahl, D.A., Triffitt J.T., and Czernuska, J.T. 2008. The impact of critical point drying with liquid carbon dioxide on collagen-hydroxyapatite composite scaffolds. *Acta Biomater* 4:1322–1331.

Samadikuchaksaraei, A., Gholipourmalekabadi, M., Ezadyar, E.E. et al. 2016. Fabrication and in vivo evaluation of an osteoblast-conditioned nano-hydroxyapatite/gelatin composite scaffold for bone tissue regeneration. *Biomed Mater Res Part A* 104A:2001–2010.

Sartuqui, J., Gravina, A.N., Rial, R. et al. 2016. Biomimetic fiber mesh scaffolds based on gelatin and hydroxyapatite nano-rods: Designing intrinsic skills to attain bone reparation abilities. *Colloids Surface B* 145:382–391.

Schneiders, W., Reinstorf, A., Pompe, W. et al. 2007. Effect of modification of hydroxyapatite/collagen composites with sodium citrate, phosphoserine, phosphoserine/RGD-peptide and calcium carbonate on bone remodeling. *Bone* 40:1048–1059.

Shen, S., Fu, D., Xu, F., Long, T., Hong, F., and Wang, J. 2013. The design and features of apatite-coated chitosan microspheres as injectable scaffold for bone tissue engineering. *Biomed Mater* 8:025007 (10pp.).

Tanaka, T., Hirose, M., Kotobuki, N., Ohgushi, H., Furuzono, T., and Sato, J. 2007. Nano-scaled hydroxyapatite/silk fibroin sheets support osteogenic differentiation of rat bone marrow mesenchymal cells. *Mater Sci Eng C: Biomim* 27:817–823.

Tazi, N., Zhang, Z., Messaddeq, Y. et al. 2012. Hydroxyapatite bioactivated bacterial cellulose promotes osteoblast growth and the formation of bone nodules. *AMB Express* 2(61):1–10.

TenHuisen, K.S., Martin, R.I., Klimkiewicz, M., and Brown, P.W. 1995. Formation and properties of a synthetic bone composite: Hydroxyapatite-collagen. *J Biomed Mater Res* 29(7):803–810.

Wahl, D. and Czernuszka, J.T. 2006. Collagen–hydroxyapatite composites for hard tissue repair. *Eur Cells Mater* 11:43–56.

Wang, J. and Liu, C. 2014. Biomimetic collagen/hydroxyapatite composite scaffolds: fabrication and characterizations. *J Bionic Eng* 11:600–609.

Wang, X., Wang, X., Tan, Y., Zhang, B., Gu, Z., and Li, X. 2009. Synthesis and evaluation of collagen-chitosan-hydroxyapatite nanocomposites for bone grafting. *J Biomed Mater Res* 89A:1079–1087.

Wopenka, B. and Pasteris, J.D. 2005. A mineralogical perspective on the apatite in bone. *Mater Sci Eng C* 25:131–143.

Wu, T.-J., Huang, H.-H., Lan, C.-W., Lin, C.-H., Hsu, F.-Y., and Wang, Y.-J. 2004. Studies on the microspheres comprised of reconstituted collagen and hydroxyapatite. *Biomaterials* 25:651–658.

Xia, Z., Yu, X., Jiang, X., Brody, H.D., Rowe, D.W., and Wei, M. 2013. Fabrication and characterization of biomimetic collagen–apatite scaffolds with tunable structures for bone tissue engineering. *Acta Biomater* 9:7308–7319.

Xu, H.H.K. and Quinn, J.B. 2002. Calcium phosphate cement containing resorbable fibers for short-term reinforcement and macroporosity. *Biomaterials* 23:193–202.

Yamauchi, K., Goda, T., Takeuchi, N., Einaga, H., and Tanabe, T. 2004. Preparation of collagen/calcium phosphate multilayer sheet using enzymatic mineralization. *Biomaterials* 25:5481–5489.

Yaylaoglu, M.B., Korkusuz, P., Ors, U., Korkusuz, F., and Hasirci, V. 1999. Development of a calcium phosphate-gelatin composite as a bone substitute and its use in drug release. *Biomaterials* 20(8):711–719.

Yunoki, S., Ikoma, T., Monkawa, A. et al. 2006. Fabrication of three-dimensional porous hydroxyapatite/collagen composite with rubber-like elasticity. *Mater Sci Eng C*, doi: 10.1016/j.msec.2006.11.011.

Yunoki, S., Marukawa, E., Ikoma, T. et al. 2007. Effect of collagen fibril formation on bioresorbability of hydroxyapatite/collagen composites. *J Mater Sci Mater Med* 18:2179–2183.

Zimmermann, K.A., LeBlanc, J.M., Sheets, K.T., Fox, R.W., and Gatenholm, P. 2011. Biomimetic design of a bacterial cellulose/hydroxyapatite nanocomposite for bone healing applications. *Mater Sci Eng C: Biomim* 31:43–49.

7

Stimuli-Responsive Polymeric Biomaterials

Maria Bercea, Mirela Teodorescu, and Simona Morariu

CONTENTS

7.1 Introduction

The increasing requirements for a healthy life and environmental protection in parallel with the economic and technical progress registered during the last years have induced an accelerated development of new and versatile materials. Considerable attention was focused on stimuli-responsive materials that are able to exhibit discontinuous changes in their physicochemical properties as a response to external stimuli or changes in environmental conditions. Depending on the nature of the system and intensity of the stimulus, the nonlinear response can be very different from the swelling/collapsing of polymeric networks (Figure 7.1) to their disintegration. Thus, new multifunctional materials presenting a high versatility and tunable sensitivity are continuously reported. Smart polymeric materials that respond to stimuli found in the human body have received increased attention as suitable platforms for developing a large variety of advanced soft biomaterials of high interest: controlled drug delivery systems, cancer diagnosis and therapy, tissue engineering scaffolds, injectable depot systems, sensors and actuators, bioseparation devices, and so on.

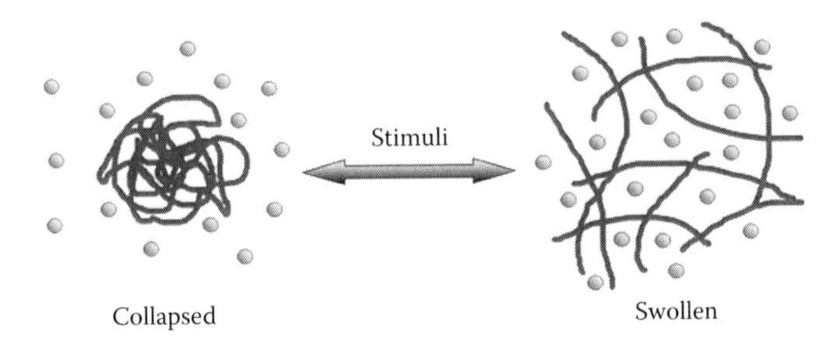

FIGURE 7.1
Schematic representation of the limiting states adopted by stimuli-responsive polymeric networks.

Researchers' interest in the topic of "stimuli-responsive" biomaterials registered a tremendous boost during the last two decades, culminating in a fruitful period after 2014, when the number of publications, as well as citations, recorded a high increase.

The physical and/or chemical cross-linked networks as smart systems present great potential for a variety of practical applications (Bercea 2013; Urban 2011). Hydrogels are generally physical or chemical cross-linked polymeric materials that are able to incorporate a large amount of water. Many efforts are now focused on stimuli-responsive hydrogels with tailored properties for targeted biomaterials (Ciobanu et al. 2015a; Koetting et al. 2015; Nita et al. 2015; Urban 2011). Beside some required properties, such as good biocompatibility and biological functionality, nontoxicity, and biodegradability, these biomaterials possess some distinct features under the action of different stimuli, each within a narrow range of sensitivity, allowing the customization of materials as a function of a particular application. Thus, smart multiresponsive hydrogels can be obtained by a synergistic combination of two or more natural/synthetic macromolecular structures with different functionalities, either by chemical or physical procedures. Generally, two types of stimuli having physiological importance are taken into account (Cheng et al. 2013; Singh and Amiji 2016):

1. Stimuli from outside the body (external stimuli), whose duration and intensity can be spatially and temporally controlled: temperature, light, magnetic or electric field, ultrasound.
2. Stimuli from inside the body (internal stimuli) such as pH, redox processes, presence of enzymes (proteases), or other factors able to regulate the drug delivery process or the recovery of different bodily functionalities. The action of such stimuli is wholly dependent on the physiological state and cannot be externally controlled.

This chapter deals with the recent developments as well as some future trends in stimuli-responsive biomaterials.

7.2 Temperature-Responsive Polymeric Biomaterials

Temperature-responsive polymers exhibit a sol–gel transition by changing the temperature when a viscous fluid becomes a network with elastic properties. From a thermodynamic point of view, the ability of macromolecular chains to change their properties as a function of temperature, in the presence of small molecules, originates from the phase diagram. By passing the cloud point temperature, the hydrogen bonds or other interactions favoring the dissolution are broken, hydrophobic polymer–polymer interactions become stronger, and the entropy term in the Gibbs equation is dominant. Thus, the polymers in solutions exhibiting upper critical solution temperature (UCST) shrink when the temperature is below UCST, and the polymer–polymer interactions are favored. For temperatures above the lower critical solution temperature (LCST), the polymer chains contract and the polymer–polymer interactions are preponderant, determining the formation of supramolecular structures such as micelles (Bercea et al. 2015c; Ciobanu et al. 2015a; Cui et al. 2011; Gradinaru et al. 2012a,b; Trong et al. 2008) or hydrogels (Bercea et al. 2011, 2014, 2015c; Ciobanu et al. 2015a,b; Gradinaru et al. 2012a,b).

The following LCST polymers (and their derivatives) are of significant interest for their applications as biomaterials:

- Poloxamers, copolymers of poly(ethylene oxide) (PEO) and poly(propylene oxide) (PPO) known as Pluronics, for which the sol–gel transition temperature can vary from room to body temperature or higher, depending on the copolymer composition and concentration (Trong et al. 2008)
- Poly(*N*-substituted acrylamide)s, mainly poly(*N*-isopropylacrylamide), (PNIPAAm) with LCST in aqueous solution around 32.7°C–33.1°C (Shen et al. 2006), and its copolymers with hydroxyethylacrylamide (Bucatariu et al. 2014; Fundueanu et al. 2010, 2013; Shen et al. 2006)
- Poly[2-(dimethylamino) ethyl methacrylate] (PDMAEMA) of different architectures (Plamper et al. 2007a,b)
- Triblock copolymer poly(DL-lactide-*co*-glycolide-*b*-ethylene glycol-*b*-DL-lactide-*co*-glycolide) as an injectable platform for drug delivery in peritoneal ovarian cancer (carrying paclitaxel, rapamycin, and LS301) (Cho and Kwon 2014; McKenzie et al. 2016)
- Hydroxypropylcellulose (HPC) (Carotenuto and Grizzuti 2006)
- Amphiphilic diblock copolymer of poly(ethylene glycol) (PEG), the hydrophilic part, and poly(*N*-acryloyl-2,2-dimethyl-1,3-oxazolidine), as the acid-labile hydrophobic part, structures able to organize into micelles, which can form aggregates with multicore structures when the temperature increases (Cui et al. 2011)

The polymer systems with LCST near physiological conditions are of potential interest for injectable hydrogels or implants (Ciobanu et al. 2015a; Morariu et al. 2015). In order to obtain polymeric biomaterials, the customization of the transition temperature and an improvement of other hydrogel properties can be realized by changing the polymer structure and architecture, the molecular weight and/or concentration, or the hydrophilic/hydrophobic balance through copolymerization (Cui et al. 2011) or physical mixing (Bercea et al. 2011, 2013).

Pluronic F127, a triblock copolymer consisting of 70% PEO and 30% PPO, presents high potential for biomedical applications with high solubility in water at low temperatures attributed to excessive hydrogen bonding between water molecule and ethereal oxygen of the polymer. By applying a controlled heating/cooling, the solutions are reversibly transformed from low-viscosity solutions into micelles, polymicellar structures, and solid hydrogels. An illustration of the thermoreversible behavior of Pluronic F127 aqueous systems is given in Figure 7.2 (Bercea et al. 2013). The copolymer response to the thermal stimulus is very fast, and the gel–sol and sol–gel transitions occur nearly instantly.

The presence of a few long xanthan chains changes the viscosity profile with successive changes in temperature (Figure 7.3). At 37°C, Pluronic F127 responds in the first few seconds and the network structure evolves during the next 1000 s. Such a delayed answer was attributed to long xanthan macromolecules. Then, the reversible gel–sol transition is compromised, and the network structure is maintained by the xanthan chains, which keep together the copolymer micelles even when the temperature is decreased again to 5°C. Further increases in temperature strengthen the physical network (Bercea et al. 2013). In acidic medium, xanthan chains are always in a double helix conformation, whereas in neutral or alkaline medium, xanthan chains exhibit a partial conformation transition to coils, which is favorable above room temperature (Brunchi et al. 2016).

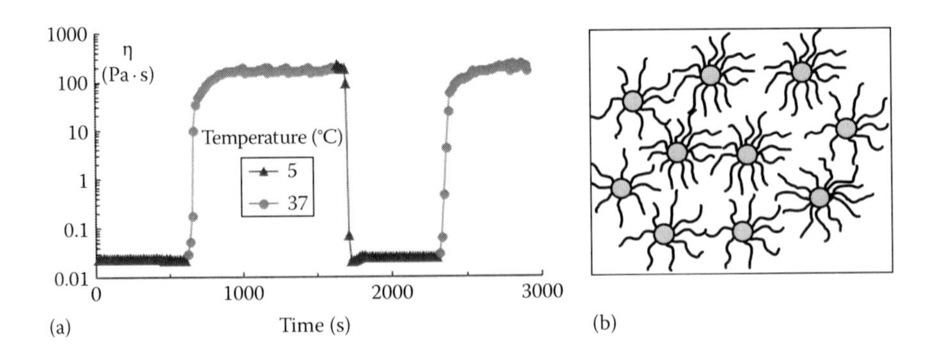

FIGURE 7.2
(a) Viscosity of 13% Pluronic F127 at successive temperature changes (5°C–37°C–5°C–37°C); (b) schematic presentation of micellar structure in Pluronic F127 hydrogel. (From Bercea, M. et al., *Rev. Roum. Chim.*, 58(2–3), 189, 2013. With permission.)

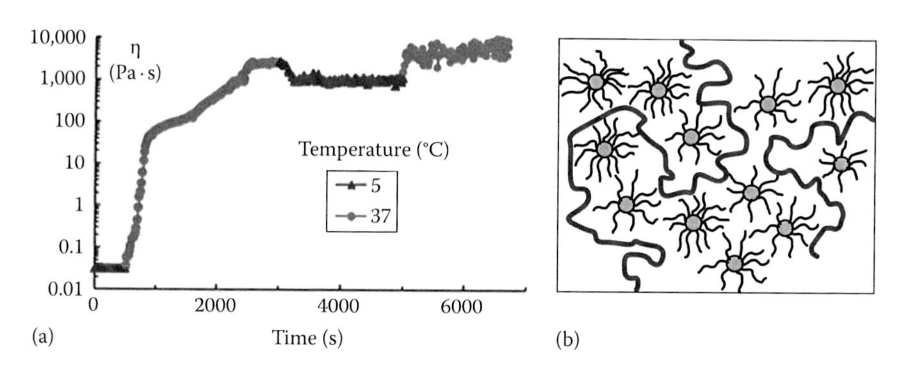

FIGURE 7.3
(a) Viscosity of 13% Pluronic F127 in presence of 0.05% xanthan at successive temperature changes (5°C–37°C–5°C–37°C); (b) schematic presentation of Pluronic F127/xanthan hydrogel structure. (From Bercea, M. et al., *Rev. Roum. Chim.*, 58(2–3), 189, 2013. With permission.)

Thermo-sensitive polymers are important for different biomaterials, such as controlled drug delivery carriers, injectable depot systems, tissue engineering, imaging and diagnostics, wound dressing, and other applications (Gradinaru et al. 2015, 2016; Prabaharan and Mano 2006). These systems, which are in sol state at low temperature and undergo physical reversible gelation when temperature increases to a physiological one, are potential candidates for different biomaterials, especially for injectable drug delivery (Bercea et al. 2011, 2013, 2015c; Ciobanu et al. 2015a; Cui et al. 2011; Gradinaru et al. 2012a,b, 2016; Morariu et al. 2015). As drug delivery vehicles, smart polymeric systems must possess a high drug-loading level because they have to deliver the drug to the pathological sites in the body or target cells without drug leakage on the way or undesirable side effects.

The rheological measurements highlight the *in situ* sol–gel behavior. When the solution presents a predominant viscous behavior (sol state), the elastic modulus (G′) is lower than the viscous one (G″) and the loss tangent (tan δ) is close to 100; as the supramolecular structure starts to appear, the viscoelastic moduli increase and, above the transition point, G′ exceeds G″ and tan δ becomes lower than unity. When the hydrogel structure is formed, the viscoelastic parameters remain nearly constant showing solid-like behavior (Figure 7.4).

Thermoreversible hydrogels with gelation points near body temperature were obtained from aqueous solutions of Pluronic F127/poly(vinyl alcohol) (PVA) mixtures (Bercea et al. 2011, 2014, 2015c), Pluronic F127/xanthan (Bercea et al. 2013), amphiphilic polyurethanes (Ciobanu et al. 2015a) or polyurethane derivatives functionalized with citric acid or succinic acid and ethyl ester L-lysine diisocyanate (Gradinaru et al. 2012a), and poly(*N*-isopropylacrylamide-*co*-*N*-hydroxymethyl acrylamide) grafted onto PVA microspheres modified with succinic anhydride (Fundueanu et al. 2010).

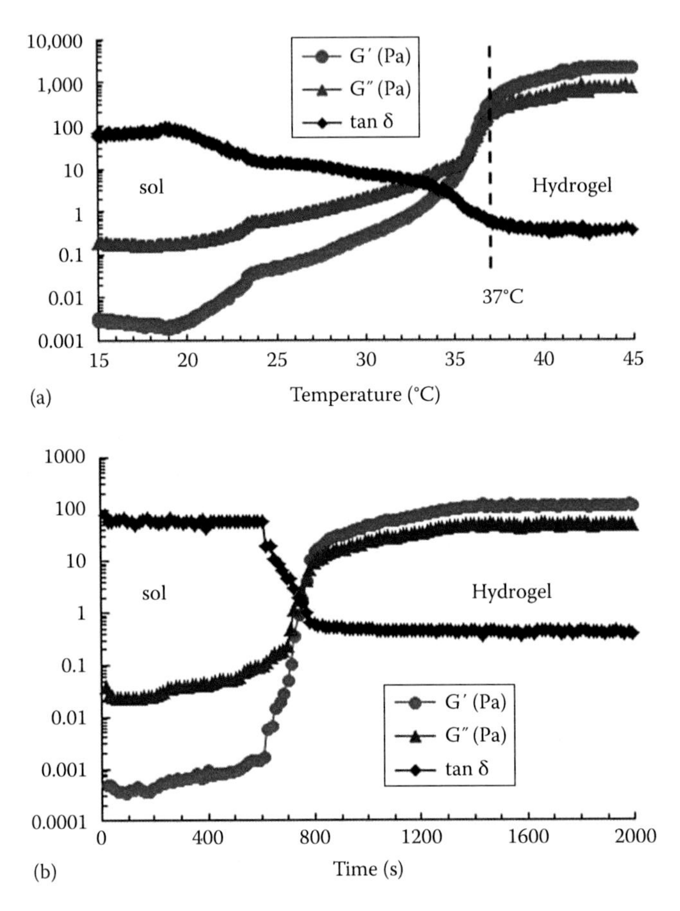

FIGURE 7.4
The typical viscoelastic behavior during sol–gel transition. The curves were obtained for 75% PVA/25% Pluronic F127 in aqueous solutions (15%) (a) during a temperature sweep test with a heating rate of 0.5°C/min at 1 rad/s and 1 Pa; and (b) at 37°C, in the presence of bovine serum albumin. (From Bercea, M. et al., *Rev. Roum. Chim.*, 60(7–8), 787, 2015a. With permission.)

The thermoreversible gelation of HPC aqueous solutions is more complex. A two-step mechanism was proposed: first, a precipitation occurs, which is then followed by the network formation (Carotenuto and Grizzuti 2006). The HPC–water interactions decrease as the temperature increases and the hydrophobic interactions determine the precipitation at a well-established temperature, which is independent of concentration; further increase in temperature determines the formation of a weak gel for high HPC concentrations.

The hydrophobic/hydrophilic balance is influenced by the structure of the functional groups and dictates the sol–gel transition, gelation point, and the gel structure induced by temperature changes.

7.3 Light-Responsive Polymeric Biomaterials

Light is a particularly attractive external stimulus because its intensity and wavelength can be well controlled for a targeted behavior in macromolecule assemblies. Light-sensitive biomaterials, mainly polymers with photochromic groups, undergo chemical or structural changes in response to light exposure, which is of high interest to drug delivery systems, information storage, holographic techniques, microdevices, imaging and diagnostics, multicomponent surface patterning for advanced cell assays, tissue engineering, viscosity controllers, photomechanical transduction/actuation, protein bioactivity modulation, and other applications (Katz and Burdick 2010; Nor et al. 2007; Urban 2011).

In order to obtain light-responsive polymeric biomaterials, specific chemical moieties are incorporated into the polymer structure, such as azobenzene, *o*-nitrobenzene, stilbene, spiropyran, and diarylethene, anthracene, pyrene, or coumarin derivatives (Katz and Burdick 2010; Nor et al. 2007; Qu et al. 2015). These moieties are responsive in the ultraviolet (UV) or visible spectral domains, when the light is able to trigger either reversible photoisomerization or irreversible photocleavage (Feng et al. 2016; Nor et al. 2007; Wang et al. 2015) or sol–gel transition (Priya et al. 2014). UV-induced ionization/deionization influences the swelling/collapsing behavior of the networks incorporating light-sensitive groups (Mamada et al. 1990) or the light is transformed into thermal energy and triggers the gelation of the thermo-responsive hydrogel (Suzuki and Tanaka 1990).

The most widely investigated light-responsive polymers are azobenzene derivatives containing an azo-chromophore group, which presents a light *cis*-to-*trans* isomerization, accompanied by a change of electronic structure, polarity, and macromolecular architecture.

Lee and Tae (2007) studied thermo-sensitive diacrylated Pluronic F127, which was subjected to UV irradiation before injecting into the target site, where the structure evolved into a tridimensional network. The gelation time was optimized by monitoring the viscoelastic parameters and should be longer than the required UV irradiation time. The disadvantage of this system is the traces of toxic unreacted monomer or a release rate decreasing in time (Priya et al. 2014).

Encapsulated drugs that use light-responsive biomaterials as carriers could be activated or released after irradiation with a well-controlled light intensity and wavelength, these systems being very promising for triggering drug release. For *in vivo* conditions, the response is expected to be limited to the near-infrared region (NIR) for bioimaging (Au et al. 2011), diagnosis (Tao et al. 2015), controlled drug release in deep tissues (Cao et al. 2013), tumor ablation (Vogel and Venogopalan 2003), or for curing inflammatory diseases or regulating enzymatic reactions (Wang et al. 2015).

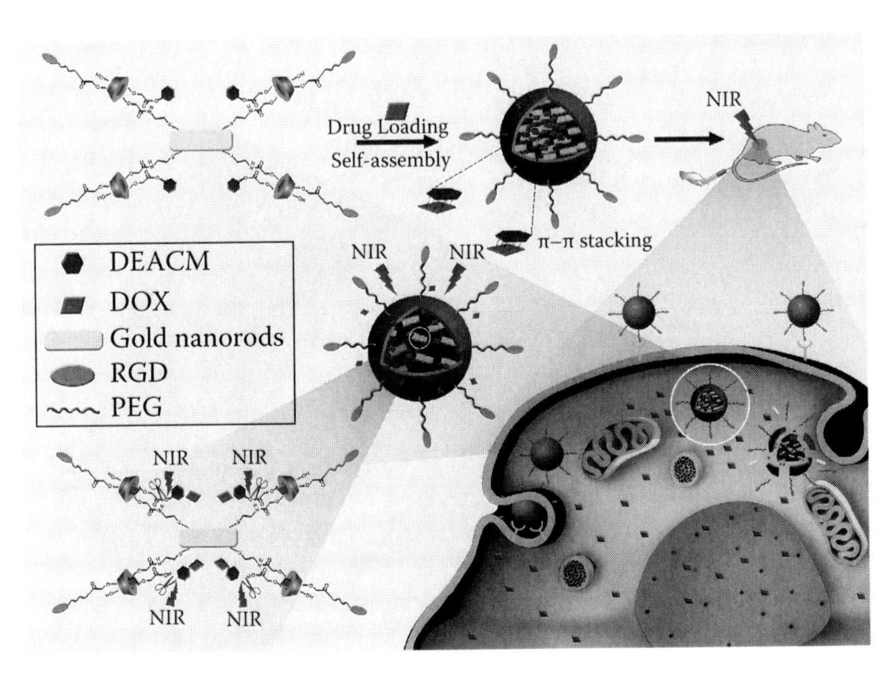

FIGURE 7.5
Schematic illustration of NIR-responsive materials for cancer therapy. DEACM, 7 (diethylamino)-4-(hydroxymethyl)-2*H*-chromen-2-one (light-responsive chromophore); DOX, doxorubicin; RGD, arginylglycylaspartic acid (tripeptide); PEG, poly(ethylene glycol). (From Liang, Y. et al., *Biomaterials*, 100, 76, 2016. With permission.)

NIR light-sensitive hybrid nanoparticles for cancer chemotherapy were recently reported (Liang et al. 2016) (Figure 7.5). The used light-responsive chromophore was a coumarin derivative chromophore moiety [7-(diethylamino)-4-(hydroxymethyl)-2*H*-chromen-2-one, DEACM], which was attached to β-cyclodextrins with gold nanorods. The DEACM bonds become cleavable for a wavelength of 808 nm. For active targeting and long circulation, PEG functionalized with a tripeptide, arginylglycylaspartic acid, was also connected to β-cyclodextrins. *In vitro* and *in vivo* anticancer activities of doxorubicin (DOX)-loaded hybrid nanoparticles with NIR sensitivity were investigated, showing a promising therapeutic effect in combination with chemotherapy and hyperthermia therapy.

Advanced nanomaterials, called image-guided systems, are promising for detecting and monitoring tumors in cancer therapy. PEGylated polyelectrolytes were reported as photosensitive carriers capable of generating reactive oxygen species for photodynamic and chemotherapy with on-demand drug release triggered by one light switch (Yuan et al. 2014). Laser was also used by activating the photosensitizers in order to produce single oxygen to kill cancer cells (Qu et al. 2015). Another new strategy recently discussed is binding photo-responsive host–guest functional systems in which the host macromolecule can recognize and bind a specific structure through noncovalent interactions, such as van der Waals forces, electrostatic interactions, hydrogen bonds, hydrophobic associations, or π–π stacking interactions. The host–guest recognition is now an attractive research area (a host system can capture and release a guest molecule in a controlled manner). Light is also able to control and modulate *in situ* chemical reactions (Qu et al. 2015).

Photo-responsive receptors for anions (Lee and Flood 2013) and cations (Natali and Giordani 2012) were explored in the area of ion recognition and separation. Rotaxanes, pseudorotaxanes, and catenanes are versatile host–guest systems, which are able to adopt various conformational and co-conformational states even in a metastable state (Farcas et al. 2015; Stefanache et al. 2013). The construction and operation of "molecular machines" represent a new challenge for nanoscience and nanotechnology. They are stimuli-responsive supramolecular structures able to perform specific mechanical movements. In this context, light-responsive rotaxanes are of interest for the construction of artificial muscles, as they are able to amplify the contraction/extension of nanoscale motion (Tsuda et al. 2006). The "molecular machines" are of interest for storing or processing information, controlling chemical or biochemical processes, directing flow into porous materials, or channel-controlling protein migration, and changing surface characteristics (Silvi et al. 2011).

7.4 Electro-Responsive Polymeric Biomaterials

Conducting polymer-based materials generally contain a high amount of water and their physical properties are close to the extracellular environment. Hydrogels that respond to an electrical stimulus have attracted high attention of researchers in the last two decades due to their potential applications as sensors and actuators in biomedical engineering, as artificial muscles, synthetic valves, and controlled drug delivery systems. The main advantages of the actuators based on polymer hydrogels are rigidity, which is closer to biological tissues, and high deformation capability, which sometimes exceeds 100%. In an electric field, some hydrogels can show either a change in volume (contraction or expansion) or a change in shape (curvature). The observed phenomena are influenced by the number of ionic groups included in the hydrogel, the nature of the ions and of the environment surrounding the hydrogel, and the reactions of the electrodes. The electro-sensitive biomaterials are based on polyelectrolytes (Yao and Krause 2003) or polymeric networks in which electro-responsive particles were incorporated (Filipcsei et al. 2000).

Electrically controllable release of drugs by using polyelectrolyte hydrogels as gel matrices, implants, or membranes for drug delivery was reviewed by Murdan (2003), Kulkarni and Biswanath (2007), and Otero et al. (2012).

Drug therapy can be electrically controlled by alternative application and removal of the electrical stimulus. The release of the drug from the hydrogel is due to the changes induced by applying an electric field: swelling, deswelling, erosion (Murdan 2003). Thus, these hydrogels are able to transform the electrical energy into mechanical energy, which is attractive for the construction of artificial muscles.

A particular interest was displayed in reactive conducting polymers such as polythyophene, PEDOT [n- and p-doped poly(3,4-ethylenedioxythiophene)], and polyfluorenes (Otero et al. 2012), which can be oxidized or reduced in the presence of electrolytes, determining changes in their properties: color (electrochromic), volume (electrochemomechanical), porosity or permselectivity (electroporosity), stored charge (electrical storage), wettability, and so on.

In some cases, the materials containing electro-responsive polymers reversibly change the electrical energy into mechanical energy and can mimic the processes in living organs during their functioning (muscles, skin, glands) (Otero 2000). New biomimetic devices were also developed from electro-responsive polymers: artificial muscles, smart windows and mirrors, smart membranes and drug delivery systems, nervous interfaces and artificial synapses, and sensors and actuators.

Most of the electro-responsive materials are in the form of polyelectrolyte hydrogels derived from polysaccharides (chitosan, hyaluronic acid, alginate) or synthetic polymers [PVA, poly(acrylonitrile), poly(aniline), poly(thiophene)s, poly(oxazolines), poly(acrylic acid), and polyacrylates)]. The deformation of a hydrogel in an electrical field depends on the applied voltage, which induces the motion of the ions existing in the solution, pH (ionic strength, ion nature, and salt concentration in the environment), network characteristics (shape and thickness), and the distance of the hydrogel to the electrodes (Urban 2011).

The sensitivity of a hydrogel to an electrical field is investigated by measuring the bending angle or bending rate. Figure 7.6 shows the behavior of a physical PVA/chitosan hydrogel obtained by the freezing/thawing method (Morariu et al. 2015). During the first cycle, the bending angle of 26° is reached in about 18 min and for $U = 0$, the hydrogel comes back in about 50 min. By applying a second voltage cycle, the bending angle of 26° reaches the same maximum value, but at a different time (22 min), and the shape of the curve is similar to the first one. During the second cycle, the return to the starting position was realized in approximately 50 min.

Generally, the biosensor devices are polymeric or organic matrices with a porous structure and a large surface area allowing the diffusion of biosubstrates and enzyme immobilization. The patterning of bioelectronics and scalable sensors can be realized by printing or spraying techniques. An overview concerning biosensors based on organic conductors and hydrogels was recently published (Li et al. 2015).

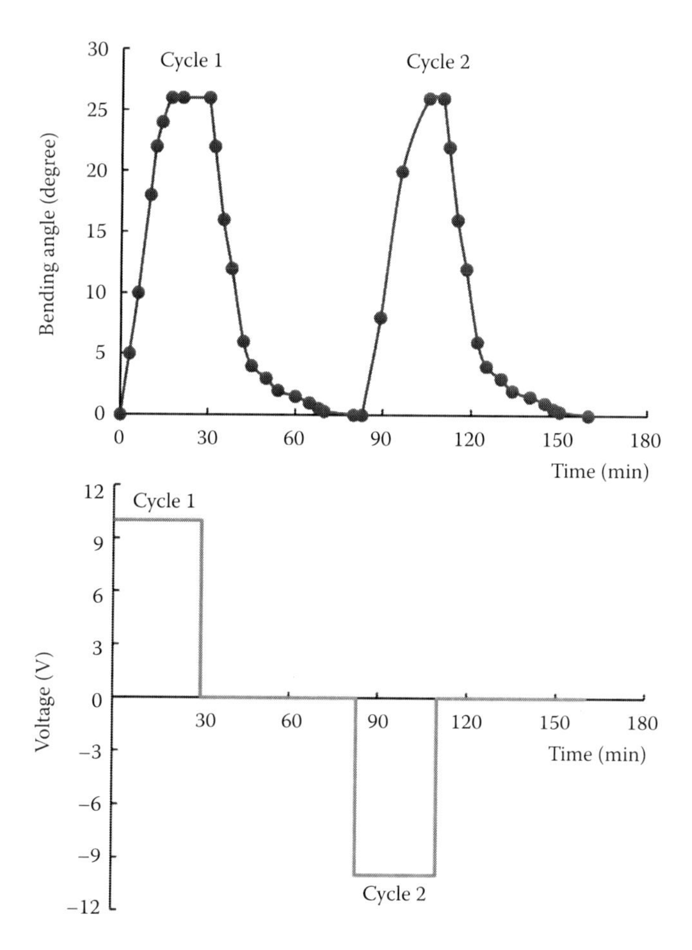

FIGURE 7.6
The bending angle of PVA/chitosan hydrogel when a voltage is applied. (From Bercea, M., *Polymer Materials with Smart Properties*, Figure 6.10, Final report, project PN-II-ID-PCE-2011-3-0199,Romanian National Authority for Scientific Research, CNCS-UEFISCDI, Iasi, 2016.)

7.5 Magnetic-Responsive Polymeric Biomaterials

Magnetic-responsive biomaterials can contain polymer chains, which are either free in solution, immobilized to a surface, or part of a physical/chemical network. Most studies refer to gels swollen in complex fluids, which are able to produce a rapid response in the presence of a magnetic field. Magnetic nanoparticles are often incorporated into delivery systems in order to impart magnetic properties to them. Delivery systems that are sensitive to magnetic fields can offer an imaging modality (by magnetic resonance) for better control of drug delivery efficiency. Typical magnetic field–responsive hydrogels were prepared by incorporating the magnetic particles into cross-linked PNIPAAm (Xulu et al. 2000), PVA (Zélis et al. 2013), Pluronic F127 (Qin et al. 2009), or gelatin (Liu et al. 2006) hydrogels.

In the case of PNIPAAm, the thermo-sensitivity is not affected by the presence of magnetite and, in a uniform magnetic field, a straight chain-like structure is formed. If the applied magnetic field is nonhomogeneous, the electromagnetic force that is oriented toward the highest field intensity determines an aggregation of gel beads, determining their separation from the environment (Xulu et al. 2000). Thermo-sensitive PNIPAAm shell, coating the core of magnetic nanoparticles and loaded with specific drugs, presented high interest in cancer therapies. Loaded with DOX, these nanoparticles revealed a slow release bellow LCST and a rapid release above LCST due to hyperthermia induced by the magnetic field. *In vivo* magnetically guided studies on buffalo rats have shown how DOX is released into hepatocellular carcinoma (Purushotham et al. 2009). PVA matrices obtained either by physical methods (by applying several freezing/thawing cycles) or by chemical cross-linking with glutaraldehyde presented similar magnetic properties (Zélis et al. 2013). The hydrogels prepared by freezing/thawing method present the advantage of easy preparation and the lack of toxic impurities that can arise from the used chemical cross-linker.

Superparamagnetic iron oxide nanoparticles inside the Pluronic F127 hydrogel (also called ferrogel) did not change the micellar structure or the size of micelles (approximately 13 nm for concentrations higher than 20%) (Qin et al. 2009). A hydrophobic drug, such as indomethacin, was faster released in the case of magnetic nanoparticles embedded in the Pluronic F127 hydrogels (the half-time was reduced from 3195 to 1500 min). When subjected to a magnetic field, the magnetic particles from the ferrogel are attracted and pull the polymeric matrix, determining a decrease in volume (approximately 35%) and an enhancement of the drug release.

Smart magnetic hydrogels based on ferrite incorporated into chemically cross-linked gelatin with different amounts of genipin were tested as potential drug delivery systems (Liu et al. 2006). The authors have investigated the release of vitamin B12 from this magnetic-sensitive hydrogel by consecutively switching the magnetic field in the *on* and *off* positions. During the switching *on* mode, the swelling/deswelling rate decreases, while in the switching *off* mode, the original state is recovered. Porosity of the ferrogel decreased during the switching *on* due to aggregation of the Fe_3O_4 particles determining a considerable decrease of the swelling and drug release rate, and during switching *off* the porosity increased and drug release rate was higher (Figure 7.7). By reducing the genipin content, stronger magnetic-responsive properties were obtained for the weak cross-linked network.

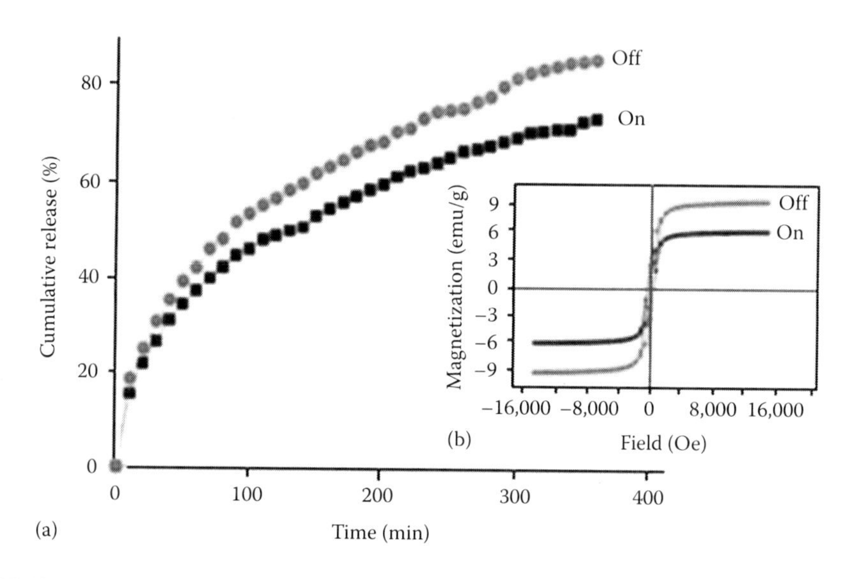

FIGURE 7.7
(a) The kinetics of vitamin B12 release from gelatin hydrogel by switching *on* or *off* the magnetic field; (b) hysteresis loop analysis by using the vibrating sample magnetometer. (From Liu, T.-Y. et al., *J. Magn. Magn. Mater.*, 304(1), e397, 2006. With permission.)

Core–shell nanoparticles with tailored properties were obtained by attaching polymers onto the iron oxide surface. Majewski et al. (2012) have reported dual-responsive (pH and temperature) magnetic core–shell nanoparticles for selective isolation of the transfected cells. The hybrid nanoparticles prepared from PDMAEMA and γ-Fe_2O_3 undergo reversible phase transition as a function of pH and temperature in a magnetic field. The magnetic properties acquired by transfected cells allow their selective isolation.

7.6 Ultrasound-Responsive Polymeric Biomaterials

The major requirements for the drug and gene delivery systems are to improve the drug efficiency in the targeted organ or tissue, to diffuse easily across the endothelial lining without negatively affecting the health of the tissues and organs, and to lack toxicity. Biocompatible materials were used for ultrasound microbubble contrast enhancement, acting as molecular imaging agents in perfusion monitoring.

Microbubbles are of interest for ultrasound-mediated drug delivery applications and they are similar in composition and action to thermo-responsive materials. They can be lipids, albumin, or polymer systems, which are liquids at low temperature and, after intravenous injection, change the phase at physiological temperature. The microbubbles can be destroyed by ultrasound irradiation, ensuring the selectivity of the drug action by focusing the ultrasonic field onto a small targeted region on the body and increasing the ultrasound intensity. The drug lipo- and hydrophilicity influence the rate of the drug release process. Weak interactions of polymer fragments with the hydrophilic drug can be easily destroyed by ultrasound, and the rate of drug release is high. Hydrophobic drugs are gradually released from the fragments of polymeric materials.

It was demonstrated that DNA delivery and tissue transfection were improved by applying ultrasound, after intravascular administration of plasmid DNA in the presence of microbubbles, which act as cavitation nuclei and favor the energy accumulation in the tissues and cells (Hernot and Klibanov 2008).

The main advantage of polymeric microbubbles is that their structure allows the incorporation of both hydrophobic and hydrophilic drugs. Biocompatible and biodegradable polymeric microbubbles with a high loading capacity were prepared from poly(lactide-*co*-glycolide) or poly(lactide-*co*-ethylene glycol) and used for an efficient encapsulation of proteins (enzymes, hormones) without altering them after release (Blanco and Alonso 1998; El-Sherif et al. 2004; Li et al. 2000, 2001). The bubbles gradually degrade in the aqueous media, and in dry lyophilized state, they can be stored in sealed vials for a long period.

7.7 Polymeric Biomaterials Responsive to pH Change

Environmentally sensitive polymeric materials are of high interest, especially for site-specific controlled drug delivery. Among them, pH-sensitive coupled with thermo-sensitive or biomolecule-sensitive systems were intensively investigated and tested as potential candidates for various biomedical applications.

pH-responsive materials have attracted special attention due to the significant differences in pH inside the body: 1–3 in stomach; 5 in duodenum; 6 in jejunum; 7 in colon. The metabolic glycolysis and lactic acid production make the pH in the tumor tissue 0.5–1 units lower, compared with the value in surrounding normal tissue. pH is different at cellular level: lysosomes 4–4.5; endosomes 5.5–6; cytosol 7.4. In addition, the microorganisms' presence changes the biological environment (Karimi et al. 2016; Singh and Amiji 2016).

Hydrogels made up of cross-linked polyelectrolytes display considerable differences in swelling properties depending on the pH of the environment. Their macromolecules have ionizable groups along the macromolecular chains, either acidic (carboxylic or sulfonic acids) or basic (ammonium) groups able to release or accept protons in response to changes in environmental pH. These pH-sensitive hydrogels have huge potential for application as oral delivery of insulin (Liu et al. 2016).

Another possibility in designing pH-sensitive biomaterials is to prepare supramolecular structures as interpolymer complexes (Nita et al. 2014) or (semi)interpenetrated networks. For example, networks of chitosan with PEO swell at low pH (stomach conditions) and can be used for the delivery of amoxicillin or metronidazole in the treatment of *Helicobacter pylori* (Qiu and Park 2001).

Polymeric micelles with a core–shell structure, as pH and redox dual stimuli-responsive materials, were obtained from poly(aspartic acid) derivatives (PEG grafted as hydrophilic part of polyaspartamide functionalized with *N*-(3-aminopropyl)-imidazole; phenyl groups were also introduced as hydrophobic segment) and tested for DOX release, as they are promising carriers for controlled drug release (Gong et al. 2016). Other core and shell self-assembled nanoparticles obtained by using different formulations were tested for intracellular targeted DOX delivery in chemotherapeutics of the tumor cells (Lu et al. 2016). Acid-cleavable PEG chains were attached to amino-functionalized mesoporous silica nanoparticles modified with TAT peptide to form a cationic core. Galactose-modified poly(allylamine hydrochloride) citraconic anhydride (Gal-PAHCit) was used as anionic shell. At pH = 7.4, PEG shells ensure the micelles' stability. A small decrease in pH to 6.5 (as in the weak acidic tumor microenvironment) determines a fast cleave and activates galactose-mediated targeted internalization by diseased cells. When pH = 5, characteristic of endosomes/lysosomes, Gal-PAHCit becomes positive and triggers nanoparticle dissociation. The exposure of TAT peptide determines DOX release at the subcellular level, to the nuclei of tumor cells. Copolymers of uncharged and charged comonomers or containing hydrophobic/hydrophilic sequences can be designed for different pH-responsive behaviors (Lin et al. 2008; Shim et al. 2008).

Due to their biocompatibility, biodegradability, and biological functionality, different polysaccharides (chitosan, alginate, carrageenan, hyaluronan, dextran derivatives), polypeptides, and proteins are frequently used as drug vehicles at targeted pH values as micelles, hydrogels, or nanogels, polymer–drug conjugate, core–shell nanoparticle, and so on (Cardoso et al. 2016; Prabaharan and Mano 2006; Qiu and Park 2001). pH-sensitive hydrogels are also of interest for biosensors and permeation controllers.

Chitosan-based materials, as physical (Bercea et al. 2015b) or chemical (Bercea et al. 2015a) networks, are efficient pH-sensitive systems producing a sharp response to small changes in pH. At high pH value (above 6.5), the amine groups of chitosan are deprotonated and reactive, whereas at low pH value (below 6.5), the amine groups become protonated and chitosan behaves as a polycation (Morariu et al. 2012; Shukla et al. 2013).

A pH-responsive hydrogel with elastic properties, stable in the acidic environment that exists in the stomach, but which can be dissolved in neutral pH conditions as in the small and large intestines, was reported by Zhang et al. (2015). In acidic conditions, the elastic network is formed by intermolecular hydrogen bonds between carboxyl groups (which are not deprotonated) and amide units from linear poly(methacrylic acid-*co*-ethyl acrylate) and poly(acryloyl 6-aminocaproic acid). In alkaline or neutral environments, the carboxyl groups become deprotonated and the intermolecular hydrogen bonds are destroyed, determining a rapid dissolution.

The protonation and adsorption of proteins in pH-responsive hydrogels are considered as being the results of different contributions: chemical equilibrium, the manifestation of physical interactions, as well as a supramolecular organization at nanoscale (Longo and Szleifer 2016). The acid–base equilibrium (and, as a consequence, the pH value) of hydrogel is modified in a complex way by protein adsorption due to environmental changes caused by a specific amino acid structure. pH-sensitive hydrogels are frequently used in protein chromatography. Redox-responsive hydrogels containing peptide are able to encapsulate enzymes without affecting their activity and the resulting materials become sensitive to a variety of physiologically significant biomolecules (Ikeda et al. 2014).

In this chapter, we have discussed only a few recent researches. Extensive information concerning pH-responsive materials is widely reported in recent reviews (Kanamala et al. 2016; Karimi et al. 2016; Li et al. 2015; Longo and Szleifer 2016; Mercado et al. 2016; Shukla et al. 2013).

7.8 Outlook

This chapter has attempted a brief presentation of some recent advances performed in the field of stimuli-responsive polymeric biomaterials. A huge progress was registered during the last years in the conception and design of smart systems that are sensitive to discrete variations of a given stimulus. Thus, the newly developed stimuli-responsive polymeric biomaterials offer targeted solutions to different diseases (diabetes, cancer), delivering the drugs in spatial-, temporal-, and dosage-controlled modes.

Of high interest are biocompatible materials that demonstrate a particular behavior or, in response to a specific stimulus, undergo a protonation, a hydrolytic cleavage, or a (supra)molecular conformational change. The specific stimuli are either exogenous (variations in temperature, magnetic field, ultrasound intensity, light or electric pulses) or endogenous (changes in pH, enzyme concentration, or redox gradients), or the targeted action is a combination of them. The wide range of stimuli and the diversity of polymeric materials able to assemble in various architectures justify the high interest in this topic. The area of applications of stimuli-responsive biomaterials is very broad, such as drug (gene) delivery carriers and in the tissue regeneration processes, biosensors, and actuators. Many concepts were tested *in vitro*, but fewer were tested *in vivo* and it is a long way until it is proven that they meet the conditions for clinical applications.

Acknowledgments

The authors acknowledge the financial support for this research through the European Regional Development Fund, Project POINGBIO, ID P_40_443, Contract no. 86/8.09.2016.

References

Au, K.M., Lu, Z., Matcher, S.J., and Armes, S.P. Polypyrrole nanoparticles: A potential optical coherence tomography contrast agent for cancer imaging. *Adv. Mater.* 23(48) (2011): 5792–5795.

Bercea, M. (Ed.). *Polymer Materials with Smart Properties*. New York: Nova Science Publishers, Inc., 2013.

Bercea, M. *Polymer Materials with Smart Properties,* Figure 6.10, Final report, project PN-II-ID-PCE-2011-3-0199. Iais: Romanian National Authority for Scientific Research, CNCS-UEFISCDI, 2016.

Bercea, M., Bibire, E.-L., Morariu, S., and Carja, G. Chitosan/poly(vinyl alcohol)/LDH biocomposites with pH-sensitive properties. *Int. J. Polym. Mater. Polym. Biomater.* 64(12) (2015a): 628–636.

Bercea, M., Bibire, E.-L., Morariu, S., Teodorescu, M., and Carja, G. pH influence on rheological and structural properties of chitosan/poly(vinyl alcohol)/layered double hydroxide composites. *Eur. Polym. J.* 70 (2015b): 147–156.

Bercea, M., Darie, R.N., and Morariu, S. Rheological investigation of xanthan/Pluronic F127 hydrogels. *Rev. Roum. Chim.* 58(2–3) (2013): 189–196.

Bercea, M., Darie, R.N., Nita, L.E., and Morariu, S. Temperature responsive gels based on Pluronic F127 and poly(vinyl alcohol). *Ind. Eng. Chem. Res.* 50(7) (2011): 4199–4206.

Bercea, M., Morariu, S., Nita, L.E., and Darie, R.N. Investigation of poly(vinyl alcohol)/Pluronic F127 physical gels. *Polym. Plast. Technol. Eng.* 53(13) (2014): 1354–1361.

Bercea, M., Nita, L.E., Morariu, S., and Chiriac, A.P. *In-situ* gelling system based on Pluronic F127 and poly(vinyl alcohol) for smart biomaterials. *Rev. Roum. Chim.* 60(7–8) (2015c): 787–795.

Blanco, D. and Alonso, M.J. Protein encapsulation and release from poly(lactide-*co*-glycolide) microspheres: Effect of the protein and polymer properties and of the co-encapsulation of surfactants. *Eur. J. Pharm. Biopharm.* 45(3) (1998): 285–294.

Brunchi, C.-E., Bercea, M., Morariu, S., and Dascalu, M. Some properties of xanthan gum in aqueous solutions: Effect of temperature and pH. *J. Polym. Res.* 23(123) (2016): 1–8.

Bucatariu, S., Fundueanu, G., Prisacaru, I. et al. Synthesis and characterization of thermosensitive poly(N-isopropylacrylamide-*co*-hydroxyethylacrylamide) microgels as potential carriers for drug delivery. *J. Polym. Res.* 21(580) (2014): 1–12.
Cao, J., Huan, S., Chen, Y. et al. Near-infrared light-triggered micelles for fast controlled drug release in deep tissue. *Biomaterials* 34(26) (2013): 6272–6283.
Cardoso, M.J., Costa, R.R., and Mano, J.F. Marine origin polysaccharides in drug delivery systems. *Mar. Drugs* 14(34) (2016): 1–27.
Carotenuto, C. and Grizzuti, N. Thermoreversible gelation of hydroxypropylcellulose aqueous solutions. *Rheol. Acta* 45(4) (2006): 468–473.
Cheng, R., Meng, F., Deng, C., Klok, H.-A., and Zhong, Z. Dual and multi-stimuli responsive polymeric nanoparticles for programmed site-specific drug delivery. *Biomaterials* 34(14) (2013): 3647–3657.
Cho, H. and Kwon, G.S. Thermosensitive poly-(D,L-lactide-*co*-glycolide)-*block*-poly(ethylene glycol)-*block*-poly-(D,L-lactide-*co*-glycolide) hydrogels for multi-drug delivery. *J. Drug Target.* 22(7) (2014): 669–677.
Ciobanu, C., Gradinaru, L.M., Drobota, M. et al. Injectable thermoreversible hydrogels based on amphiphilic polyurethanes: Structure-property correlations *J. Hydrogels* 1(1) (2015a): 12–24.
Ciobanu, C., Gradinaru, L.M., Drobota, M. et al. Influence of diisocyanate structure on properties of some thermoreversible polyurethane hydrogels. *J. Hydrogels* 1(1) (2015b): 41–49.
Cui, Q., Wu, F., and Wang, E. Thermosensitive behavior of poly(ethylene glycol)-based block copolymer (PEG-*b*-PADMO) controlled via self-assembled microstructure. *J. Phys. Chem. B* 115(19) (2011): 5913–5922.
El-Sherif, D.M., Lathia, J.D., Le, N.T., and Wheatley, M.A. Ultrasound degradation of novel polymer contrast agents. *J. Biomed. Mater. Res.* 68A(1) (2004): 71–78.
Farcas, A., Tregnago, G., Resmerita, A.-M., Aubert, P.-H., and Cacialli, F. Synthesis and photophysical characteristics of polyfluorene polyrotaxanes. *Beilstein J. Org. Chem.* 11 (2015): 2677–2688.
Feng, Y., Dai, C., Lei, J., Ju, H., and Cheng, Y. Silole-containing polymer nanodot: An aqueous low-potential electrochemiluminescence emitter for biosensing. *Anal. Chem.* 88(1) (2016): 845–850.
Filipcsei, G., Fehér, J., and Zrínyi, M. Electric field sensitive neutral polymer gels. *J. Mol. Struct.* 554(1) (2000): 109–117.
Fundueanu, G., Constantin, M., and Ascenzi, P. Poly(vinyl alcohol) microspheres with pH- and thermosensitive properties as temperature-controlled drug delivery. *Acta Biomater.* 6(10) (2010): 3899–3907.
Fundueanu, G., Constantin, M., Asmarandei, I. et al. Poly(N-isopropylacrylamide-*co*-hydroxyethylacrylamide) thermosensitive microspheres: The size of microgels dictates the pulsatile release mechanism. *Eur. J. Pharm. Biopharm.* 85(3) (2013): 614–623.
Gong, C., Shan, M., Li, B., and Wu, G. A pH and redox dual stimuli-responsive poly(amino acid) derivative for controlled drug release. *Colloids Surf. B Biointerfaces* 146 (2016): 396–405.
Gradinaru, L.M., Ciobanu, C., Vlad, S., Bercea, M., and Popa, M. Synthesis and rheology of thermoreversible polyurethane hydrogels. *Cent. Eur. J. Chem.* 10(6) (2012a): 1859–1866.
Gradinaru, L.M., Ciobanu, C., Vlad, S., Bercea, M., and Popa, M. Thermoreversible poly(isopropyl lactate diol)-based polyurethane hydrogels: Effect of isocyanate on some physical properties. *Ind. Eng. Chem. Res.* 51(38) (2012b): 12344–12354.

Gradinaru, L.M., Ciobanu, C., Vlad, S., and Bercea, M. Rheological investigation of thermoreversible polyurethane hydrogels. *Rev. Roum. Chim.* 61(4–5) (2016): 413–419.

Gradinaru, L.M., Ciobanu, C., Vlad, S. et al. Thermal behavior, surface energy analysis, and hemocompatibility of some polycarbonate urethanes for cardiac engineering. *High Perform. Polym.* 27(5) (2015): 637–645.

Hernot, S. and Klibanov, A.L. Microbubbles in ultrasound-triggered drug and gene delivery. *Adv. Drug Deliv. Rev.* 60(10) (2008): 1153–1166.

Ikeda, M., Tatsuya, T., Tatsuyuki, Y. et al. Installing logic-gate responses to a variety of biological substances in supramolecular hydrogel-enzyme hybrids. *Nat. Chem.* 6(6) (2014): 511–518.

Kanamala, M., Wilson, W.R., Yang, M., Palmer, B.D., and Wu, Z. Mechanisms and biomaterials in pH-responsive tumour targeted drug delivery: A review. *Biomaterials* 85 (2016): 152–167.

Karimi, M., Eslami, M., Sahandi-Zangabad, P. et al. pH-sensitive stimulus-responsive nanocarriers for targeted delivery of therapeutic agents. *WIREs Nanomed. Nanobiotechnol.* 8(5) (2016): 696–716.

Katz, J.S. and Burdick, J.A. Light-responsive biomaterials: Development and applications. *Macromol. Biosci.* 10(4) (2010): 339–348.

Koetting, M.C., Peters, J.T., Steichen, S.D., and Peppas, N.A. Stimulus-responsive hydrogels: Theory, modern advances, and applications. *Mater. Sci. Eng. R Rep.* 93 (2015): 1–49.

Kulkarni, R.V. and Biswanath, S. Electrically responsive smart hydrogels in drug delivery: A review. *J. Appl. Biomater. Biomech.* 5(3) (2007): 125–139.

Lee, S. and Flood, A.H. Photoresponsive receptors for binding and releasing anions. *J. Phys. Org. Chem.* 26(2) (2013): 79–86.

Lee, S.-Y. and Tae, G. Formulation and *in vitro* characterization of an *in situ* gelable, photo-polymerizable Pluronic hydrogel suitable for injection. *J. Control. Release* 119(3) (2007): 313–319.

Li, L., Shi, Y., Pan, L., Shi, Y., and Yu, G. Rational design and applications of conducting polymer hydrogels as electrochemical biosensors. *J. Mater. Chem. B* 3(25) (2015): 2920–2930.

Li, X., Deng, X., and Huang, Z. *In vitro* protein release and degradation of poly-DL-lactide-poly(ethylene glycol) microspheres with entrapped human serum albumin: Quantitative evaluation of the factors involved in protein release phases. *Pharm. Res.* 18 (2001): 117–124.

Li, X., Zhang, Y., Yan, R. et al. Influence of process parameters on the protein stability encapsulated in poly-DL-lactide-poly(ethylene glycol) microspheres. *J. Control. Release* 68(1) (2000): 41–52.

Liang, Y., Gao, W., Peng, X. et al. Near infrared light responsive hybrid nanoparticles for synergistic therapy. *Biomaterials* 100 (2016): 76–90.

Lin, S., Du, F., Wang, Y. et al. An acid-labile block copolymer of PDMAEMA and PEG as potential carrier for intelligent gene delivery systems. *Biomacromolecules* 9(1) (2008): 109–115.

Liu, T.-Y., Hu, S.-H., Liu, K.H., Dean-Mo, L., and Chen, S.-Y. Preparation and characterization of smart magnetic hydrogels and its use for drug release. *J. Magn. Magn. Mater.* 304(1) (2006): e397–e399.

Liu, X., Li, X., Zhang, N., Zhao, Z., and Wen, X. Bioengineering strategies for the treatment of Type I diabetes. *J. Biomed. Nanotechnol.* 12(4) (2016): 581–601.

Longo, G.S. and Szleifer, I. Adsorption and protonation of peptides and proteins in pH responsive gels. *J. Phys. D Appl. Phys.* 49(32) (2016): 323001-1–323001-16.

Lu, H., Cui, T., and Chunhua, Y. pH-responsive core-shell structured nanoparticles for triple-stage targeted delivery of doxorubicin to tumors. *ACS Appl. Mater. Interfaces* 8(36) (2016): 23498–23508.

Majewski, A.P., Schallon, A., Jérôme, V. et al. Dual-responsive magnetic core-shell nanoparticles for nonviral gene delivery and cell separation. *Biomacromolecules* 13(3) (2012): 857–866.

Mamada, A., Tanaka, T., Kungwatchakun, D., and Irie, M. Photoinduced phase transition of gels. *Macromolecules* 23(5) (1990): 1517–1519.

McKenzie, M., Betts, D., Suh, A. et al. Proof-of-concept of polymeric sol-gels in multidrug delivery and intraoperative image-guided surgery for peritoneal ovarian cancer. *Pharm. Res.* 33(9) (2016): 2298–2306.

Mercado, S.A., Orellana-Tavra, C., Chen, A., and Slater, N.K.H. The intracellular fate of an amphipathic pH-responsive polymer: Key characteristics towards drug delivery. *Mater. Sci. Eng. C Mater. Biol. Appl.* 3(69) (2016): 1051–1057.

Morariu, S., Bercea, M., and Brunchi, C.-E. Effect of cryogenic treatment on the rheological properties of chitosan/poly(vinyl alcohol) hydrogels. *Ind. Eng. Chem. Res.* 54(45) (2015): 11475–11482.

Morariu, S., Brunchi, C.-E., and Bercea, M. The behaviour of chitosan in solvents with different ionic strengths. *Ind. Eng. Chem. Res.* 51(39) (2012): 12959–12966.

Murdan, S. Electro-responsive drug delivery from hydrogels. *J. Control. Release* 92(1–2) (2003): 1–17.

Natali, M. and Giordani, S. Molecular switches as photocontrollable "smart" receptors. *Chem. Soc. Rev.* 41(10) (2012): 4010–4029.

Nita, L.E., Chiriac, A., and Bercea, M. Effect of pH and temperature upon self-assembling process between poly(aspartic acid) and Pluronic F127. *Colloids Surf. B Biointerfaces* 119 (2014): 47–54.

Nita, L.E., Chiriac, A., Mititelu-Tartau, L. et al. Patterning poly(maleic anhydride-*co*-3,9-divinyl-2,4,8,10-tetraoxaspiro (5.5) undecane) copolymer bioconjugates for controlled release of drugs. *Int. J. Pharm.* 493(1–2) (2015): 328–340.

Nor, I., Enea, R., Hurduc, V., and Bercea, M. Rheological study of some photo-response stimuli azo-polysiloxanes. *J. Optoelectron. Adv. Mater.* 9(11) (2007): 3639–3644.

Otero, T.F. Biomimicking materials with smart polymers. In: Elices, M. (Ed.), *Structural Biological Materials. Design and Structure-Properties Relationships*, pp. 187–220. Pergamon, Elsevier, Amsterdam, Netherlands, 2000.

Otero, T.F., Martinez, J.G., and Arias-Pardilla, J. Biomimetic electrochemistry from conducting polymers. A review. Artificial muscles, smart membranes, smart drug delivery and computer/neuron interfaces. *Electrochim. Acta* 84(1) (2012): 112–128.

Plamper, F.A., Ruppel, M., Schmalz, A. et al. Tuning the thermoresponsive properties of weak polyelectrolytes: Aqueous solutions of star-shaped and linear poly (N,N-dimethylaminoethyl methacrylate). *Macromolecules* 40(23) (2007a): 8361–8366.

Plamper, F.A., Schmalz, A., Ballauff, M., and Müller, A.H.E. Tunning the thermo-responsiveness of weak polyelectrolytes by pH and light: Lower and upper critical-solution temperature of poly (N,N-dimethylaminoethyl methacrylate). *J. Am. Chem. Soc.* 129(47) (2007b): 14538–14539.

Prabaharan, M. and Mano, J.F. Stimuli-responsive hydrogels based on polysaccharides incorporated with thermo-responsive polymers as novel biomaterials. *Macromol. Biosci.* 6(12) (2006): 991–1008.

Priya, J.H., John, R., Alex, A., and Anoop, K.R. Smart polymers for the controlled delivery of drugs—A concise overview. *Acta Pharm. Sin. B* 4(2) (2014): 120–127.

Purushotham, S., Chang, P.-E.J., Rumpel, H. et al. Thermoresponsive core-shell magnetic nanoparticles for combined modalities of cancer therapy. *Nanotechnology* 20(30) (2009): 305101-1–305101-11.

Qin, J., Asempah, I., Laurent, S. et al. Injectable superparamagnetic ferrogels for controlled release of hydrophobic drugs. *Adv. Mater.* 21(13) (2009): 1354–1357.

Qiu, Y. and Park, K. Environment-sensitive hydrogels for drug delivery. *Adv. Drug Deliv. Rev.* 53(3) (2001): 321–339.

Qu, D.-H., Wang, Q.-C., Zhang, Q.-W., Ma, X., and Tian, H. Photoresponsive host-guest functional systems. *Chem. Rev.* 115(15) (2015): 7543–7588.

Shen, Z., Terao, K., Maki, Y. et al. Synthesis and phase behavior of aqueous poly(N-isopropylacrylamide-*co*-acrylamide), poly(N-isopropylacrylamide-*co*-N,N-dimethylacrylamide) and poly(N-isopropylacrylamide-*co*-2-hydroxyethyl methacrylate). *Colloid Polym. Sci.* 284(9) (2006): 1001–1007.

Shim, Y.-H., Bougard, F., Coulembier, O., Lazzaroni, R., and Dubois, P. Synthesis and characterization of original 2-(dimethylamino)ethyl methacrylate/poly(ethyleneglycol) star-copolymers. *Eur. Polym. J.* 44(11) (2008): 3715–3722.

Shukla, S.K., Mishra, A.K., Arotiba, O.A., and Mamba, B.B. Chitosan-based nanomaterials: A state-of-the-art review. *Int. J. Biol. Macromol.* 59 (2013): 46–58.

Singh, A., and Amiji, M.M. *Stimuli-responsive Materials as Intelligent Drug Delivery Systems*, 2016. http://www.sigmaaldrich.com/technical-documents/articles/materials-science/stimuli-responsive-materials.html. Accessed on November 14, 2016.

Silvi, S., Venturi, M., and Credi, A. Light operated molecular machines. *Chem. Commun.* 47(9) (2011): 2483–2489.

Stefanache, A., Stoica, I., Resmerita, A.-M., and Farcas, A. Some photophysical and morphological properties of polyrotaxane based on fluorene derivatives. *Rev. Roum. Chim.* 58(2–3) (2013): 197–202.

Suzuki, A., and Tanaka, T. Phase transition in polymer gels induced by visible light. *Nature* 346 (1990): 345–347.

Tao, P., Shang, W., Song, C. et al. Bioinspired engineering of thermal materials. *Adv. Mater.* 27(3) (2015): 428–463.

Trong, L.C.P., Djabourov, M., and Ponton, A. Mechanisms of micellization and rheology of PEO-PPO-PEO triblock copolymers with different architectures. *J. Colloid Interface Sci.* 328(2) (2008): 278–287.

Tsuda, S., Aso, Y., and Kaneda, T. Linear oligomers composed of a photochromically contractible and extendable Janus [2]rotaxane. *Chem. Commun.* 29 (2006): 3072–3074.

Urban, M.W. (Ed.). *Handbook of Stimuli-Responsive Materials*. Weinheim, Germany: Wiley, 2011.

Vogel, A. and Venogopalan, V. Mechanisms of pulsed laser ablation of biological tissues. *Chem. Rev.* 103(2) (2003): 577–644.

Wang, J., Zhao, J., Li, Y. et al. Enhanced light absorption in porous particles for ultra-NIR-sensitive biomaterials. *ACS Macro Lett.* 4(4) (2015): 392–397.

Xulu, P.M., Filipcsei, G., and Zrínyi, M. Preparation and responsive properties of magnetically soft poly(N-isopropylacrylamide) gels. *Macromolecules* 33(5) (2000): 1716–1719.

Yao, L. and Krause, S. Electromechanical responses of strong acid polymer gels in DC electric fields. *Macromolecules* 36(6) (2003): 2055–2065.

Yuan, Y., Liu, J., and Liu, B. Conjugated-polyelectrolyte-based polyprodrug: Targeted and image-guided photodynamic and chemotherapy with on-demand drug release upon irradiation with a single light source. *Angew. Chem. Int. Ed.* 53(28) (2014): 7163–7168.

Zélis, M.P., Muraca, D., Gonzalez, J.S. et al. Magnetic properties study of iron-oxide nanoparticles/PVA ferrogels with potential biomedical applications. *J. Nanopart. Res.* 15(1613) (2013): 1–12.

Zhang, S., Bellinger, A.M., Glettig, D.L. et al. A pH-responsive supramolecular polymer gel as an enteric elastomer for use in gastric devices. *Nat. Mater.* 14(10) (2015): 1065–1071.

8

Intelligent Amide- and Imide-Based Polymeric Materials for Biomedical Applications

Radu Dan Rusu, Mariana Dana Damaceanu, and Catalin Paul Constantin

CONTENTS

8.1 Introduction

More than 50 years after accessing the market of high-performance polymers, polyamides (PAs) and polyimides (PIs) (in their aliphatic and aromatic forms) are still a key topic of enduring research in academia and industry, due to a remarkable amalgam of high thermal resistance and superior mechanical properties, long-term use, and inexpensive synthetic pathways (García et al. 2010, Liaw et al. 2012). These robust macromolecular architectures are unable to unlock a plethora of alluring features for advanced technologies: highly ordered systems, strength, durability, interesting optical properties, excellent electrical attributes, and chemical stability, among others (Rusu et al. 2010, Damaceanu et al. 2011, 2013, 2014, 2016).

The innate beauty of the molecular structures and commercially relevant traits of these related families of biocompatible and biostable/biodegradable polymers generate a real interest from the medical field. They also present plenty of possibilities for processing and functionalization in order to fulfill a handful of complex requirements of current biomedical topics (Teo et al. 2016).

The successful use of polymeric materials based on amidic and imidic building blocks in various biomedical applications has been widely explored in recent decades, with emphasis on the synthesis of new functionalized materials, with different rates of biodegradation and multiple processing openings; micropatterned cell substrates; biomedical fibers; antimicrobial materials; controlled drug release; gene therapy; tissue engineering; neuronal and electrocardiographic sensors; and others. This chapter attempts to touch on some deep insights into the considerable potential of these polymeric materials in several biomedical areas, by reviewing some of the new concepts of molecular design, physical and chemical features of interest for the envisaged area, functionalization potential, processing opportunities, and some clinical trials.

8.2 Aliphatic Polyamides

Aliphatic PAs (frequently referred to as nylons) are remarkable engineering materials that found their way into the biomedical field due to a plethora of outstanding mechanical features. Nylons are already available on the biomarket as sutures, wound dressings, medical tubing, and implants, further proof of their biocompatibility for applications with short-, mid-, and long-term contact with the human body. PAs are linear semicrystalline, thermoplastic macromolecules that generally consist of saturated alkyl segments connected through amide groups, the number of C atoms dividing the

N ones being responsible for a particular kind of nylon (PA6, PA46, PA66, PA11, etc.). Any variation in the number of C atoms leads to different properties in terms of toughness, hardness, softness, and resilience (Negoro 2005). Even if generally considered immune to microbial and enzymatic actions, PAs do slowly hydrolyze. The low biodegradation rate is determined by the regular, rather short repeating units, organized into highly ordered structures held together by strong hydrogen interchain interactions (Bianco et al. 1997). Any mutation in this high order (flexible units, hydrophilic motifs, various main-chain substituents) alters the stability toward hydrolysis.

8.2.1 Antimicrobial Materials

Antimicrobial nylon-based macromolecular architectures are a family of new advanced bioactive materials fueled by two main health care–related industries: wound dressings and antimicrobial textiles. The most-used approach to generate antimicrobial features of aliphatic PAs is the inclusion of specific bioactive compounds in the polymer matrix by using different chemical and physical tools, from covalent connection in the early stages to blending or coating in the finishing ones. The main antimicrobial agents used for nylons are (Morais et al. 2016) metals and metallic salts (Ag, ZnO, TiO_2), triclosan, polybiguanidines, quaternary ammonium compounds, N-halamines, and chitosan. They display different action modes and specific advantages and drawbacks. Industrial research in the field developed commercial products like X-STATIC®, SilveR.STAT®, Meryl® Skinlife, and Nylcare®, generally using Ag as the bioactive agent.

Recent years have seen the rise of new nylon-like structures as clinically relevant materials, namely, membrane-active cationic polymeric antimicrobials. The most active in this field are Gellman and coworkers, their intensive research in modulating the structural features of cationic nylon 3-based polymers leading to a new genre of effective, broad-spectrum antimicrobial aliphatic PAs (Ganewatta and Tang 2015). They developed PAs with robust bioactivity and proper biocompatibility, by employing (different, analogous, or isomeric) cyclic and/or acyclic hydrophobic subunits in the relatively easy construction of protein-like polymeric backbones and binary or tertiary sequence-random copolymers. Some of their materials display a concentration-dependent antimicrobial action: at low concentrations, nylon 3 polymers permeate the membrane of the bacteria, bind to intracellular DNA, and impart cell death without lysis; membrane lysis comes into play when moving to high concentrations. The group thoroughly investigated the effect of similar structural units, chain length, and chain end on the bioactivity of their PAs. Binary copolyamides containing cyclohexane hydrophobic groups were then prepared by anionic ring-opening polymerization and showed the capacity to surpass the difficulty of achieving similar activities against fungi compared to bacteria while still being hemocompatible. The group functionalized the N and C termini of the random amidic copolymers and studied the impact on biological activity, obtaining better selectivity for the N-terminal modification and higher hemolysis for the C ones. They have also optimized the selectivity of their cationic–hydrophobic copolymers by incorporating homoglycine and honoserine in tertiary nylon 3 systems and modulating the ration between hydrophobic, hydrophilic, and cationic motifs.

8.2.2 Sutures

Nylons are leading biomaterials in the surgical sutures market, due to a handful of desirable features like excellent mechanical properties, good handling, knot security, low tissue reactivity, and low cost (Maitz 2015), and have been used for almost 50 years now as nonabsorbable (or rather, very slowly absorbable) sutures for slow-healing or highly mechanically exposed tissues, like skin or tendons. PA6 and PA66 are the most preferred materials from this family, along with other homopolymers like PA 610, PA12, and PA61 (Gupta et al. 2008). PAs with molecular weights around 5 kDa and tensile strengths of 900–1000 MPa are usually used, and the polymeric material can be structured so as to maintain certain strength along a complete particular healing process. Commercial nylon sutures are available in different physical configurations of the threads (monofilament or braided), which impact key biological effects, especially wound infection (Chu 2008). Some of the most common trade names are monofilament Dermalon™, Monosof™, Ethilon™, Nylene®, Surulon®, Supramid®, braided Surgilon®, Nurolon®, and the core-sheath (a twisted PA66 core and a PA6 jacket) Supramid Extra®. The only downside of nylon wound closure materials is their relatively high packaging memory (the innate propensity to return to the original shape after usage), a feature related to their stiffness, especially in the monofilament case. This issue is tackled in surgical practice by additional knots.

The hottest topic in the field is the incorporation of bioactive agents in nylons to achieve various antimicrobial properties. A wide range of chemical tools were employed to impart a destructive or inhibiting behavior toward microorganisms growth, from nanostructuration (Kim and Michielsen 2015) and I_2 or Ag (Gupta et al. 2008, Pant et al. 2012, Kleyi et al. 2014) doping to drug binding or antibiotics immobilization (Gupta et al. 2008) to the internal or outer structure of nylon sutures.

8.2.3 Catheters

Aliphatic PAs and block copolymers made therefrom are the star polymers in the field of medical tubing. The tensile strength that they are able to provide to these load-bearing devices makes them the materials of choice in the catheter market, from urology catheters to angioplasty, stent delivery, or balloon catheters (Maitz 2015). Several drawbacks associated with the use of intravascular catheters in diagnostic or interventional maneuvers, like structural integrity, specific functional properties, or delamination issues (Pruitt and

Furmanski 2009), lead to consecutive design evolutions, from single polymeric materials (like nylon, polyethylene, or polyethylene terephthalate) to quite intelligent polymeric systems. One example is the so-called polyether-block-amides (PEBAS), block copolymers that combine through ester bridges the rigidity of aliphatic PAs (usually PA11) with the softness of polyethers (usually polytetramethylene oxide) (Todros et al. 2013). They covalently blend hard polyamidic domains containing interchain hydrogen bonding with flexible polyether areas where loose dipole–dipole forces come into play. The final material allows a wide range of flexibility by manipulating the soft block content, together with prime mechanical and chemical resistance and excellent processing ease. Biocompatible thermoplastic elastomers of this type, marketed by Arkema under the trade name Pebax®, are widely used in medical tubing and standard cardiovascular devices. The same producer commercializes tougher, still flexible polyamidic materials, known as Rilsan®MED (PA11 and PA12), which are designed for similar applications in which "pushability" and burst strength are top requirements.

Intensive research in the field of electrospun PA6 nanofibers loaded with metal ions (mostly Ag) (Pant et al. 2012, Kleyi et al. 2014) developed materials with a broad spectrum of antimicrobial properties, which could be used to dress the surface of catheters or other medical tubing.

8.2.4 Implants

Nylon-type biomaterials are also suitable for implant-related applications, especially prostheses. Nevertheless, special attention has to be paid to their hydrolytic degradation and subsequent infections. A documented case (Dang et al. 2014) is related to PA6 intrauterine contraceptive devices prone to hydrolytic and stress-cracking deterioration leading to several types of inflammation.

Biocompatible nylon in combination with a thermoplastic resin has been used for more than 60 years under the Valplast® brand for flexible partial dental prosthesis, providing a resistant, esthetic, and functional choice for traditional metal-based removable partial dentures. Nylon-based Supramid foils are considered safe and effective implant materials for the restoration of orbital fractures with a low complication rate (Timoney et al. 2014). Supramid meshes have been successfully used for more than three decade as synthetic facial implants (Quatela and Chow 2008) but are guilty of a foreign body response and chronic inflammation, paving the way for extra research.

Due to time-related issues in the field, computational methods are widely used to evaluate the performance of nylon-based materials as efficient prosthesis. For example, highly cold-drawn, twisted PA66 fibers were tested *in silico* as artificial muscles (Sharafi and Li 2015), the obtained mechanistic insights serving as useful tools for the design and development of nylon-based polymeric muscles. Carbon fiber/PA12/hydroxyapatite composites were tested *in silico* as hip stems, being predicted to display superior features to their metallic counterparts (Scholz et al. 2011). Several studies (Huang et al. 2014) have confirmed *in vivo* the potential of hydroxyapatite/PA composites to be applied in redressing bone defects. Moreover, Riel and coworkers (Scholz et al. 2011) used fiberglass/nylon composites to build a prosthetic arm kit successfully used by a Canadian cyclist at the 2008 Paralympic Games.

The rising field of 3D printing also considers nylons and their composites to build unique, patient-specific implants. A team from the Welsh Centre for Printing and Coating has used Taulman Nylon 645 filament (a copolymer of PA 69, PA 6, and PA 6T) to print cartilage joint replacements with several intricate chambers for bone attachment, which under extensive stress testing showed zero delamination (Thomas 2014). The same team used a new material called Samsonium (nylon/titanium composite) for 3D printed, more durable knee implants. The impact-absorbing material brings an excellent tensile strength in a new 3D printing filament and is a feasible replacement for collagen fibers and matrix, which downgrade due to arthritis (Millsaps 2015).

8.2.5 Tissue Engineering

Aliphatic PAs, PA6 in particular, have proven to be suitable candidates for hard tissue engineering, especially as scaffolds for osteoblasts and bone repair, since PA6 and collagen have similar chemical structures (Abdal-hay et al. 2013a,b). Hybrid nylon composites induce greater functionality and performance as compared to the pure organic polymer and are able to solve several issues like low hydrophilicity and insufficient bone biocompatibility. Therefore, several pathways were followed by using different proper inorganic/organic constituents and various preparation (mostly electrospinning) methods. Nirmala et al. have produced ultrafine, homogeneous porous fibers of PA6/lecithin composites as osteoblasts scaffolds and tested them in bone regeneration. They showed some mechanical drawbacks but proved worthy in engineering hard tissue *in vitro* for further transplantation. The same team developed PA6/chitosan high-aspect ratio nanofibers with a distinct spider-net-like structure to be used as cell culture scaffolds (Nirmala et al. 2011). Kim et al. have also used natural chitosan to impart hydrophilicity and cellular recognition sites (Shrestha et al. 2016) and studied *in vitro* the optimal biopolymer concentration (20 wt%) so as to provide biomimetic and biocompatible electrospun nanofibrous scaffolds. Kim et al. used chitin butyrate to coat the surface of PA6 nanofibers by single-spinneret electrospinning and obtained various phase-separated morphologies suitable for bone cell culture (Pant et al. 2013a). Lim and coworkers tried to mimic the extracellular matrix of bone tissue by nucleating and uniformly coating PA6 electrospun fibers with aligned, ultrafine bone-like apatite nanorods through a hydrothermal approach (Abdal-hay et al. 2013a). The method modified the crystallinity of the nylon and received a promising biological response. When spherical hydroxyapatite and PA66 were used, the obtained composites displayed a compressive strength close to natural bone and suitable cell growth, proliferation, and differentiation (Zhang et al. 2014). Core–shell structured PA6/lactic acid nanofibers have also shown increased bone biocompatibility as compared to the single polymer (Pant et al. 2013b) and a good proliferation capacity of the composite mat (Pant et al. 2013c). When Lim et al. (Abdal-hay et al. 2013b) used the simple CaP motif to coat the surface of PA6 nanofibers so as to mimic the mineralized hard tissue, they obtained an efficient cell proliferation response, depending upon the coating technique. Migliaresi et al. showed that even PA6/multiwalled carbon nanotube composites show favorable features for osteoblasts cultures, like induced cell cytoskeleton alignment, short-term enhanced cell proliferation, and proper mechanical properties (Volpato et al. 2011).

Nylons can also be used as scaffolds for ligament, tendon (Maitz 2015), and skin (Patel and Fisher 2008) repair, some materials even being on the market, like Biobrane® (biocomposite of nylon, silicone, and porcine collagen) or TransCyte® (human fibroblast cells cultured on nylon mesh).

8.2.6 Drug Delivery

Nylons have also made it into the wide field of drug delivery, being already commercially available in the form of transdermal therapeutic systems that operate as drug reservoirs. An example is the Smopex® 108 fiber (a polyethylene backbone grafted with PAs), an ion-exchange fiber incorporating therapeutic agents for targeted delivery (Zhu and Yu 2008). In the quest for more efficient drug performances, many researchers are dealing with the modification of aliphatic PAs to be used in various therapeutic systems.

Neuse and coworkers synthesized linear PAs integrating an ethylene ligand system to be used as water-soluble Pt conjugates (Neuse et al. 1996). They also enhanced polyamidic backbones (aspartamides and amidoamines) with several pairs of carboxylic side groups for Pt binding, in order to use them as antiproliferative agents for cancerous diseases (Komane et al. 2008). These polymers showed cytotoxic activities above *cisplatin* or simple Pt-coordinating polymeric standards but require extended screening to gain commercial relevance.

Mager et al. structured a stimuli-responsive PA nanogel by employing a self-assembling, amphiphilic PA backbone containing glutamic acid and putrescine and ethyleneglycol/thiopropionic acid side-chain motifs (Prasad et al. 2015). These versatile gels are able to impound hydrophobic bioactive agents and release them under the action of glutathione.

Pillai et al. built a copolyamide incorporating spermine and aspartic acid and connected it to polyethylene glycol so as to obtain nonviral gene delivery vehicles (Viola et al. 2008). They condensed different DNAs on this water-soluble polycationic structure and obtained several block ionomer complexes with various charge ratios, which displayed compact, nano-/micrometer-sized particles essential for gene delivery.

8.3 Aromatic Polyamides

One of the most important factors that differentiate biomaterials from others is their ability to ensure responsive contact with human tissues, biocompatibility being a basic concept within biomaterials science. Aromatic moieties play a key role in this regard, producing π–π interactions with, for example, unsaturated fatty acids which differentiate microbial and human cytoplasmic membranes (Yeaman and Yount 2003). Furthermore, aromatic rings are known bioisosteres of polyunsaturated fatty acids, which are involved in inflammatory processes and have antimicrobial activity, being primarily effective against gram-positive bacteria (Knapp and Melly 1986, Bergsson et al. 2001, Kelsey et al. 2006, Seo et al. 2012). As a consequence, aromatic PAs are important players in the field, having outstanding antimicrobial activity (Liu et al. 2004).

8.3.1 DNA-Interactive Applications

DNA-targeting drugs are widely used in human cancer treatment, considerable evidence being provided for the binding of these agents to preferred DNA sequences. However, the ability of some agents to recognize specific DNA sequences has not previously been considered a significant factor in their anticancer activity. Kotecha et al. recently showed that a PA directed against the binding site of NF-Y in the topoisomerase IIa promoter was able to inhibit NF-Y binding and alter gene expression in confluent cells (Kotecha et al. 2008). Other studies have shown that PAs can modulate gene expression *in vivo* (Matsuda et al. 2006). By all criteria used (electrophoretic mobility shift assays (EMSA), deoxyribonuclease (DNase) I footprint, chromatin immunoprecipitation (ChIP), and expression analysis), the di-butyl phthalate (PBD)–PA conjugate GWL-78 (a pyrrolobenzodiazepine-poly(N-methylpyrrole) conjugate) shown in Figure 8.1 displays the ability to inhibit specific DNA-protein interactions. Its cellular penetration and consequent modulation of gene transcription suggest that such agents can target the cellular transcription machinery. The balance between the cytotoxicity and transcriptional effects will be a critical factor in their therapeutic application and needs further investigation.

Another direction in DNA-interactive applications is the development of chemical approaches for the regulation of gene expression in cell culture.

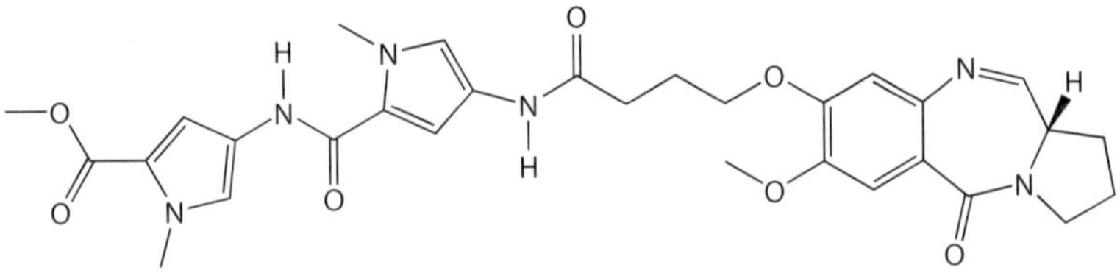

FIGURE 8.1
GWL-78, a PBD–polyamide conjugate which inhibits specific DNA-protein interactions.

PAs bind specific DNA sites in a model nucleosome substrate with little loss in affinity and specificity (Gottesfeld et al. 2001, Suto et al. 2003). However, it is unclear how the sequence-specific binding of PAs is affected by both higher-order chromatin structures and the large excess of competing genomic DNA sites in the cell nucleus.

Dudouet et al. revealed that the pyrrole–imidazole PAs shown in Figure 8.2 bind DNA with affinities comparable to those of transcriptional regulatory proteins and inhibit the DNA-binding activities of components of the transcription apparatus (Dudouet et al. 2003).

If PAs are to be useful for the regulation of gene expression in cell culture experiments, one pivotal issue is the accessibility of specific sites in nuclear chromatin. The kinetics of uptake and subcellular distribution of PAs in lymphoid and myeloid cells were firstly determined by using fluorescent PA–bodipy conjugates and deconvolution microscopy. Cells were then incubated with a PA–chlorambucil conjugate, and the sites of specific DNA cleavage in the nuclear chromatin were assayed by ligation-mediated polymerase chain reaction (PCR). In addition, DNA microarray analysis revealed that two different PAs generated distinct transcription profiles. Remarkably, the PAs affected only a limited number of genes.

8.3.2 Antimicrobial Activity

Specific modification of polymeric backbones via incorporation of known antimicrobial compounds is an efficient pathway to generate antimicrobial activity. Recently, N-halamines have attracted considerable interest as antimicrobial materials. An N-halamine may be defined as a compound containing one or more nitrogen-halogen covalent bonds. The biocidal action of N-halamines was believed to be a manifestation of a chemical reaction involving the direct transfer of positive halogens from the N-halamines to appropriate receptors and/or following oxidative reactions in the microorganism cells (Worley and Sun 1996).

Sun et al. chose a simple approach by chlorinating commercial aromatic PAs such as Kevlar or Nomex (Sun and Sun 2004). Chlorinated Nomex demonstrated potent antimicrobial efficacy against both *E. coli* and *S. aureus*. The materials provide a total kill of 10^6–10^7 CFUs/mL bacteria at a contact time of only 10 min, the strongest antibacterial activity among all the reported hydrophobic biocidal fabrics (Sun and Sun 2001a,b).

Sulfonamide derivatives have been reported to show substantial antitumor activity *in vitro* and/or *in vivo* (Abbate et al. 2004, Ghorab et al. 2006), HIV protease inhibition (Zhao et al. 2008), and cell entry (Lu et al. 2009). Polysulfonamides are active agents which shield toxic polycations. Sulfonamide-containing copolymers possess higher activity toward fungi than bacteria, being more gram-positive rather than gram-negative as is common. Hassan et al. reported the synthesis of nanosized PAs containing various bioactive pendent structures as shown in Figure 8.3 (Hassan et al. 2015). PAs containing

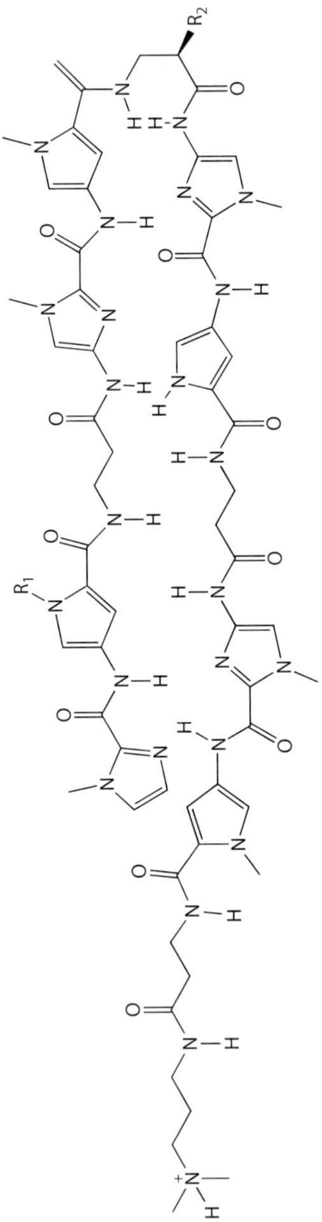

FIGURE 8.2
General structure of DNA-binding pyrrole-imidazole polyamides.

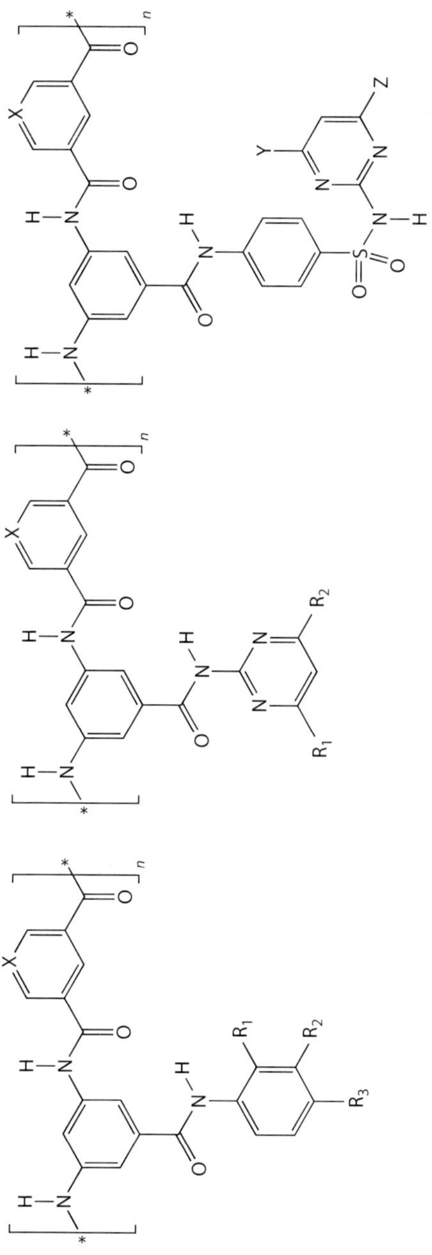

FIGURE 8.3
Aromatic polyamides with various bioactive pendant structures.

both sulfonamide and chlorinated substituents showed higher antimicrobial activity against all fungi and gram-positive bacteria. The presence of such bioactive groups in a polymeric motif plays a key role in catalyzing both biological and chemical systems.

Synthesized chloro-aromatic PAs played a vital role in the development of different bioactive agents since chlorine is electronegative and therefore oxidizes the peptide linkages and denatures proteins. Exposure of strains of *E. coli*, *Pseudomonas* spp., and *Staphylococcus* spp. to lethal doses causes a decrease in adenosine triphosphate (ATP) production. Sulfonamidopyrimidine-containing PAs analogs exhibited high antibacterial activity against gram-negative bacteria. It is noteworthy that one PA exhibited comparable antibacterial activity against gram-negative bacteria relative to the reference antibiotic gentamicin. Pyrimidine-containing PAs exhibited high antifungal activity against *A. fumigatus* and, interestingly, the observed activities were more potent than those of the reference *Amphotericin B.* bacteria.

8.3.3 Cellular Adhesion Processes

Nonthrombogenic biomaterials have created great interest in the development of medical devices and implants in recent decades. When coming in contact with blood or internal organs, the material surface of a device should avoid the initiation of any process leading to thrombosis.

Nagase et al. describe the preparation of high-molecular-weight aromatic copolyamides (Figure 8.4) containing phosphorylcholine (PC) group, a polar component of phospholipid molecules which cover the surface of cell membranes (Nagase et al. 2007). They confirmed that synthetic polymer-based materials containing PC groups exhibit wide biocompatibility, including blood compatibility (Gong et al. 2005). The quantitative analysis of adhered platelets revealed the strict difference in the thrombogenic properties of the copolymer films. Thus, the PC unit plays an important role in the blood compatibility of the polymeric systems. In addition, being hard materials, these copolyamides are useful for artificial bones or joints.

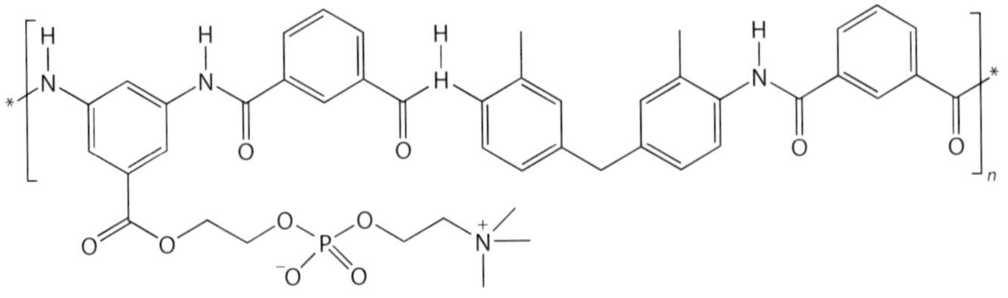

FIGURE 8.4
A typical example of an aromatic copolyamide containing PC motifs.

8.4 Aromatic Polyimides

In production since the 1950s, polyimides (PIs) are commercially available polymers widely used in the automotive, electronics, and military industries, and, within the last 30 years, also in biomedical applications. A great variety of applications are known for PIs and refer to their use as adhesives, insulating film and coatings, flexible cables, advanced composites, asbestos substitutes, advanced fabrics and nonwoven materials, protective and sport clothing, and medical tubing, among others (Liaw et al. 2012). Their success is due to some key properties like thermoxidative stability, high mechanical strength, excellent insulating properties, and superior chemical inertness (Rusu et al. 2010, Damaceanu et al. 2012, 2014, Barzic et al. 2014).

8.4.1 Bio- and Hemocompatibility

While PIs are generally regarded as biocompatible (Richardson et al. 1993), their safety in biological systems has been poorly explored. More often, the implanted materials and devices based on PIs were evaluated with regard to their *in vitro* cytotoxicity and *in vivo* histological response. The broad variability of PI formulations can lead to important differences in their performance relative to more stringent factors of biocompatibility, such as thrombogenicity, interaction with versatile cells or tissues, and stability. These factors require investigation of the PIs' biocompatibility in new research fields. *In vitro* studies with mouse fibroblasts (Richardson et al. 1993, Sun et al. 2009), rat neurons (Lacour et al. 2008), or human and rat retinal epithelial cells (Seo et al. 2004) showed a negligible cytotoxicity. In addition, the inflammatory response to implanted PI in *in vivo* neural or retinal studies proved to be minimal (Lago et al. 2005, Jiang et al. 2013). Recently, the biocompatibility of PIs with human endothelial cells has been assessed on the basis of ISO 10993-5 standards for evaluating medical devices. Thus, an experimental blood pressure transducer based on two structurally different PIs shown in Figure 8.5 was developed. Little to no cytotoxicity or stress induction *in vitro* was observed, suggesting its suitability for short-term intravascular operation (Starr et al. 2016).

Protein adsorption is one of the most important features in designing a biomedical polymer. It was found that albumin adsorption on the surface of fluorinated PIs (Figure 8.5b and c) was strongly dependent on the annealing temperature and time, and decreased with annealing temperature that induced a higher hydrophobicity and reduced polar and hydrogen-bonding components on the PI surfaces (Kawakami et al. 2001). A PI containing alicyclic units (Figure 8.5e) was investigated in comparison with a fully aromatic one (Figure 8.5a) with regard to the structural, rheological, and surface properties, to check their suitability as hemocompatible polymer films. The compatibility of PI surfaces with blood was assessed by calculating the

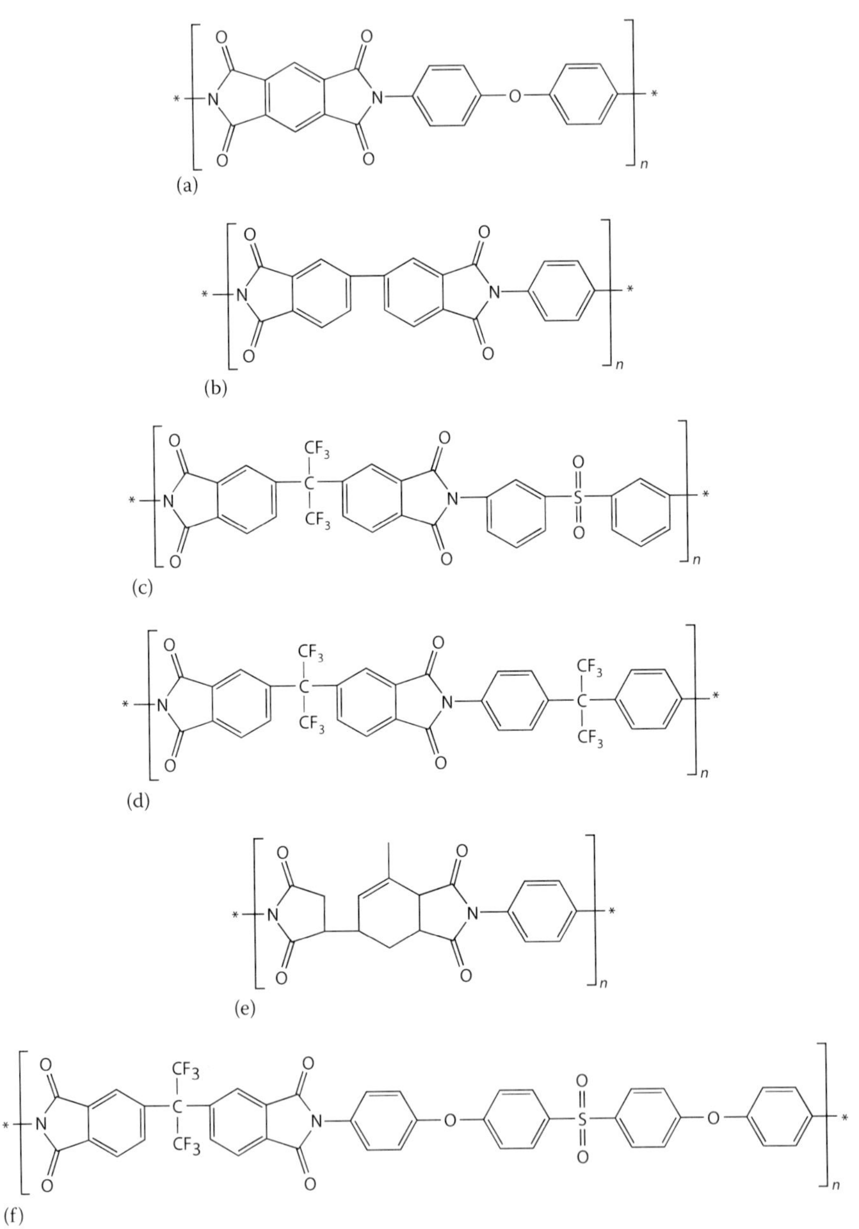

FIGURE 8.5
Chemical structures of the most investigated bio- or hemocompatible PIs. Generally used abbreviations: (a) PMDA-ODA, (b) BPDA-PPD, (c) 6FDA-DDS, (d) 6FDA-6FAP, (e) EPICLON-PPD, and (f) 6FDA-APPS.

spreading work of some basic blood cells and proteins. The results indicated that the sample containing alicyclic units is more suitable for applications that require good hemocompatibility (Buruiana et al. 2016).

Surface modification of materials to enhance the final biocompatibility and/or the cell-interactive behavior of implants has proved to be of increasing interest over recent decades (Vepari et al. 2010). Thus, biocompatible implant PI films (Pyralin PI 2611) were surface-functionalized with reactive succinimidyl ester group or cross-linkable vinyl groups and gelatin was immobilized on the PI surface after the surface modification (Van Vlierberghe et al. 2010, Sirova et al. 2014). The subcutaneous implantation in mice suggested that the proposed modification strategy led to a biocompatible material, inducing only limited cellular infiltration to the surrounding tissue.

To enhance the biocompatibility of PI-based neural electrodes, Heo et al. realized an anti-inflammatory drug loading by soaking the PI (VTEC PI-1338) in the drug-loaded solvent and investigated their inhibitory effects on inflammation under *in vitro* and *in vivo* conditions. The drug-loaded PI films were subcutaneously implanted in a rat model. Relative to the control and nontreated PI film, they showed better short-term biocompatibility when analyzed using cytotoxicity assays, RT-PCR, and H&E staining (Heo et al. 2016).

8.4.2 Supports for Cell Cultures

Due to superior heat resistance, mechanical strength, and chemical stability, PIs are able to withstand the high temperatures required for sterilization and their films can be used as supports for cell cultures. Microstructures on cell-cultured PI sheets were fabricated by hot embossing, followed by cultivation of OP9 stromal marrow cells on them. The PI proved to be optimal for cell culture, and, interestingly, the cells adhered in slight alignment to the fabricated fine structure (Maenosono et al. 2014). In another study, cell adhesion, proliferation, and orientation on the surface of a fluorinated PI (Figure 8.5d) film modified by thermal treatment and rubbing were investigated using a continuous cell line of human epithelial cells (adherent HeLa). The key finding was the alignment of the cells on the PI surface along the rubbing direction, while the cells proliferated randomly on the unrubbed surface (Nagaoka et al. 2002).

Ilmarinen et al. investigated the suitability of ultrathin and porous PI as carrier for subretinal transplantation of human embryonic stem cell–derived retinal pigment epithelial (RPE) cells in rabbits (Ilmarinen et al. 2015). The PI film was well tolerated in the subretinal area while maintenance of the outer nuclear layer was noted even 3 months after transplantation.

The cylindrical PI capillary described in Figure 8.6 has been used for the directly internal culture of *Aplysia californica* neurons (Lee et al. 2016). The neuron-in-capillary platform proved to be robust and easily integrated with capillary-based analytical tools. The addition of a particle-embedded monolith allowed mass spectrometric characterization of released neuropeptide and monitoring of the chemical signals between live neurons.

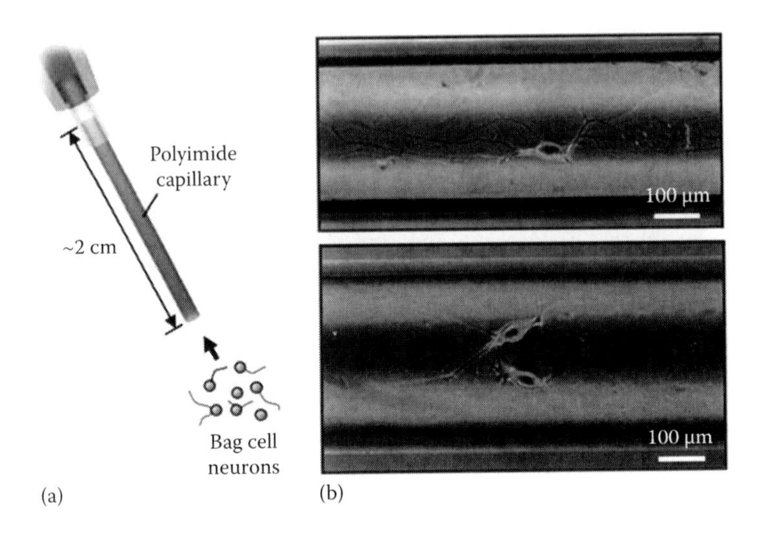

FIGURE 8.6
(a) Neuron in PI capillary platform. (b) Individual (top, 5 days *in vitro* [DIV]) and network-forming (bottom, 3 DIV) bag cell neurons of *Aplysia* in a bare polyimide capillary. (Adapted from Lee, C.Y. et al., *Sci. Rep.*, 6, 26940, 2016.)

8.4.3 Protective Sheets in Medical Applications

As PIs are the most common known insulating materials or passivation layers, providing protection for circuitry and metals from effects such as corrosion, ion transport, humidity uptake, or physical damage, they attracted particular interest from the medical device industry for encapsulation and insulation of active implants. For example, a PI was used as a protective sheath since it provides suitable protection and can be custom-fabricated with micro apertures to accelerate diffusion of gas during sterilization of the device leads (Thota et al. 2015). A thorough study was conducted by Rubehn and Stieglitz to evaluate the *in vitro* long-term survivability of three commercially available PIs (PI2611—HD-Microsystems, U-Varnish-S—UBE, and Durimide 7510) as materials for neural implants (Rubehn and Stieglitz 2010). The application of the PI material in neural prostheses demands its stability in the body environment for many years. The PI films were stored in phosphate-buffered saline at 37°C (body temperature) and much higher temperatures (60°C and 85°C) to accelerate aging. The results mentioned no decrease of the PIs' mechanical properties with respect to the reference, proving their long-term stability.

8.4.4 Microelectrode Arrays

Advanced micro- and nanotechnologies offer new opportunities for the development of active implants throughout the body. Functional electrical stimulation offers the possibility to neurologically rehabilitate different organs that are irreversibly damaged, when neurons or muscles are electrically excited in order to affect muscles or senses such as vision or hearing. This can be achieved under current and/or voltage pulses across an electrode array (Feili et al. 2006). The PI materials have been widely used as flexible substrates in implantable neuronal interfaces as well as in coating silicon-based implants providing chemical barriers and electrical insulation layers (Cheung et al. 2007). Thus, Seo et al. reported on the *in vitro* biocompatibility of PI (PI 2525, HD Micro Systems) microelectrode array tested by coculture with human RPE cells and *in vivo* biocompatibility in rabbit eyes, being suitable for the fabrication of retinal stimulator in visual prosthesis systems (Seo et al. 2004). A photosensitive PI, Durimide 7510 (Arch Chemicals, Norwalk, CT), has also been tested with the thin-film microelectrode arrays presented in Figure 8.7 for use as epiretinal implants, being fabricated based on microelectro-mechanical system (MEMS) processing and microfabrication techniques (Jiang et al. 2013).

PI 2525 from HD Micro Systems was used in the fabrication of a microelectrode array with 16 electrodes (5 μm-thick and 16 μm in radius) for use

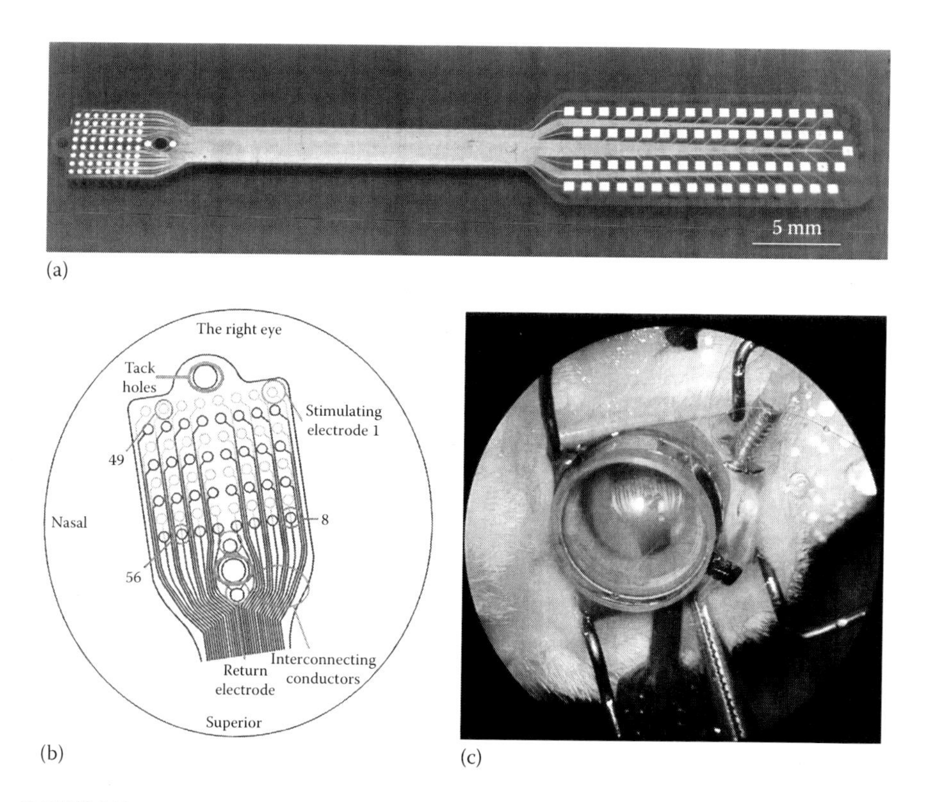

FIGURE 8.7
The 64-channel dual-metal-layer thin PI film microelectrode array. (a) The whole array structure; (b) expanded view of the stimulating electrodes implanted on the surface of rabbit retina; (c) placement of the stimulating array in rabbit eye. (From Jiang, X. et al., *J. Neuroeng. Rehabil.*, 10, 48, 2013.)

in neural recording and repeatable electrolytic lesion in rat brain (Chen et al. 2009). High signal-to-noise ratio during chronic neural recordings and high reusability for electrolytic lesions were obtained upon surveying its performance in chronic *in vivo* recordings in rodents.

Although PI microelectrode array technology has progressed rapidly, its practical applications are limited by packaging technologies, especially regarding system interconnections. Baek et al. developed a simple packaging method for preparing thin PI multichannel microelectrodes (Baek et al. 2012). Simple connections were implemented by making via-holes at the interconnection pad between the thin PI electrodes with a soldering process. An electroplated Ni ring through the via-hole was constructed to achieve stable soldering and strong adhesion of the electrode to the printed circuit board. Studies were carried out for high-resolution recording from the skull of a rat. The *in vivo* and *in vitro* tests suggested that the packaged PI electrode is a good candidate for the continuous measurement of biosignals or for neural prosthetics.

As technology pushes toward miniaturization, efforts are being made to integrate multiple laboratory procedures into a compact portable microlaboratory for DNA diagnostics (Pancrazio et al. 1998). Generally, such a microlaboratory encompasses several functions that include sample preparation, amplification, hybridization, and detection. The first prototypes of a three-dimensional, electrophoretically driven microlaboratory were constructed by Forster et al. from laminated layers of flexible PI for the analysis of proteins and DNA (Forster et al. 2001). They proved that the biased electrodes preserve the integrity of the DNA by performing an electronic reverse-dot blot hybridization assay after electrophoretic transport of the target oligonucleotides. Another procedure developed to immobilize DNA probes on a microarray patterned on a flexible polymer substrate involved the chemical activation of a thin-film surface by introduction of the amine functionality via a silanization step, the coupling of an adequate crosslinker, followed by the immobilization of the DNA probe. After immobilization in patterned pixels, the DNA probes were allowed to hybridize with complementary target DNA labeled with a fluorescent molecule. A prototype array consisting of thin-film pixels of SiO_2 functionalized by silanization deposited on a PI substrate was demonstrated (Fixe et al. 2002).

8.5 Conclusions

Aliphatic, semialiphatic, and aromatic amide- and imide-type polymers form related families of synthetic, biocompatible, and biostable or biodegradable polymorphic macromolecular compounds, which are able to provide some of the missing pieces in the great puzzle of unsolved synthetic challenges and necessary features in the envisaged area. They display many interesting traits and processing and functionalization possibilities capable of fulfilling a handful of complex requirements of current and future biomedical topics.

Acknowledgments

The authors acknowledge the financial support of this research through the European Regional Development Fund, Project POINGBIO, ID P_40_443, Contract no. 86/8.09.2016.

References

Abbate, F., Casini, A., Owa, T., Scozzafava, A., and Supuran, C. T. 2004. Carbonic anhydrase inhibitors: E7070, a sulfonamide anticancer agent, potently inhibits cytosolic isozymes I and II, and transmembrane, tumor-associated isozyme IX. *Bioorg. Med. Chem. Lett.* 14:217–223.

Abdal-hay, A., Lim, J., Hassan, M. S., and Lim, J. K. 2013a. Ultrathin conformal coating of apatite nanostructures onto electrospun nylon 6 nanofibers: Mimicking the extracellular matrix. *Chem. Eng. J.* 228:708–716.

Abdal-hay, A., Tijing, L. D., and Lim, J. K. 2013b. Characterization of the surface biocompatibility of an electrospun nylon 6/CaP nanofiber scaffold using osteoblasts. *Chem. Eng. J.* 215–216:57–64.

Baek, D. H., Han, C. H., Jung, H. C. et al. 2012. Soldering-based easy packaging of thin polyimide multichannel electrodes for neuro-signal recording. *J. Micromech. Microeng.* 22:115017.

Barzic, A. I., Rusu, R. D., Stoica, I. and Damaceanu, M. D. 2014. Chain flexibility versus molecular entanglement response to rubbing deformation in designing poly(oxadiazole-naphthylimide)s as liquid crystal orientation layers. *J. Mater. Sci.* 49:3080–3098.

Bergsson, G., Arnfinnsson, J., Steingrimsson, O., and Thormar, H. 2001. Killing of Gram-positive cocci by fatty acids and monoglycerides. *APMIS* 109:670–678.

Bianco, B., Castaldo, L., del Gaudio, A. et al. 1997. Biocompatible α-aminoacids based aliphatic polyamides. *Polym. Bull.* 39:279–286.

Buruiana, L. I., Barzic, A. I., Stoica, I., and Hulubei, C. 2016. Evaluation of blood cells and proteins spreading on imidic polymers containing alicyclic sequences. *J. Polym. Res.* 23:217.

Chen, Y. Y., Lai, H. Y., Lin, S. H. et al. 2009. Design and fabrication of a polyimide-based microelectrode array: Application in neural recording and repeatable electrolytic lesion in rat brain. *J. Neurosci. Methods* 182:6–16.

Cheung, K. C., Renaud, P., Tanila, H., and Djupsund, K. 2007. Flexible polyimide microelectrode array for in vivo recordings and current source density analysis. *Biosens. Bioelectron.* 22:1783–1790.

Chu, C. C. 2008. Types and properties of surgical sutures. In *Biotextiles as Medical Implants*, M. W. King, B. S. Gupta, and R. Guidoin (Eds.). Cambridge, U.K.: Woodhead Publishing Limited.

Damaceanu, M. D., Rusu, R. D., and Bruma, M. 2012. Six-member polyimides incorporating redox chromophores. *J. Mater. Sci.* 47:6179–6188.

Damaceanu, M. D., Constantin, C. P., Bruma, M., and Pinteala, M. 2013. Tuning of the color of the emitted light from new polyperyleneimides containing oxadiazole and siloxane moieties. *Dyes Pigm.* 99:228–239.

Damaceanu, M. D., Rusu, R. D., Cristea, M., Musteata, V. E., Bruma, M., and Wolinska-Grabczyk, A. 2014. Insights into the chain and local mobility of some aromatic polyamides and their influence on the physicochemical properties. *Macromol. Chem. Phys.* 215:1573–1587.

Damaceanu, M. D., Rusu, R. D., Nicolescu, A., and Bruma, M. 2011. Blue fluorescent polyamides containing naphthalene and oxadiazole rings. *J. Polym. Sci. Polym. Chem.* 49:893–906.

Damaceanu, M. D., Sava, I., and Constantin, C. P. 2016. The chromic and electrochemical response of $CoCl_2$-filled polyimide materials for sensing applications. *Sens. Actuators B Chem.* 234:549–561.

Dang, T. T., Nikkhah, M., Memic, A., and Khademhosseini A. 2014. Polymeric biomaterials for implantable prostheses. In *Natural and Synthetic Biomedical Polymers*, S. Kumbar, C. Laurencin, and M. Deng (Eds.), pp. 309–331. Oxford, U.K.: Elsevier.

Dudouet, B., Burnett, R., Dickinson, L. A. et al. 2003. Accessibility of nuclear chromatin by DNA binding polyamides. *Chem. Biol.* 10:859–867.

Feili, D., Schuettler, M., Doerge, T., Kammer, S. K., Hoffmann, P., and Stieglitz, T. 2006. Flexible organic field effect transistors for biomedical microimplants using polyimide and parylene C as substrate and insulator layers. *J. Micromech. Microeng.* 16:1555–1561.

Fixe, F., Faber, A., Gongalves, D. et al. 2002. Thin film micro arrays with immobilized DNA for hybridization analysis. *MRS Proc.* 723:125.

Forster, A. H., Krihak, M., Swanson, P. D., Young, T. C., and Ackley, D. E. 2001. A laminated, flex structure for electronic transport and hybridization of DNA. *Biosens. Bioelectron.* 16:187–194.

Ganewatta, M. S. and Tang, C. 2015. Controlling macromolecular structures towards effective antimicrobial polymers. *Polymer* 63:1–29.

García, J. M., García, F. C., Serna, F., and de la Peña, J. L. 2010. High-performance aromatic polyamides. *Prog. Polym. Sci.* 35:623–686.

Ghorab, M. M., Noaman, E., Ismail, M., Heiba H. I., Ammar, Y. A., and Sayed, M. Y. 2006. Novel antitumor and radioprotective sulfonamides containing pyrrolo [2,3-d]pyrimidines. *Arzneim.-Forsch.* 56:405–413.

Gong, Y. K., Luo, L., Petit, A. et al. 2005. Adhesion of human U937 macrophages to phosphorylcholine-coated surfaces. *J. Biomed. Mater. Res. Part A* 72A:1–9.

Gottesfeld, J. M., Melander, C., Suto, R. K., Raviol, H., Luger, K., and Dervan, P. B. 2001. Sequence-specific recognition of DNA in the nucleosome by pyrrole-imidazole polyamides. *J. Mol. Biol.* 309:615–629.

Gupta, B., Grover, N., Viju, S., and Saxena, S. 2008. Polyester and nylon based textiles in biomedical engineering. In *Polyesters and Polyamides*, B. L. Deopura, R. Alagirusamy, M. Joshi, and B. Gupta (Eds.), pp. 441–504. Cambridge, U.K.: Woodhead Publishing Limited.

Hassan, A. M., Mansour, E. M. E., Abou-Zeid, A. M. S., El-Helow, E. R., Elhusseiny, A. F., and Soliman, R. 2015. Synthesis and biological evaluation of new nano-sized aromatic polyamides containing amido- and sulfonamidopyrimidines pendant structures. *Chem. Cent. J.* 9:44.

Heo, D. N., Ko, W. K., Lee, W. J. et al. 2016. Enhanced biocompatibility of polyimide film by anti-inflammatory drug loading. *J. Nanosci. Nanotechnol.* 16:8800–8804.

Huang, D., Niu, L., and Wei, Y. 2014. Interfacial and biological properties of the gradient coating on polyamide substrate for bone substitute. *J. R. Soc. Interfaces*, article number 11:20140101.

Ilmarinen, T., Hiidenmaa, H., Kööbi, P. et al. 2015. Ultrathin polyimide membrane as cell carrier for subretinal transplantation of human embryonic stem cell derived retinal pigment epithelium. *PLoS One* 10:e0143669.

Jiang, X., Sui, X., Lu, Y. et al. 2013. In vitro and in vivo evaluation of a photosensitive polyimide thin-film microelectrode array suitable for epiretinal stimulation. *J. Neuroeng. Rehabil.* 10:48.

Kawakami, H., Takahashi, T., Nagaoka, S., and Nakayama, Y. 2001. Albumin adsorption to surface of annealed fluorinated polyimide. *Polym. Adv. Technol.* 12:244–252.

Kelsey, J. A., Bayles, K. W., Shafii, B., and McGuire, M. A. 2006. Fatty acids and monoacylglycerols inhibit growth of *Staphylococcus aureus*. *Lipids* 41:951–961.

Kim, J. R. and Michielsen, S. 2015. Photodynamic antifungal activities of nanostructured fabrics grafted with rose bengal and phloxine B against *Aspergillus fumigatus*. *J. Appl. Polym. Sci.* 132:42114.

Kleyi, P., Frost, C. L., Tshentu, Z. R., and Torto, N. 2014. Electrospun nylon-6 nanofibers incorporated with 2-substituted N-alkylimidazoles and their silver(I) complexes for antibacterial applications. *J. Appl. Polym. Sci.*, article number 131:39783.

Knapp, H. R. and Melly, M. A. 1986. Bactericidal effects of polyunsaturated fatty acids. *J. Infect. Dis.* 154:84–94.

Komane, L. L., Mukaya, E. H., Neuse, E. W., and van Rensburg, C. E. J. 2008. Macromolecular antiproliferative agents featuring dicarboxylato-chelated platinum. *J. Inorg. Organomet. Polym.* 18:111–123.

Kotecha, M., Kluza, J., Wells, G. et al. 2008. Inhibition of DNA binding of the NF-Y transcription factor by the pyrrolobenzodiazepine-polyamide conjugate GWL-78. *Mol. Cancer Ther.* 7:1319–1328.

Lacour, S. P., Atta, R., FitzGerald, J. J., Blamire, M., Tarte, E., and Fawcett, J. 2008. Polyimide micro-channel arrays for peripheral nerve regenerative implants. *Sens. Actuators A Phys.* 147:456–463.

Lago, N., Ceballos, D., Rodriguez, J., Stieglitz, F., and Navarro, T. X. 2005. Long term assessment of axonal regeneration through polyimide regenerative electrodes to interface the peripheral nerve. *Biomaterials* 26:2021–2031.

Lee, C. Y., Fan, Y., Rubakhin, S. S., Yoon, S., and Sweedler, J. V. 2016. A neuron-in-capillary platform for facile collection and mass spectrometric characterization of a secreted neuropeptide. *Sci. Rep.* 6:26940.

Liaw, D. J., Wang, K. L., Huang, Y. C., Lee, K. R., Lai, J. Y., and Ha, C. S. 2012. Advanced polyimide materials: Syntheses, physical properties and applications. *Prog. Polym. Sci.* 37:907–974.
Liu, D. H., Choi, S., Chen, B. et al. 2004. Nontoxic membrane-active antimicrobial arylamide oligomers. *Angew. Chem. Int. Ed.* 43:1158–1162.
Lu, R. J., Tucker, J. A., Pickens, J. et al. 2009. Heterobiaryl human immunodeficiency virus entry inhibitors. *J. Med. Chem.* 52:4481–4487.
Maenosono, H., Saito, H., and Nishioka, Y. 2014. A transparent polyimide film as a biological cell culture sheet with microstructures. *J. Biomater. Nanobiotechnol.* 5:17–23.
Maitz, M. F. 2015. Applications of synthetic polymers in clinical medicine. *Biosurf. Biotribol.* 1:161–176.
Matsuda, H., Fukuda, N., Ueno, T. et al. 2006. Development of gene silencing pyrrole-imidazole polyamide targeting the TGF-h1 promoter for treatment of progressive renal diseases. *J. Am. Soc. Nephrol.* 17:422–432.
Millsaps, B. B. 2015. Samsonium: Scientists develop nylon titanium material for 3D printed knee implants, 10x the strength of ABS or PLA. https://3dprint.com/77305/samsonian-nylon-titanium, accessed on November 14, 2016.
Morais, D. S., Guedes, R. M., and Lopes, M. A. 2016. Antimicrobial approaches for textiles: From research to market. *Materials*, article number 9:498 .
Nagaoka, S., Ashiba, K., and Kawakami, H. 2002. Biomedical properties of nanofabricated fluorinated polyimide surface. *Artif. Organs* 26:670–675.
Nagase, Y., Oku, M., Iwasaki, Y., and Ishihara, K. 2007. Preparations of aromatic diamine monomers and copolyamides containing phosphorylcholine moiety and the biocompatibility of copolyamides. *Polym. J.* 39:712–721.
Negoro, S. 2005. Biodegradation of nylon and other synthetic polyamides. *Biopolymers*, 9:395–401.
Neuse, E. W., Caldwell, G., and Perlwitz, A. G. 1996. Carrier polymers for cisplatin-type anticancer drug models. *Polym. Adv. Technol.* 7:867–872.
Nirmala, R., Park, H. M., Navamathavan, R., Kang, H. S., Newehy, M. H. E., and Kim, H. Y. 2011. Lecithin blended polyamide-6 high aspect ration nanofiber scaffolds via electrospinning for human osteoblast cell culture. *Mater. Sci. Eng. C* 31:486–493.
Pancrazio, J. J., Bey, P. P. Jr., Cuttino, D. S. et al. 1998. Portable cell-based biosensor system for toxin detection. *Sens. Actuators B Chem.* 53:179–185.
Pant, B., Pant, H. R., Pandeya, D. R., Panthi, G., Nam, K. T., Hong, S. T., Kim, C. S., and Kim, H. Y. 2012. Characterization and antibacterial properties of Ag NPs loaded nylon-6 nanocomposites prepared by one-step electrospinning process. *Colloids Surf. A* 395:94–99.
Pant, H. R., Kim, H. J., Bhatt, L. R. et al. 2013a. Chitin butyrate coated electrospun nylon-6 fibers for biomedical applications. *Appl. Surf. Sci.* 285:538–544.
Pant, H. R., Risal, P., Park, C. H., Tijing, L. D., Jeong, Y. J., and Kim, C. S. 2013b. Synthesis, characterization, and mineralization of polyamide-6/calcium lactate composite nanofibers for bone tissue engineering. *Colloids Surf. B* 102:152–157.
Pant, H. R., Risal, P., Park, C. H., Tijing, L. D., Jeong, Y. J., and Kim, C. S. 2013c. Core–shell structured electrospun biomimetic composite nanofibers of calcium lactate/nylon-6 for tissue engineering. *Chem. Eng. J.* 221:90–98.
Patel, M. and Fisher, J. P. 2008. Biomaterial scaffolds in pediatric tissue engineering. *Pediatr. Res.* 63:497–501.

Prasad, P., Molla, M. R., Cui, W. et al. 2015. Polyamide nanogels from GRAS components and their toxicity in mouse pre-implantation embryos. *Biomacromolecules* 16:3491–3498.

Pruitt, L. and Furmanski, J. 2009. Polymeric biomaterials for load-bearing medical devices. *JOM* 61:14–20.

Quatela, V. C. and Chow, J. 2008. Synthetic facial implants. *Facial Plast. Surg. Clin. N. Am.* 16:1–10.

Richardson, R., Jr., Miller, J., and Reichert, W. 1993. Polyimides as biomaterials: Preliminary biocompatibility testing. *Biomaterials* 14:627–635.

Rubehn, B. and Stieglitz, T. 2010. In vitro evaluation of the long-term stability of polyimide as a material for neural implants. *Biomaterials* 31:3449–3458.

Rusu, R. D., Damaceanu, M. D., Marin, L., and Bruma, M. 2010. Copoly(peryleneimide)s containing 1,3,4-oxadiazole rings: Synthesis and properties. *J. Polym. Sci. Polym. Chem.* 48:4230–4242.

Scholz, M. S., Blanchfield, J. P., Bloom, L. D. et al. 2011. The use of composite materials in modern orthopaedic medicine and prosthetic devices. *Compos. Sci. Technol.* 71:1791–1803.

Seo, J. M., Kim, S. J., Chung, H., Kim, E. T., Yu, H. G., and Yu, Y. S. 2004. Biocompatibility of polyimide microelectrode array for retinal stimulation. *Mater. Sci. Eng. C* 24:185–189.

Seo, M. D., Won, H. S., Kim, J. H., Mishig-Ochir, T., and Lee, B. J. 2012. Antimicrobial peptides for therapeutic applications: A review. *Molecules* 17:12276–12286.

Sharafi, S. and Li, G. 2015. A mutliscale approach for modeling actuation response of polymeric artificial muscle. *Soft Matter* 11:3833–3843.

Shrestha, B. K., Mousa, H. M., Tiwari, A. P., Ko, S. W., Park, C. H., and Kim, C. S. 2016. Development of polyamide-6,6/chitosan electrospun hybridnanofibrous scaffolds for tissue engineering application. *Carbohydr. Polym.* 148:107–114.

Sirova, M., Van Vlierberghe, S., Matyasova, V. et al. 2014. Immunocompatibility evaluation of hydrogel-coated polyimide implants for applications in regenerative medicine. *J. Biomed. Mater. Res. A* 102A:1982–1990.

Starr, P. C., Agrawal, M., and Bailey, S. 2016. Biocompatibility of common polyimides with human endothelial cells for a cardiovascular microsensor. *J. Biomed. Mater. Res. A* 104A:406–412.

Sun, Y., Lacour, S., Brooks, R., Rushton, N., Fawcett, J., and Cameron, R. 2009. Assessment of the biocompatibility of photosensitive polyimide for implantable medical device use. *J. Biomed. Mater. Res. A* 90:648–655.

Sun, Y. and Sun, G. 2001a. Novel rgenerable N-halamine polymeric biocides. I: Synthesis, characterization and antimicrobial activity of hydantoin-containing polymers. *J. Appl. Polym. Sci.* 80:2457–2460.

Sun, Y. and Sun, G. 2001b. Novel regenerable N-halamine polymeric biocides. II: Grafting hydantoin-containing monomers onto cotton cellulose. *J. Appl. Polym. Sci.* 81:617–624.

Sun, Y. and Sun, G. 2004. Novel refreshable N-halamine polymeric biocides: N-chlorination of aromatic polyamides. *Ind. Eng. Chem. Res.* 43:5015–5020.

Suto, R. K., Edayathumangalam, R. S., White, C. L. et al. 2003. Effects of ligand binding on structure and dynamics of the nucleosome core particle. *J. Mol. Biol.* 326:371–380.

Teo, A. J. T., Mishra, A., Park, I., Kim, Y. J., Park, W. T., and Yoon, Y. J. 2016. Polymeric biomaterials for medical implants & devices. *ACS Biomater. Sci. Eng.* 2:454–472.

Thomas, D. 2014. New polymers set to revolutionize 3D printed implants. www.engineering.com/3DPrinting/3DPrintingArticles/ArticleID/9051/New-Polymers-Set-to-Revolutionize-3D-Printed-Implants.aspx, accessed on November 14, 2016.

Thota, A. K., Kuntaegowdanahalli, S., Starosciak, A. K. et al. 2015. A system and method to interface with multiple groups of axons in several fascicles of peripheral nerves. *J. Neurosci. Methods* 244: 78–84.

Timoney, P. J., Krakauer, M., Wilkes, B. N., Lee, H. B., and Nunery, W. R. 2014. Nylon foil (supramid) orbital implants in pediatric orbital fracture repair. *Ophthal. Plast. Reconstr. Surg.* 30:212–214.

Todros, S., Natali, A. N., Pace, G., and Di Noto, V. 2013. Correlation between chemical and mechanical properties in renewable poly(ether-blockamide)s for biomedical applications. *Macromol. Chem. Phys.* 214:2061–2072.

Van Vlierberghe, S., Sirova, M., Rossmann, P. et al. 2010. Surface modification of polyimide sheets for regenerative medicine applications. *Biomacromolecules* 11:2731–2739.

Vepari, C., Matheson, D., Drummy, L., Naik, R., and Kaplan, D. L. 2010. Surface modification of silk fibroin with poly(ethylene glycol) for antiadhesion and antithrombotic applications. *J. Biomed. Mater. Res. A* 93A:595–606.

Viola, B. M., Abraham, T. E., Arathi, D. S. et al. 2008. Synthesis and characterization of novel water-soluble polyamide based on spermine and aspartic acid as a potential gene delivery vehicle. *Express Polym. Lett.* 2:330–338.

Volpato, F. Z., Ramos, S. L. F., Motta, A., and Migliaresi, C. 2011. Physical and in vitro biological evaluation of a PA 6/MWCNT electrospun composite for biomedical applications. *J. Bioact. Compat. Polym.* 26:35–47.

Worley, S. D. and Sun, G. 1996. Biocidal polymers. *Trends Polym. Sci.* 11:364–370.

Yeaman, M. R. and Yount, N. Y. 2003. Mechanisms of antimicrobial peptide action and resistance. *Pharmacol. Rev.* 55:27–55.

Zhang, X., Lu, M., Wang, Y., Su, X., and Zhang, X. 2014. The development of biomimetic spherical hydroxyapatite/polyamide 66 biocomposites as bone repair materials. *Int. J. Polym. Sci.*, article number 2014:579252.

Zhao, Z. J., Wolkenberg, S. E., Lu, M. Q. et al. 2008. Novel indole-3-sulfonamides as potent HIV non-nucleoside reverse transcriptase inhibitors (NNRTIs). *Bioorg. Med. Chem. Lett.* 18:554–559.

Zhu, L. M. and Yu, D. G. 2008. Drug delivery systems using biotextiles. In *Biotextiles as Medical Implants*, M. W. King, B. S. Gupta, and R. Guidoin (Eds.), pp. 213–231. Cambridge, U.K.: Woodhead Publishing Limited.

9

Tailoring Protein-Based Materials for Regenerative Medicine and Tissue Engineering

Mioara Drobota, Maria Butnaru, and Magdalena Aflori

CONTENTS

9.1 Introduction

Protein coatings are applied to a range of biomaterial surfaces. This chapter addresses the need for coating applications for skin regeneration. We illustrate the coating methods used in biomedical applications. Applications for surfaces involve processes using photochemical methods to generate hydrophilic surfaces, and addition of protein immobilization technologies is outlined.

A selection of polymers commonly employed in commercially available coatings is discussed, and their interaction with growth cells in the context of the application area is described.

Tissue engineering is a viable alternative domain in the medical field in our days. This application is intended to enable tissue reconstruction by addressing the need of those who are affected and require biological replacement (Orlando et al. 2012). Therefore, biomaterial cells are used for replacement therapy, especially for implantation. Many of these biomaterials are easily accepted as biological components outside the body and are also easier to achieve considering the biological phenomenon of rejection of foreign biological substitutes.

The important aim in the application of tissue engineering is the investigation of the cutaneous skin regeneration and all the factors that contribute to reconstruction, without allowing infection and others complications to set in (Mandal et al. 2012). Thus, different strategies were taken into consideration such as replacement with artificial skin substitutes or the use of various cellular growth therapies in order to implement skin reconstruction.

These areas often use biomaterials as carriers for cell delivery to skin sites (such as collagen or fibrin) for direct cell growth and regeneration (Kirker et al. 2002, Sun et al. 2011). Ultimately, the choice of biomaterial has a defining effect on the clinical manifestation, and on the investigations that incorporate more natural components.

Scaffolds for tissue engineering are usually obtained with protein components from different animal tissues (Muyonga et al. 2004). Collagen is mainly a biological component and an important protein for structural support intended to be used in many tissue engineering applications.

The skin is the organ that covers the entire body and is therefore considered to be the greatest. This organ is the first to interact with the environment and is in a state of permanent stress with different factors (pathogenic, mechanical, thermal, chemical). Recent research has made many discoveries and substituents have been created to mimic human skin (MacNeil 2007). These skin substitutes were obtained with the help of advanced tissue engineering for clinical applications that promote the healing of different wounds (Kitano et al. 2008). Many methods are used in the functioning of polymeric structures (Lan et al. 2010, Ciobanu et al. 2011, 2012, Ding et al. 2014) but because some of them present disadvantages, new approaches need to be found. This function can be performed by developing new artificial self-assembling peptides or different bioactive substances that are not found together in nature.

The biological components are used as alternatives for tissue engineering. They are already present in nature; therefore, the field of synthetic biology is focused on designing new architectures that can replace the ones that are already degenerate. Successful developments using cell transplant are influenced by the ability to substitute tissues in favorable conditions as long as they eliminate malfunctions deriving from here. More specifically, accurate assessment is the key ability of grafted tissue regeneration. The aim of this study was to evaluate the ultraviolet (UV) functionalization of surface polymers and the interaction of the modified polymer support with molecular solutions like collagen, BSA, and gelatin, in order to obtain new supports for the immobilization of biologically active molecules that could be used in medical applications as patches.

9.2 Surface Modification of Polymer Film

UV light was used to promote activated surfaces with new functional groups. This study aims at identifying an alternative method to chemical functionalization. Polyethylene terephthalate (PET) films of 20 μm were placed and exposed to a UV lamp (Philips lamps from Holland TUV 30 W G30T8) by a polychrome emission spectrum ranging from 200 to 400 nm for surface modification. PET surface samples were first treated with UV light for different lengths of time (i.e., 0, 2, and 6 h). For better agreement, the samples were immobilized with collagen.

PET-2H-col and PET-6H-col after being UV-irradiated for 2 and 6 h, respectively; BSA PET-2H-BSA and PET-6H-BSA after being UV-irradiated for 2 and 6 h, respectively; gelatin with PET-2H-Gel and PET-6H-Gel after being UV-irradiated for 2 and 6 h, respectively. Figure 9.1 shows schematic machine for functionalization film and protein immobilization.

The polymer films were irradiated in atmospheric air and the mechanism of surface photooxidation during UV exposure in the presence of oxygen was presented by Drobota et al. (2015a).

This process provides matrix conditions for stimulating and anchoring proteins and cells that can be subsequently recognized by the biological actions of the biomaterials. Under UV irradiation, the surface of the polymers generates polar groups such as –COO–, –OCO–, –HCO, or –OH. Therefore, the molecules anchored onto the sample were obtained by immersing the

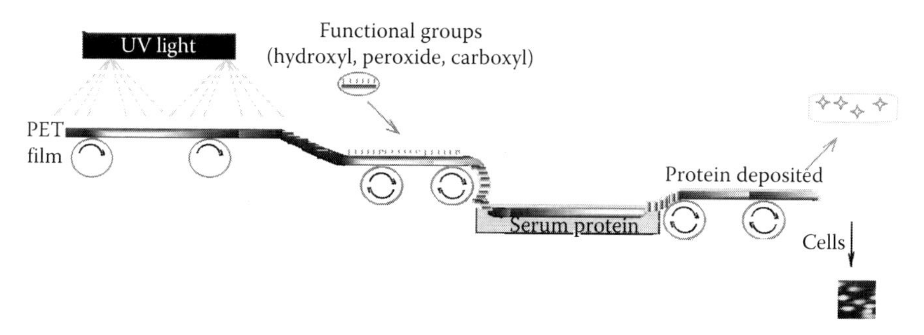

FIGURE 9.1
Schematic illustration of smart materials with immobilized surface for regenerative tissues.

films after irradiation in three solutions with collagen, BSA, and gelatin at the same concentration. For immobilization, the activated films were incubated in solutions of biomolecules previously mentioned (with a concentration of 1 mg/mL in PBS) for 24 h at 37°C.

After UV irradiation, the contact angle of the surface film decreases to 45°, and all other physicochemical properties of the surface are highlighted by Drobota et al. (2015b). Based on results obtained from previous treatment, the behavior and evolution of the attached molecules on the surface of the polymer support are confirmed by the presence of new surface groups, known as polar groups, which induce the morphology of the molecules.

9.3 Characterization of Immobilized Polymeric Film

The chemical composition and the geometrical structure obtained from the surface of the immobilized PET and pristine PET films, respectively, were monitored by attenuated total reflectance–Fourier transform infrared (ATR-FTIR) and scanning electron microscopic (SEM) analysis. The compatibility of the immobilized films was checked through cytotoxicity tests, and the population was analyzed with fibroblast cell culture.

9.3.1 Investigation Methods

9.3.1.1 Scanning Electron Microscopy

SEM micrographs were obtained with a Quanta 200 scanning probe microscope, and the samples were fixed on Al conducting supports and on sputter coated with gold.

9.3.1.2 ATR-FTIR Spectroscopic Analysis

ATR-FTIR spectra of the surface-modified PET membranes were obtained from a Bruker Vertex 70 spectrophotometer equipped with a reflectance device (ATR with diamond crystal, single reflection, and an incident angle of 45°). Each spectrum was collected by cumulating 64 scans at a resolution of 2 cm^{-1} in the 600–4000 cm^{-1} range.

9.3.2 Results and Discussion

9.3.2.1 Surface Chemical Property

After irradiation, the surface becomes more hydrophilic due to the unstable radicals as carboxyl, carbonyl, and peroxides, which form a polar layer at the surface of these groups. The results from ATR-FTIR spectra indicate

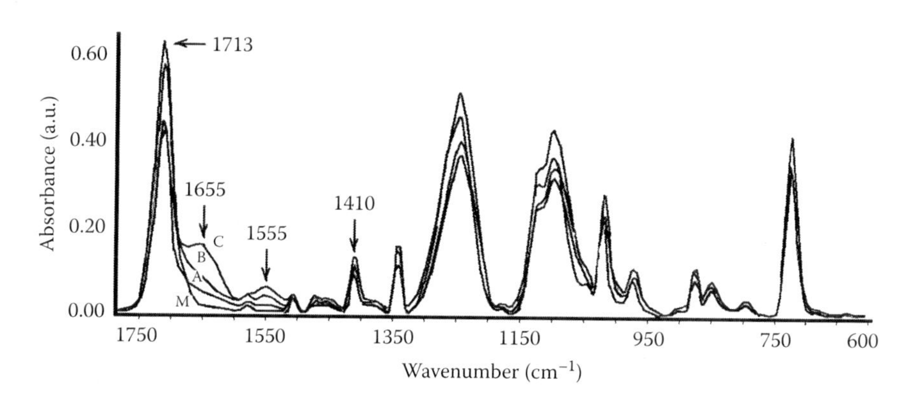

FIGURE 9.2
The ATR-FTIR spectra for untreated PET (M) and immobilized sample: (A) PET-6H-BSA, (B) PET-6H-Gel, and (C) PET-6H-col.

that these surface groups react with the amine group from the solution. Collagen and BSA are proteins that contain peptides in their structure and hence all the biomolecules have molecules with N groups that have a repetitive structure of amino acid. These biomolecules interact with the surface in order to form protonated structures (Wang et al. 2012). Gelatin is a denaturated biomolecule, derived from collagen molecules, which contain peptide in their structure.

In Figure 9.2 (M), ATR-FTIR spectra present the PET film with characteristic absorption peaks located at 1713 cm^{-1} (C=O stretching band characteristic from ester group), the vibration of the aromatic ring evidenced at 1410, 1018, and 865 cm^{-1}, and the bending vibration characteristic of $–CH_2$ groups at 1340 cm^{-1}. The structure of PET was confirmed by the absorption bands located at 1655 cm^{-1} (stretching vibration, νC=O) and at 1555 cm^{-1} (NH bending vibration δNH from the formation of amide I and II bands).

After immobilization, it was demonstrated that functional groups containing nitrogen from biomolecules were attached to the PET film surface. The conformational changes of biomolecules (Tamm and Tatulian 1997) depended on the characteristics of molecule structure, the surface support, and the environment involved.

FTIR data highlighted the molecules' presence in any structural changes after interaction with the polymer surface (Taravel and Domard 1995). This spectrum shows the interaction that occurs when the anchoring molecules (collagen, BSA, gelatin) are adsorbed onto the support. In this study, FTIR data show that the biomolecule chains dramatically change their secondary structure after contact with the functionalized substrate. A quantitative analysis of the protein's secondary structure for biomolecules immobilized onto films can be observed in amide I at the most sensitive probe in order to detect different changes in the protein's secondary structure (Bourassa et al. 2011).

Its absorption band was located at 1700–1600 cm^{-1} (Figure 9.3).

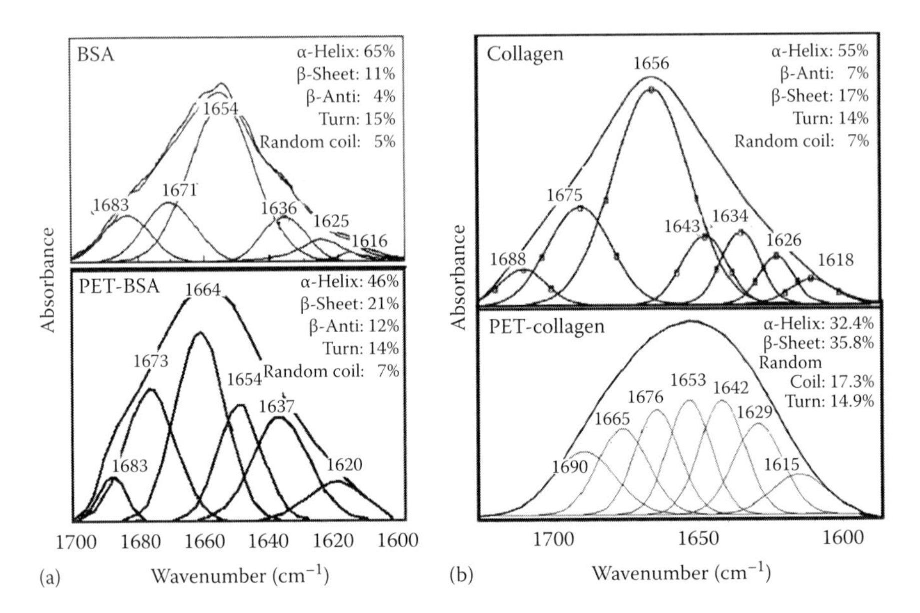

FIGURE 9.3
Second derivative resolution enhancement and curve-fitted amide I region (1700–1600 cm^{-1}) of FTIR spectra for (a) BSA and PET-BSA and (b) collagen and PET-collagen.

By comparing the spectra from this region of the sample with and without the presence of biomolecules attached on the polymer, some information about the different types of secondary structures, such as α-helix, β-sheets, turns, and random coil, has been obtained.

The fitting curve of the original broad amide I band was used as input parameters (Goormaghtigh et al. 2006).

The profile of each spectrum was deconvoluted at the peaks in the 1700–1600 cm^{-1} region using the Gaussian/Lorentzian equation. The fitting curve of the original broad amide I band was used as input parameters (Krimm and Bandekar 1986).

Amide I is a complex band that contains stretch and partly N–H bending vibrations. Proteins have a high level of α-helix, β-sheet, and undetermined or random structures in different proportions of the amide 1 band at 1645–1657 cm^{-1}, 1665–1680 cm^{-1}, or 1660 cm^{-1}, respectively. The profile of each spectrum was deconvoluted for the peaks in the 1700–1600 cm^{-1} region using the Gaussian/Lorentzian equation.

Because collagen and BSA are proteins, these biomolecules were evaluated by the secondary structures conformation.

First, the collagen secondary structure anchors onto a primarily parallel β-sheet conformation (amide I peak at 1656 cm^{-1}). After interaction with the substrate, the amide I peaks were moved to the central peak at 1653 cm^{-1}. This distinctive interaction is characteristic of the turn structure, but no other significant changes were observed in the rest of the contents.

The complex secondary structure of the molecules undergoes greater changes upon interaction with a polymer surface, especially because of its native collagen-binding sequence, which is described by the amide I peak. The content of the α-helix structure is increased because of some changes in the β-sheet structure (highlighted through the amide II peak as well) (Jayakumar et al. 2014). This demonstrates that molecules have a primarily α-helical secondary structure after adsorption of collagen on the surface with a strong β-sheet structure (Walton et al. 2010) due to the electrostatic and hydrogen binding. Figure 9.3a and b with the spectra of amide I bands presents differences in the conformation chains of the secondary structure, and the deconvolution bands present an organized structure (Petibois and Deleris 2006). The amide I adopted band depends on the hydrogen bonding from the conformation of the protein structure (Frushour and Koenig 1975).

The surface interactions present changes in the secondary conformation and in the triple helix configuration due to the electrostatic interactions and the hydrophobic and hydrogen bonds. The results indicate that hydrophobic interactions increased and competed with hydrogen bonding when the concentration increased. Hydrophobic interactions, as nonspecific interactions, are the major driving force for protein folding and possibly the cause of chain aggregation. The strength of the electrostatic repulsion between charged residues is enhanced in the hydrophobic region, favoring the formation of a β-sheet structure, which causes the extension of molecular chains.

First, the conformation of the BSA secondary structure anchors onto the primarily parallel β-sheet (an amide I peak at 1654 cm^{-1}). After interaction with the substrate, the peaks of amide I were moved to the central peak at 1664 cm^{-1}. This distinctive interaction is characteristic of the turn structure, but no other significant changes were observed in the rest of the contents. A progressive growth of the amide bands was seen when the solutions of BSA interacted with the polymer surface (Sethuraman and Belfort 2005, Xu et al. 2009).

The secondary structures, calculated from ATR-FTIR, showed that the original BSA has an α-helix content of 66%, β-sheet content of 17%, as well as turn and random content of 25.2%. In interacting with the polymer, the content in the α-helix decreased and the turn and random content increased. This explanation suggests the formation of a hydrogen bond, and the BSA structure becomes packed by folding (Kumaran and Ramamurthy 2014). From the secondary conformation, the rearrangement of the molecules of BSA adopts a rich α-helix structure with packed refolding. The increase in the hydrophobic interactions competes with the hydrogen bonding, determining the major driving force for protein folding and the possible cause of its aggregation. In the case of gelatin, it was observed that the major spectral shift was in the amide I band at 1654 cm^{-1} (mainly C=O stretch) and in the amide II band at 1555 cm^{-1} (C–N stretching coupled with N–H bending modes).

9.3.2.2 Surface Morphology Property

SEM data confirmed the superior properties of the adsorption molecules on modified films after physical immobilization procedures.

Figure 9.4 shows the smooth morphology of the pristine PET. Figure 9.4A and A1 demonstrates how gelatin immobilization has a flattening effect on the surface morphology after surface functionalization. However, the data for the stiffer polymer are pale and for softer areas are dark (Hudon et al. 2003, Tremblay et al. 2005). The images evidence topographical data on the surface where a pale film appears as high spots and the dark areas appear as low spots (Gelman et al. 1979, Gale et al. 1995). Types of aggregation include

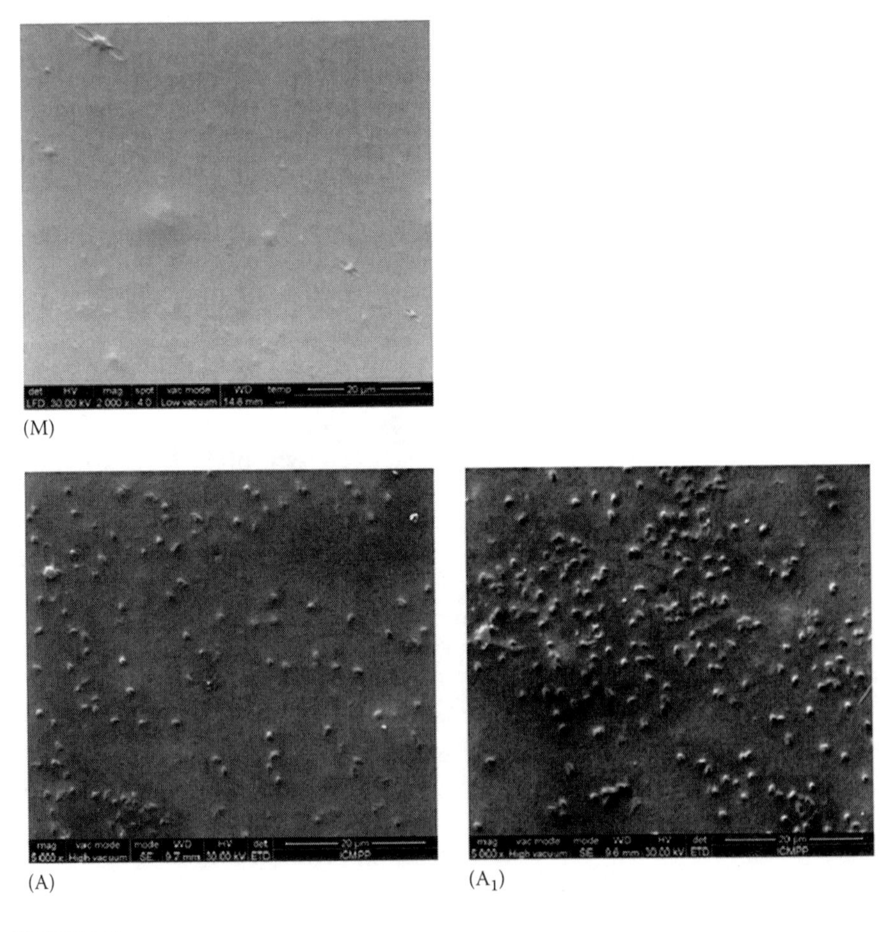

FIGURE 9.4
SEM images from pristine PET: (M) and (A) PET-2H-Gel PET and (A_1) PET-6H-Gel PET.
(Continued)

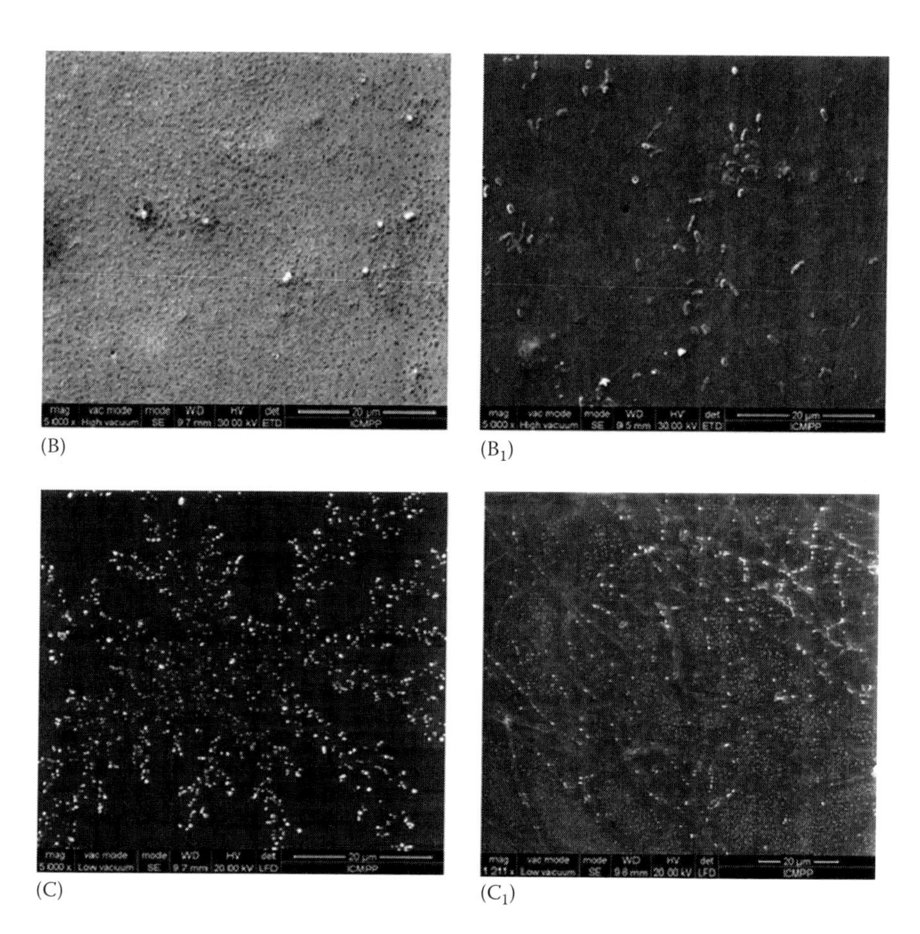

FIGURE 9.4 **(*Continued*)**
SEM images from pristine PET: (B) PET-2H-BSA and (B$_1$) PET-6H-BSA; (C) PET-2H-col and (C$_1$) PET-6H-col.

irregular aggregates, network aggregates, and the surface structure with a knotted cloth aspect. If the concentration is increased, the hydrophobic interactions of the macromolecular chains become intense (Maeda et al. 1995, Tsukida et al. 1996, Vackier et al. 1999).

Studies have concluded that hydrophobic interactions play an important role and are correlated with the diameter of the aggregates. When these interactions are intensive the diameter of the aggregates is larger.

Gelatin presents an optical activity in both secondary conformations, namely coil and helix. In the helix conformation, gelatin has higher optical activity than in the coil conformation (Tsukida et al. 1996).

A triple helix is formed using a two-stage mechanism: first, a nucleus is induced from two helical strands that are meandering and is then packed

(Vackier et al. 1999, Bergo et al. 2013); and second, a new coil segment is packed around the initial nucleus in order to get a triple helix. When the triple helix forms a chain, it remains stable. Thus, the triple helix contains two chains loops and a third loop from the same chain or belonging to another chain (Liang et al. 2003).

In this investigation, we observed that collagen is a molecule that exhibits a propensity to form natural structures in the form of alternating lamellar sheets of fibrils (Figure 9.4C and C_1). The images presented in Figure 9.4 show a crowd of collagen molecules that can be induced as a template, and the high-aspect ratio determined by the structure or the organization of small high-aspect ratio objects. The surface is formed by small aggregates or a network of native collagen fibrils after adsorptive immobilization. The SEM images present the film modified at 2 h, when the molecules are immobilized in small aggregates, and at 6 h, when the network of collagen fibrils cover the surface homogeneously. Images with collagen molecules demonstrated the presence of some individual fibrils between the network formations. In general, fibrils are small and have a polydisperse diameter distribution, with numerous fused and irregular fibrils (Parry and Craig 1977). This observation is derived from the triple helix in atelo-collagen, a coded form with long chains of structural information displaying restricted behavior and a simple concentration that produces the organization of collagens (Paige et al. 1998, 2001, Woodcock et al. 2005).

The cluster from the surface adhesion has a more aggregated aspect. The BSA molecules presented in Figure 9.4B and B_1 are protonated and attached to surfaces and are therefore reduced compared to collagen molecules and gelatin. The fact that the reduction in protein adsorption coincides approximately with the protonation level suggests that protonation of the groups with nitrogen by a protonic acid results in a proportional reduction in the number of protein adsorption sites (Goh et al. 1997). This affinity is probably due to the hydrophobic–hydrophilic interaction of the BSA molecules with the surface containing both hydrophobic and hydrophilic portions.

The amount of adsorbed BSA increases with the number of acid groups present on the polymer surface (Cui et al. 2004). Therefore, this confirms previous data that reports that the number of acid groups increased due to hydrogen bonding. The interactions between BSA molecules play an important role in controlling the adsorption process (Shirahama and Suzawa 1985, Qian et al. 2000, Huang and Gupta 2004). At high concentrations, between 1.0 and 5.0 mg/mL, the adsorption area increases, while no significant changes were observed in the morphology when the BSA concentration was increased from 0.001 to 5.0 mg/mL (Green et al. 1999, Kumaran and Ramamurthy 2014). The results indicate that the stability of functional groups and the selectivity of protein adsorption on the surfaces increase significantly when the treatment time is longer for all biomolecules used.

9.4 Cytocompatibility Test

9.4.1 Cytotoxicity Test

Cytotoxicity of the materials was tested using the direct contact method. The membranes were sterilized with 70% alcohol solution for 30 min, then cut into small (3 × 3 mm) fragments and incubated for 24 h in Dulbecco's modified eagle medium (DMEM) culture at 37°C.

Briefly, for the MTT (3-(4,5-dimethyl-2-thiazolyl)-2,5-diphenyl-2*H*-tetrazolium bromide) test, the culture media from control and experimental wells were replaced with 400 μL of MTT work solution in DMEM, without bovine fetal serum and penicillin/streptomycin/neomycin (P/S/N) (0.25 mg/mL). The culture plates with MTT solution were incubated for 3 h at 37°C under humid and dark conditions. After the incubation period, the MTT solution from each well was replaced with 500 μL of isopropanol, to solubilize the insoluble formazan crystals. The absorbance of the blue formazan solution was measured at 570 nm wavelength, using Tecan UV–VIS plate reader. The cell viability was calculated by normalizing absorbance results for experimental wells to the control, in which cells without any sample were incubated.

Results of the MTT assay from all these materials have a noncytotoxicity composition. The materials do not affect cell viability by direct contact or through degradation of the products. All samples analyzed maintained viability of more than 90% of the cells, even after 72 h of incubation. MTT results indicate that the membranes are biocompatible and can be used as a support for the growth of cells.

Cell viability results obtained in fibroblasts are presented in Figure 9.5. The viability values obtained for PET immobilized fibroblasts ranged from 90.8% to 99.2%, showing an increase in cell viability. The new materials obtained are composed of nontoxic products with excellent biocompatibility (Wang et al. 2000, Ding et al. 2013). These results could be attributed to the fact that these immobilized molecules resulted in significantly greater viability for collagen and gelatin, and less viability for BSA.

9.4.2 Cell Seeding Experiment

A cell seeding experiment was conducted on thawed Albino rabbit dermal primary fibroblasts at passage 3. Population of the materials was performed using sterile membrane discs with 8 mm diameter. Before cell seeding, the materials were placed at the bottom of the 48-well culture plates, covered with 500 μL of culture medium and pre-equilibrated at cell culture condition for 24 h. The materials were populated at 2 × 104/cm^2 cell density and evaluated after 72 and 96 h after seeding.

Population efficiency was evaluated by fluorescence microscopy after Calcein-AM staining of the live cells.

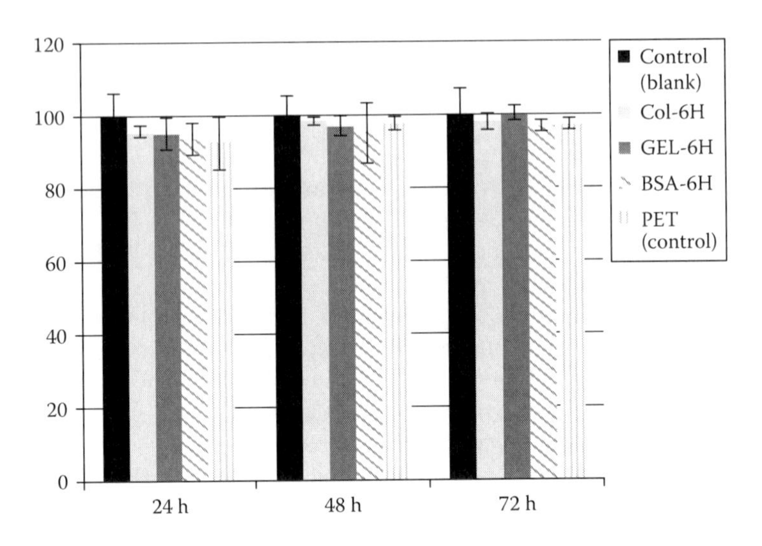

FIGURE 9.5
MTT activity for cytotoxicity test on pristin PET (control) and immobilized films for 6H action collagen (Col-6H), gelatin (GEL-6H), and BSA (BSA-6H).

The cell study was performed to evaluate the immobilization on the support surface of molecules from collagen, gelatin, and BSA. Figure 9.6 with the cell adhesion and proliferation surfaces clearly shows that the modified films present a higher number of viable cells, compared to the nonmodified pristine film, after 72 h of culture. After 96 h of incubation, it is observed that the cell populations are significantly expanded and have a good evolution. This improvement in the cell number may be attributed to the increase in the biomolecules' hydrophilicity as well as the cells' properties. In particular, molecules of collagen and gelatin have a better evolution compared to BSA molecules, because they stimulate cell adhesion and proliferation.

Biocompatibility is a decisive criterion for the ideal skin substitute. Cells that are typically derived from a reduced biopsy require a 3-week culture period in order to proliferate to the needed population size.

On the other hand, cells offer availability and secrete bioactive molecules and components that play an important role in wound healing.

The selection activity was verified by supplying a supportive environment that allows the cellular components of biofabricated constructs to freely reorganize themselves. Their environment is ultimately important for the long-term development of functional tissues, which can be applied as dermal patches. The therapy utilized a biomaterial to induce and conduct host cell proliferation, migration, and *in situ* regeneration. Therefore, for all applications, the biomaterial plays a central role in regenerative skin tissue engineering as an artificial biophysical and biochemical micromedium for cellular behavior and function.

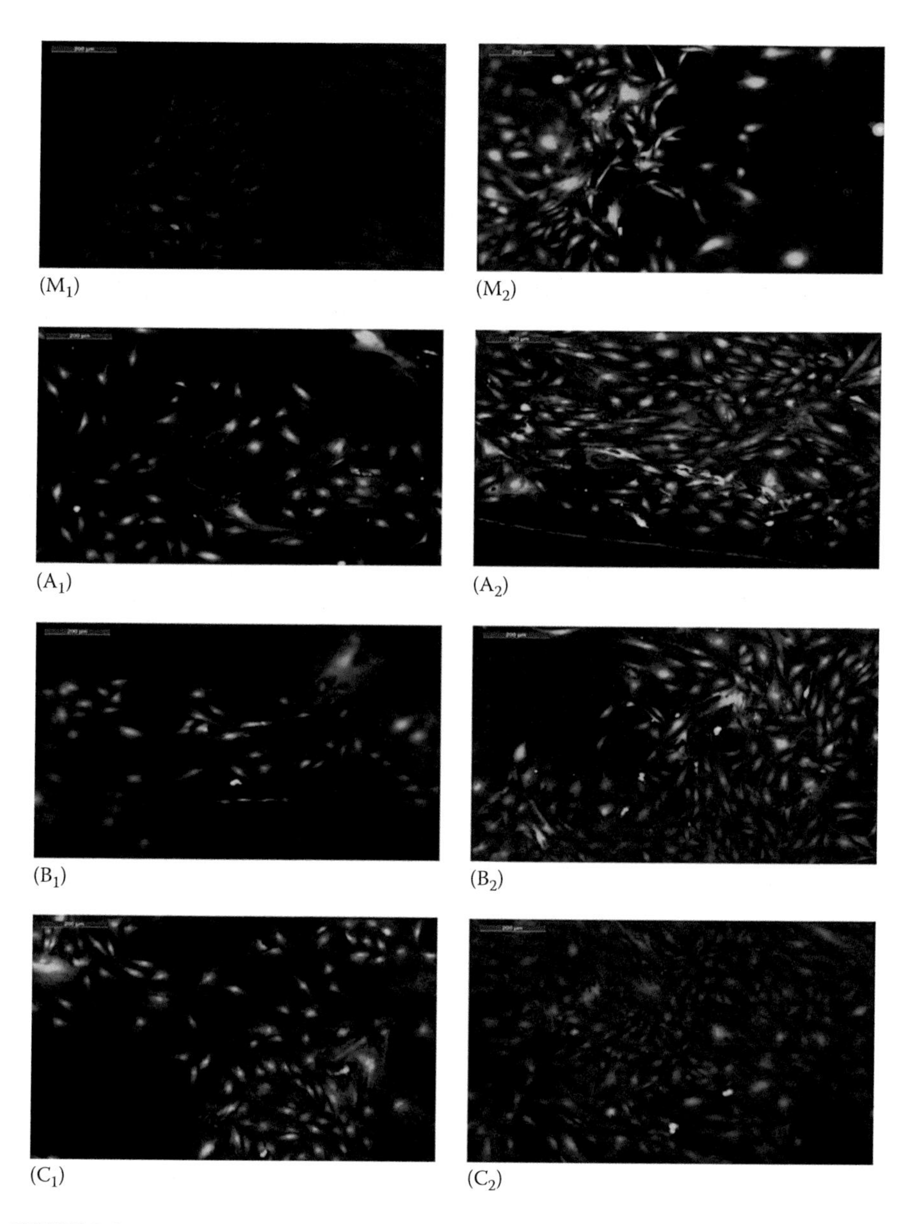

FIGURE 9.6
Results incubation of fibroblasts after 72 h on untreated PET (M_1) and immobilized irradiated 6H-PET: with BSA (A_1), with gelatin (B_1) and collagen (C_1) and after 96 h on untreated PET (M_2) and immobilized irradiated 6H-PET: with BSA (A_2), with gelatin (B_2) and collagen (C_2).

9.5 Conclusion

Collagen, gelatin, and BSA are different natural complex biopolymers whose dissolution is influenced by many parameters. Immobilization on the synthetic polymer substratum depends on different parameters.

Surface modification of scaffolds has been used as an alternative method that accepts the strategy with the induced biological responses. The molecules in the native form or those apply in the engineering regeneration with short peptides using different functional domains have been introduced to develop new surfaces and their biomimetic properties or to improve cell adhesion. The biomimetic self-assembly processes that occur in nature should be applied for the next generation of biomaterials. Different methods of introducing molecules onto the biomaterials' surface (via physical adsorption or covalent solid bonds) can be considered, to gain the chosen functions while preserving the stability of the molecules. The development of biomaterials is of continuing interest, especially those that display multiple responsiveness. This is the improvement expected in the next generation and also the scaffolds for tissue regeneration that utilize pharmaceutical potential for diagnostic availability. To realize these tissue regenerative intelligent biomaterials and to provide multifunctionality, it is necessary to maintain cell and tissue compatibility. The given therapy utilized a biomaterial to induce and conduct host cell proliferation, migration, and *in situ* regeneration. Therefore, for all the applications, biomaterial plays a central role in regenerative skin tissue engineering as an artificial biophysical and biochemical micromedium for cellular behavior and function.

Acknowledgments

The authors acknowledge the financial support for this research through the European Regional Development Fund, Project POINGBIO, ID P_40_443, Contract no. 86/8.09.2016.

References

Bergo, P., Moraes, I. C. F., and Sobral, P. J. A. 2013. Infrared spectroscopy, mechanical analysis, dielectric properties and microwave response of pig skin gelatin films plasticized with glycerol. *Food Biosci* 1(1): 10–15.

Bourassa, P., Hasni, I., and Tajmir-Riahi, H. 2011. Folic acid complexes with human and bovine serum albumins. *Food Chem* 129: 1148–1155.

Ciobanu, C., Gradinaru, L. M., Gradinaru, R. V. et al. 2011. Bovine serum albumin adsorption onto UV-activated green polyurethane surface. *Dig J Nanomater Biostruct* 6: 1751–1761.

Ciobanu, C., Gradinaru, L. M., Gradinaru, R. V. et al. 2012. Water soluble elastin adsorption onto UV-activated green polyurethane surfaces. *Dig J Nanomater Biostruct* 7: 97–106.

Cui, F. L., Fan, J., Li, J. P. et al. 2004. Interactions between 1-benzoyl-4-*p*-chlorophenyl thiosemicarbazide and serum albumin: Investigation by fluorescence spectroscopy. *Bioorg Med Chem* 12(1): 151–157.

Ding, L., Shao, L., and Bai, Y. 2014. Deciphering the mechanism of corona discharge treatment of BOPET film. *RSC Adv* 4: 21782–21787.

Ding, L., Zhou, P., Zhan, H. et al. 2013. Systematic investigation of the toxicity interaction of ZnSe@ZnS QDs on BSA by spectroscopic and microcalorimetry techniques. *Chemosphere* 92(8): 892–897.

Drobota, M., Aflori, M., Gradinaru, L. M. et al. 2015a. Collagen immobilization on ultraviolet light-treated poly(ethylene terephthalate). *High Perform Polym* 27(5): 646–654.

Drobota, M., Gradinaru, L. M., Ciobanu, C. et al. 2015b. Collagen immobilization on poly(ethylene terephthalate) and polyurethane films after UV functionalization. *J Adhes Sci Technol* 29(20): 2208–2219.

Frushour, B. G. and Koenig, J. L. 1975. Raman scattering of collagen, gelatin, and elastin. *Biopolymers* 14(2): 379–391.

Gale, M., Pollanen, M. S., Markiewicz, P. et al. 1995. Sequential assembly of collagen revealed by atomic force microscopy. *Biophys J* 68(5): 2124–2128.

Gelman, R. A., Williams, B. R., and Piez, K. A. 1979. Collagen fibril formation: Evidence for a multistep process. *J Biol Chem* 254(1): 180–186.

Goh, M. C., Paige, M. F., Gale, M. A. et al. 1997. Fibril formation in collagen. *Phys A Stat Mech Appl* 239(1–3): 95–102.

Goormaghtigh, E., Ruysschaert, J. M., and Raussens, V. 2006. Evaluation of the information content in infrared spectra for protein secondary structure determination. *Biophys J* 90(8): 2946–2957.

Green, R. J., Hopkinson, I., and Jones, R. A. L. 1999. Unfolding and intermolecular association in globular proteins adsorbed at interfaces. *Langmuir* 15(15): 5102–5110.

Huang, Y. W. and Gupta, V. K. 2004. A SPR and AFM study of the effect of surface heterogeneity on adsorption of proteins. *J Chem Phys* 121(5): 2264–2271.

Hudon, V., Berthod, F., Black, A. F. et al. 2003. A tissue-engineered endothelialized dermis to study the modulation of angiogenic and angiostatic molecules on capillary-like tube formation in vitro. *J Dermatol* 148(6): 1094–1104.

Jayakumar, G. C., Usharani, N., Kawakami, K. et al. 2014. Studies on the physico-chemical characteristics of collagen–pectin composites. *RSC Adv* 4: 63840–63849.

Kirker, K. R., Luo, Y., Nielson J. H. et al. 2002. Glycosaminoglycan hydrogel films as bio-interactive dressings for wound healing. *Biomaterials* 23(17): 3661–3671.

Kitano, H., Nagaoka, K., Tada, S. et al. 2008. Structure of water incorporated in amphoteric polymer thin films as revealed by FT-IR spectroscopy. *Macromol Biosci* 8: 77–85.

Krimm, S. and Bandekar, J. 1986. Vibrational spectroscopy and conformation of peptides, polypeptides and proteins. *Adv Protein Chem* 38(15): 181–364.

Kumaran, R. and Ramamurthy, P. 2014. Photophysical studies on the interaction of amides with bovine serum albumin (BSA) in aqueous solution: Fluorescence quenching and protein unfolding. *J Lumin* 148(5): 277–284.
Lan, C., Yu, L., Chen, P. et al. 2010. Design, preparation and characterization of self-reinforced starch films through chemical modification. *Macromol Mater Eng* 295(11): 1025–1030.
Liang, G., Ralph, H., Colby, C. et al. 2003. Whitesides kinetics of triple helix formation in semidilute gelatin solutions. *Macromolecules* 36(26): 9999–10008.
MacNeil, S. 2007. Progress and opportunities for tissue-engineered skin. *Nature* 445(7180): 874–880.
Maeda, H., Ozaki, Y., Tanaka, M. et al. 1995. Near infrared spectroscopy and chemometrics studies of temperature-dependent spectral variations of water: Relationship between spectral changes and hydrogen bonds. *J Near Infrared Spectrosc* 3: 191–201.
Mandal, A., Meda, V., and Zhang, W. J. 2012. Synthesis, characterization and comparison of antimicrobial activity of PEG/TritonX-100 capped silver nanoparticles on collagen scaffold. *Colloids Surf B Biointerfaces* 90(1): 191–196.
Muyonga, J. H., Cole, C. G. B., and Duodu, K. G. 2004. Extraction and characterization of collagen from buffalo skin for biomedical applications. *Food Chem* 86(3): 325–332.
Orlando, G., Wood, K. J., De Coppi, P. et al. 2012. Regenerative medicine as applied to general surgery. *Ann Surg* 255(5): 867–880.
Paige, M. F., Rainey, J. K., and Goh, M. C. 1998. Fibrous long spacing collagen ultrastructure elucidated by atomic force microscopy. *Biophys J* 74(6): 3211–3216.
Paige, M. F., Rainey, J. K., and Goh, M. C. 2001. A study of fibrous long pacing collagen ultrastructure and assembly by atomic force microscopy. *Micron* 32: 341–353.
Parry, D. A. D. and Craig, A. S. 1977. Quantitative electron microscope observations of the collagen fibrils in rat-tail tendon. *Biopolymers* 16(5): 1015–1031.
Petibois, C. and Deleris, G. 2006. Histological mapping of biochemical changes in solid tumors by FT-IR spectral imaging. *Trends Biotechnol* 24(10): 455–462.
Qian, W., Yao, D., Yu, F. et al. 2000. Immobilization of antibodies on ultraflat polystyrene surfaces. *Clin Chem* 46(9): 1456–1463.
Sethuraman, A. and Belfort, G. 2005. Protein structural perturbation and aggregation on homogeneous surfaces. *Biophys J* 88(2): 1322–1333.
Shirahama, H. and Suzawa, T. 1985. Adsorption of bovine serum albumin onto styrene/acrylic acid copolymer latex. *Colloid Polym Sci* 263(2): 141–146.
Sun, G., Zhang, X., Shen, Y. I. et al. 2011. Dextran hydrogel scaffolds enhance angiogenic responses and promote complete skin regeneration during burn wound healing. *Proc Natl Acad Sci USA* 108(52): 20976–20981.
Tamm, L. K. and Tatulian, S. A. 1997. Infrared spectroscopy of proteins and peptides in lipid bilayers. *Q Rev Biophys* 30(4): 365–429.
Taravel, M. N. and Domard, A. 1995. Collagen and its interaction with chitosan. II. Influence of the physicochemical characteristics of collagen. *Biomaterials* 16(11): 865–871.
Tremblay, P. L., Hudon, V., Berthod, F. et al. 2005. Inosculation of tissue-engineered capillaries with the host's vasculature in a reconstructed skin transplanted on mice. *Am J Transplant* 5(5): 1002–1010.
Tsukida, N., Maeda, Y., and Kitano, H. 1996. Raman spectroscopic study on water in aqueous gelatin gels and sols. *Macromol Chem Phys* 197(5): 1681–1690.

Vackier, M. C., Hills, B. P., and Rutledge, D. N. 1999. An NMR relaxation study on the state of water in gelatin gels. *J Magn Reson* 138(1): 36–42.
Walton, R. S., Brand, D. D., and Czernuszka, J. T. 2010. Influence of telopeptides, fibrils and crosslinking on physicochemical properties of type I collagen films. *J Mater Sci Mater Med* 21: 451–461.
Wang, N., Wu, X. S., Li, C. et al. 2000. Synthesis, characterisation, biodegradation and drug delivery application of biodegradable lactic/glycolic polymers: Synthesis and characterisation. *J Biomater Sci Polym Ed* 11: 301–318.
Wang, Q. X., Zhang, X., Zhou, T. et al. 2012. Interaction of different thiol-capped CdTe quantum dots with bovine serum albumin. *J Lumin* 132(7): 1695–1700.
Woodcock, S. E., Johnson, W. C., and Chen, Z. 2005. Collagen adsorption and structure on polymer surfaces observed by atomic force microscopy. *J Colloid Interface Sci* 292(1): 99–107.
Xu, H., Gao, S.-L., Lv, J.-B. Q. et al. 2009. Spectroscopic investigations on the mechanism of interaction of crystal violet with bovine serum albumin. *J Mol Struct* 919: 334–338.

10

Inside of the Transport Processes in Biomedical Systems

Maria Spiridon and Magdalena Aflori

CONTENTS

10.1 Introduction

Nanomedicine provides a better relevance of restrained interaction with biological systems at the molecular level leading to new pathways for the diagnosis, prevention, and treatment of human diseases and in the repair of damaged tissues in alignment with the global evolution of medicine. In other words, nanomedicine in health care is the controlled use of nanotechnology and scientists see a future in this area (Adiseshaiah et al., 2016).

Today people are suffering from many more diseases than before and one of the causes is the development and progress of human society (Irache et al., 2011).

Professor Peter Speiser, one of the pioneers in the progress and evaluation of nanoparticles for drug delivery, developed a method for the controlled release of drugs through miniaturized delivery systems (Birrenbach, 1973; Birrenbach and Speiser, 1976).

Until now diverse types of nanodevices and strategies based on nanotechnologies convenient for drug delivery had been suggested. Usually, these devices can (1) protect a drug from deterioration, (2) improve drug absorption by helping diffusion through the epithelium, (3) change pharmacokinetic and drug tissue distribution profile, and/or (4) improve intracellular diffusion and distribution (Couvreur and Vauthier, 2006).

Mathematical modeling of controlled drug delivery may improve the scientific knowledge and also the fundamental part of the mass transport mechanisms that are implicated in the control of drug release. Mathematically, it is used for designing a specific pharmaceutical system and can also be utilized to simulate the effect of the device's design parameters (geometry and composition) on the resulting drug release kinetics (Hassan and Khan, 2008).

Chemical properties of drugs are very important because they can be absorbed from the gastrointestinal tract by either passive diffusion or active transport (Manallack et al., 2013).

10.2 Active and Passive Transport

Active transport occurs when the drug is transferred against the concentration gradient from lower concentration to higher concentration. In this case, the rate of transport is significantly higher than in passive diffusion. This mode of active transport for drug entry also implicates particular carrier proteins that cross the membrane. Active transport is energy-dependent and is directed by the hydrolysis of adenosine triphosphate (Lemke et al., 2012).

The mechanisms of active transport can be split into two types:

1. Primary active transport, which directly uses a source of chemical energy for moving molecules over a membrane against their gradient
2. Secondary active transport–cotransport, which utilizes an electrochemical gradient generated by active transport as an energy source to move molecules against their gradient, and in this way does not directly need a chemical source of energy (Zhang and Rudnick, 2006)

Passive transport or passive diffusion is the process that occurs across the concentration gradient, from higher concentration to lower concentration (Fick's law). This mechanism is driven by an inside-negative membrane potential. Passive diffusion does not include a carrier. Most drugs gain entry into the body through this mechanism. Lipid-soluble drugs quickly move across most biological membranes because of their solubility in the membranes' bilayers. Water-soluble drugs pass through the cell membrane between aqueous canals or pores. Other agents can access the cells through particular transmembrane carrier proteins that help the section of large molecules. This process is commonly used as it facilitates diffusion. This class of diffusion does not need external energy, can be saturated, and may be constrained. Passive diffusion is mathematically most clearly expressed by Fick's first law of diffusion (Ravna et al., 2009).

There is significant proof of the interaction between many drugs and transporter proteins expressed along the intestine, mainly in enterocyte membranes, with the role of facilitating the absorption rate or reducing it depending on the drug type (Varma et al., 2010). Therefore, it is necessary to gauge the intestinal region-specific expression of these transporters accurately in order to be able to predict the potential impact of these transporters on the gastrointestinal drug absorption rate and regulate the dosage form (Giacomini et al., 2010).

10.3 Endocytic Processes and Persorption

Nanomedicines use diversified endocytic pathways to get into the cells. In general, drugs with small molecules enter the cells through passive diffusion or active transport, as long as nanomedicines pass into the cells by endocytosis. That's why nanomedicine supports the introduction and growth of particular cells because endocytosis is the main route of transport across membranes (Kou et al., 2013).

There are various types of endocytosis: Phagocytosis or "cell eating" is the first step in the uptake and degradation of particles larger than 0.5 μm and is utilized for the uptake of large particles like bacteria. Pinocytosis or "cell drinking" has the scope to incorporate fluid surrounding the cell, involving all substances in the fluid-phase area of invagination that are taken up at the same time (Iversen et al., 2011).

The endocytic pathway manages the transport of molecules, like receptor ligands and solutes entering the cells (Sahay et al., 2010). These pathways are obviously interdependent and many of the compartments and protein machines are common to both.

In the case of drug delivery, the endocytic pathway is most significant. New drug design requires the transfer of drugs to a particular location in the cell. Their place of activity may be particularly within the inside of a range of organelles or the agent can get away from endosomes (endosomolytic) or lysosomes (lysosomolytic) prior to reaching its target. Certainly, various systems are required to encourage early escape from endosomes in comparison with the necessity to transfer them and with the application of a lysosomal protease for delivery of a drug inside the cytosol. Usually, it is also essential that the drug is not transported from the cell following its entry into reuse or secretion pathways. For this reason, the plasma membrane and downstream organelles pose considerable limitations to drug delivery but increase the knowledge of endocytosis. In addition, the agents that disturb or manage endocytic pathways are opening fresh channels for more productive intracellular delivery (Iversen et al., 2011, Kou et al., 2013).

Current cell biology exploits a plethora of technologies to gain insight into intracellular trafficking, whose path is based on microscopy. Current evolutions in imaging technology signify that more can be produced by imaging fixed cells in terms of spatial resolution and sensitivity (Richard et al., 2005).

Common drugs that have small molecules make their entry into cells mostly through passive diffusion or sometimes through active transport. At the same time, nanomedicines enter the cells through endocytosis, which better helps these drugs to penetrate specific cells and also to accumulate there. Scientists in pharmaceutical sciences have shown a keen interest in this process and as a result of their studies some significant achievements have been made in this area. It was thus possible to classify the endocytosis pathway according to the proteins that play a role in the process. The process by which nanomedicines interact with the cytomembrane during penetration has also been explained, as well as how they travel in the cells following different pathways (Doherty and McMahon, 2009).

The cellular processes occur according to the degree of fidelity of intracellular membrane traffic. Proteins, lipids, receptor ligands, and solute molecules are taken to distinct compartments within the cell both through the biosynthetic and endocytic pathways (Rappoport, 2008).

Endocytosis comprises the multiple methods of internalization, which include clathrin-dependent endocytosis, macropinocytosis, clathrin-independent endocytosis, and internalization via caveolae (Doherty and McMahon, 2009, Pucadyil et al., 2009). Most agents that are delivered to cells are also delivered to compartments outside the classical endocytic pathway (Watson et al., 2005).

Just as endocytosis is a gateway for drug delivery, some features of the delivery direction must be resolved and these include the following: (1) the interaction of the molecule with the plasma membrane, (2) the mechanism by which it is invaginated into the cell, (3) its sorting within the highly complex endosomal sorting system, and (4) its eventual fate within the cell or whether it is recycled back into the extracellular milieu (Iversen et al., 2011, Kou et al., 2013).

10.4 Pore Transport and Mass Transfer Models

In many distinct fields of science and technology, flow and transport phenomena in porous media play a relevant role (Xiong et al., 2016).

Pore transport or convective transport is the process through which a drug of small-to-moderate molecular weight (like sugars, urea, and water) can pass rapidly through the intestinal epithelium over the water-filled pores between the cells (Crank, 1975).

When we evaluate transport in porous media, we need to study a few details such as the intricacy of the pore structure. Challenges also come into question when analyzing transport in porous media. First of all, the intricacy of the pore structure makes the transport process in porous media very complex because pores tend to have irregular surfaces. Some of them even make dead ends, and these factors influence the flow and transport behavior quite significantly. The evolution of the pore structure during service or operation, as well as other factors, makes the study of the behavior of porous media difficult (Peppas and Narasimhan, 2014).

Over the last 50 years, mathematical modeling has been utilized to design a large number of simple and complex drug delivery systems and devices, and also to anticipate the general release behavior of drugs (Khan and Shefeeq, 2009). These kinds of systems have been used to conceptualize pharmaceutical formulations and to analyze the process of drug release *in vitro* and *in vivo* (Peppas and Narasimhan, 2014).

For the most part, mathematical models have been used to anticipate the temporal release of the encapsulated cargo molecules. These models add value in terms of ensuring optimal design of pharmaceutical formulation as well as understanding release mechanisms through experimental verification (Narasimhan and Peppas, 1997).

In pharmaceutical sciences, mass transfer is an important phenomenon because it is used in different processes and mechanisms such as distribution and metabolism studies, dosage form, drug synthesis, and preformulation investigations (Narasimhan and Peppas, 1997, Peppas and Narasimhan, 2014).

Many existing models are based upon diffusion equations. Because the diffusion of drugs is an important function of the structure, the models must account for polymer morphology (Nokhodchi et al., 2012).

Controlled-release systems can be classified into drug release mechanisms as follows: (1) diffusion-controlled; (2) chemically controlled; (3) osmotically controlled; and (4) swelling- or dissolution-controlled (Nokhodchi et al., 2012).

Models range from simple yet empirical and phenomenological to probabilistic or molecular, and they also help in guiding the design of drug delivery mechanisms. Starting from the use of steady-state and transient descriptions of drug diffusion using Fick's law, the models account for chain relaxation, polymer microstructure, glassy/rubbery transitions, chain disentanglement, polymer crystallinity, environmental effects, concentration effects, multidimensional effects, nonuniform drug distributions, and device geometry (Peppas and Narasimhan, 2014).

The mathematical model equation can be utilized to create advanced systems by electing the optimal geometry, the methods of formulation, and size.

10.5 Conclusions and Future Directions

The mathematical model plays a vital role in the design of drug delivery systems; at the same time, it aids specialists to understand the drug delivery mechanism and allows physicians to make a choice regarding the optimal dose with which to treat patients. Mathematical modeling in controlled drug delivery will enable the development of new and more productive therapeutics for the treatment of diseases (Peppas and Narasimhan, 2014).

Mathematical modeling helps in anticipating drug release rates and diffusion behavior, thereby decreasing the number of experiments required. A conclusion that can be drawn is that mathematical modeling can facilitate not only the optimization of existing pharmaceutical products but also the development of new ones. The consistent use of such models can prove economical in terms of money and time. Mathematical modeling can help researchers in their process of developing highly effective drugs and plan more accurate dosages (Peppas and Narasimhan, 2014).

Yet, the steps from the lab to the clinic continue to be difficult. Important work still needs to be done for a better understanding of the different mechanisms involved in the biological interactions in order to clearly identify the toxicological implications of chronic administration of treatments based on these carriers. Some topics that might help the implementation of these new medicines are as follows: (1) the design and use of "intelligent" materials and devices, (2) the conception of new strategies that can offer various alternative routes of administration (i.e., biomimetic nanoparticles), and (3) simplification of the preparative methods to facilitate their scale-up and industrial transposition (Irache et al., 2011).

Acknowledgments

The authors acknowledge the financial support for this research through the European Regional Development Fund, Project POINGBIO, ID P_40_443, Contract no. 86/8.09.2016.

References

Adiseshaiah, P.P., Crist, R.M., Hook, S.S., McNeil, S.E. 2016. Nanomedicine strategies to overcome the pathophysiological barriers of pancreatic cancer. *Nat Rev Clin Oncol* 13:750–765.

Birrenbach, G. 1973. Uber Mizellpolymerisate, mogliche Einschlussverbindun-gen (Nanokapseln) und deren Eignung als Adjuvantien. Dissertation, Nr. 5071, ETH Zurich, Zürich, Switzerland.

Birrenbach, G., Speiser, P.P. 1976. Polymerized micelles and their use as adjuvants in immunology. *J Pharm Sci* 65:1763–1766.
Couvreur, P., Vauthier, C. 2006. Nanotechnology: Intelligent design to treat complex disease. *Pharm Res* 23(7):1417–1450.
Crank, J. 1975. *The Mathematics of Diffusion*, 2nd edn. Oxford University Press, Bristol, England.
Doherty, G.J., McMahon, H.T. 2009. Mechanisms of endocytosis. *Annu Rev Biochem* 78:857–902.
Giacomini, K.M., Huang, S.-M., Tweedie, D.J. et al. 2010. Membrane transporters in drug development. *Nat Rev Drug Discov* 9(3):215–236.
Hassan, M.I., Khsn, M. 2008. Mathematical Modeling as a tool for improving the action of drugs. *Aust J Basic&Appl Sci* 4:81–88.
Irache, J.M., Esparza, I., Gamazo, C., Agueros, M., Espuelas, S. 2011. Nanomedicine: Novel approaches in human and veterinary therapeutics. *Vet Parasitol* 180:47–71.
Iversen, T.G., Skotland, R., Sandvig, K. 2011. Endocytosis and intracellular transport of nanoparticles: Present knowledge and need for future studies. *Nano Today* 6:176–185.
Khan, M.A., Shefeeq, T. 2009. Role of mathematical modeling in controlled drug delivery. *J Sci Res* 1(3):539–550.
Kou, L., Sun, J., Zhai, Y. et al. 2013. The endocytosis and intracellular fate of nano-medicines: Implication for rational design. *Asian J Pharmacol* 8(1):1–10.
Lemke, T.L., Williams, D.A., Roche, V.F., Zito, W.S. 2012. *Foye's Principles of Medicinal Chemistry*, 7th edn. Lippincott Williams & Wilkins/Wolters Kluwer Philadelphia, PA.
Manallack, D.T., Prankerd, R.J., Yuriev, E., Oprea, T.I., Chalmers, D.K. 2013. The significance of acid/base properties in drug discovery. *Chem Soc Rev* 42(2):485–496.
Narasimhan, B., Peppas, N.A. 1997. Molecular analysis of drug delivery systems controlled by dissolution of the polymer carrier. *J Pharm Sci* 86:297–304.
Nokhodchi, A., Raja, S., Patel, P., Asare-Addo, K. 2012. The role of oral controlled release matrix tablets in drug delivery systems. *Bioimpacts* 2(4):175–187.
Peppas, N., Narasimhan, B. 2014. Mathematical models in drug delivery: How modeling has shaped the way we design new drug delivery systems. *J Control Release* 190:75–81.
Pucadyil, T.J., Schmid, S.L. 2009. Conserved functions of membrane active GTPases in coated vesicle formation. *Science* 325:1217–1220.
Rappoport, J. 2008. Focusing on clathrin-mediated endocytosis. *Biochem J* 412:415–423.
Ravna, A.W., Sager, G., Dahl, S.G., Sylte, I. 2009. Membrane transporters structure, function and targets for drug design. *Top Med Chem* 4:15–51.
Richard, J.P., Melikov, K., Brooks, H. et al. 2005. Cellular uptake of unconjugated TAT peptide involves clathrin-dependent endocytosis and heparin sulfate receptors. *J Biol Chem* 280:15300–15306.
Sahay, G., Alakhova, D.Y., Kabanov, A.K. 2010. Endocytosis of nanomedicines. *J Control Release* 145(3):182–195.
Varma, M.V., Obach, R.S., Rotter, C., Miller, H.R., Chang, G., Steyn, S.J., El-Kattan, A., Troutman, M.D. 2010. Physicochemical space for optimum oral bioavailability: Contribution of human intestinal absorption and first-pass elimination. *J Med Chem* 53:1098–1108.

Watson, P., Jones, A.T., Stephens, D.J. 2005. Intracellular trafficking pathways and drug delivery: Fluorescence imaging of living and fixed cells. *Adv Drug Deliv Rev* 57:43–61.

Xiong, Q., Baychev, T.G., Jivkov, A.P. 2016. Review of pore network modeling of porous media: Experimental characterizations, network constructions and applications to reactive transport. *J Contam Hydrol* 192:101–117.

Zhang, Y.W., Rudnick, G. 2006. The cytoplasmatic substrate permeation pathway of serotonin transporter. *J Biol Chem* 281:36213.

Index

C

D

E

N

O

P